STUDY GUIDE AND LAB MANUAL

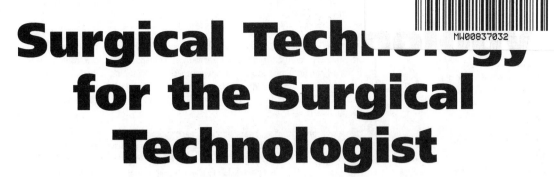

Surgical Technology for the Surgical Technologist

A POSITIVE CARE APPROACH

Third Edition Updated

Association of Surgical Technologists, Inc.

Dana Grafft, CST
Program Director/Instructor
Iowa Lakes Community College
Spencer, Iowa

William Hammer, CST
Program Director
Illinois Central College
Washington, Illinois

Mary E. (Libby) McNaron, RN, CNOR, CST, BSN, MS
Coordinator Surgical Technology/Perioperative Nursing
Gulf Coast Community College
Panama City, Florida

Additional Content Provided By:

Teri L. Junge, CST, CFA, FAST
Surgical Technology Program Director
San Joaquin Valley College
Fresno, California

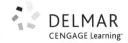

DELMAR
CENGAGE Learning

Australia • Brazil • Japan • Korea • Mexico • Singapore • Spain • United Kingdom • United States

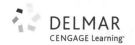

DELMAR
CENGAGE Learning

Study Guide and Lab Manual to Accompany: Surgical Technology for the Surgical Technologist, Third Edition Updated
The Association of Surgical Technologists, Dana Grafft, William Hammer, Teri L. Junge, Mary E. McNaron

Vice President, Career and Professional Editorial: Dave Garza

Director of Learning Solutions: Matthew Kane

Managing Editor: Marah Bellegarde

Executive Editor: Steve Helba

Product Manager: Jadin Babin-Kavanaugh

Vice President, Career and Professional Marketing: Jennifer McAvey

Executive Marketing Manager: Wendy Mapstone

Marketing Manager: Michele McTighe

Marketing Coordinator: Erica Ropitzky

Production Director: Carolyn Miller

Senior Content Project Manager: James Zayicek

Senior Art Director: Jack Pendleton

For product information and technology assistance, contact us at
Cengage Learning Customer & Sales Support, 1-800-648-7450

For permission to use material from this text or product,
submit all requests online at **cengage.com/permissions**
Further permissions questions can be emailed to
permissionrequest@cengage.com

Windows is a registered trademark of the Microsoft Corporation used herein under license. Macintosh and Power Macintosh are registered trademarks of Apple Computer, Inc. Used herein under license.

Library of Congress Cataloging-in-Publication Data

ISBN-13: 978-1-4354-8766-6

ISBN-10: 1-4354-8766-4

Delmar Cengage Learning
5 Maxwell Drive
Clifton Park, NY 12065-2919
USA

Cengage Learning products are represented in Canada by Nelson Education, Ltd.

For your lifelong learning solutions, visit **delmar.cengage.com**

Visit our corporate website at **cengage.com**

Notice to the Reader
Publisher does not warrant or guarantee any of the products described herein or perform any independent analysis in connection with any of the product information contained herein. Publisher does not assume, and expressly disclaims, any obligation to obtain and include information other than that provided to it by the manufacturer. The reader is expressly warned to consider and adopt all safety precautions that might be indicated by the activities described herein and to avoid all potential hazards. By following the instructions contained herein, the reader willingly assumes all risks in connection with such instructions. The publisher makes no representations or warranties of any kind, including but not limited to, the warranties of fitness for particular purpose or merchantability, nor are any such representations implied with respect to the material set forth herein, and the publisher takes no responsibility with respect to such material. The publisher shall not be liable for any special, consequential, or exemplary damages resulting, in whole or part, from the reader's use of, or reliance upon, this material.

Printed in United States of America
1 2 3 4 5 6 XXX 11 10 09

CONTENTS

SKILL ASSESSMENT LIST

TO THE SURGICAL TECHNOLOGY STUDENT

The textbook *Surgical Technology for the Surgical Technologist: A Positive Care Approach*, third edition, defines the cognitive model necessary for the surgical technologist to perform effectively and provides an innovative approach for learning the role of the surgical technologist while focusing on the knowledge and skills required. This model leads the way for the surgical technology student to remember the pertinent information using the predictive model: A POSitive Care Approach. Because the text was written by surgical technology professionals and educators, the needs of the student are the focus throughout the process. The graduate of a CAAHEP (Commission on Accreditation of Allied Health Education Programs) accredited surgical technology program will meet the eligibility requirements of the LCC-ST (Liaison Council on Certification for the Surgical Technologist) to sit for the national certifying examination to become a certified surgical technologist.

The basic steps of the cognitive process are defined by Bob Caruthers, CST, PhD, former Deputy Director, Association of Surgical Technologists. The Surgical Technologist:

- Has a mental image of normal anatomy

- Makes a mental comparison of the idealized anatomy with the actual anatomy of a specific patient

- Knows an idealized operative procedure used to correct the pathologic condition

- Makes a mental comparison of the idealized procedure with the actual procedure being performed

- Allows for a particular surgeon's variations to the idealized procedure

- Allows for variances in anatomy, pathology, and surgeons' responses to the variances

- Predicts and prepares to meet the needs of the surgeon and surgical patient prior to verbalization of the need

To facilitate the learning process, *Surgical Technology for the Surgical Technologist* has been divided into two major sections. These divisions correspond to the positive care approach and are represented by the A POSitive and CARE acronyms. The first 12 chapters are related to the CARE acronym. The CARE division is further divided into two sections: Introduction to Surgical Technology and Principles and Practice of Surgical Technology. The last 12 chapters relate to the A POSitive acronym; a brief introduction to diagnostics is followed by chapters focusing on operative procedures for various specialties.

What is the A POSitive CARE Approach? It is a systematic approach to surgical problem solving focused on the ability of the surgical technologist to predict the needs of the surgeon and patient. This approach uses two simple memory tools for systematic problem solving: APOS and CARE.

The A POSitive approach relates directly to the final 12, or procedural, chapters of the book. This approach does allow the one-to-one correlation of the procedural chapter objectives and should be used to reinforce every surgical procedure encountered by the student:

A – Anatomy

P – Pathology

O – Operative procedure

S – Specific variations

The CARE division seeks to place the technical information that dominates the field of surgical technology into the broader context of patient care:

C – Care directed toward the patient and/or surgical team

A – Aseptic principles and practice of sterile technique

R – Role of the surgical technologist

E – Environmental awareness and concern

This approach is intended to serve as a reminder to the surgical technologist that all activities ultimately affect the care given to the patient.

Features of the Third Edition Study Guide

This edition of the Study Guide has been updated to more closely follow the content in the third edition of *Surgical Technology for the Surgical Technologist*. The features of the Study Guide include the following:

- New lab activities for each chapter inspires learning in creative and practical ways

- Skill Assessments now include more detail and better tracking of performance

- Image labeling exercises build knowledge of instruments and anatomy

- Case Studies with related questions develop critical thinking skills

- Select Key Terms build technical vocabulary

In this Study Guide, you are provided with learning tools to enhance your understanding of the skills and knowledge required to become a surgical technologist. Please note that while most of the information tested in this Study Guide can be found in your textbook, you may need to consult a medical dictionary or human anatomy atlas for some items, and independent research may be required for some critical thinking activities. The authors of this study guide wish you every success in your endeavor to become a Certified Surgical Technologist.

Introduction to Surgical Technology

Orientation to Surgical Technology

OBJECTIVES

After studying this chapter, the reader should be able to:

1. Demonstrate principles of communication in the surgical setting.

2. Relate awareness of aseptic principles to the surgical technologist's role in the care of the surgical patient.

3. Trace the historical development of surgical technology.

4. Recognize members of the surgical team and their roles.

5. Compare and contrast the various roles of the surgical technologist.

6. Interpret the components of a job description for the surgical technologist.

7. Summarize the different types of health care facilities.

8. Analyze a typical hospital organizational structure.

9. Classify hospital departments and their relationship to surgical services.

Select Key Terms

Define the following, using your textbook glossary or a medical dictionary if needed:

1. acronym _____

_____

2. ambulatory surgical facility _____

_____

3. ARC-ST _____

_____

4. AST _____

_____

5. circulator _____

_____

6. competency _____

_____

7. core curriculum _____

_____

8. DO _____

_____

9. elective _____

_____

10. emergent _____

_____

11. HMO _____

_____

12. intraoperative _____

_____

13. The Joint Commission _____

_____

14. NBSTSA (formerly LCC-ST) _____

_____

15. optional _____

_____

16. postoperative _____

_____

17. preceptor _____

_____

18. preoperative _____

_____

19. professional _____

_____

20. proprietary _____

_____

21. STSR _____

_____

22. urgent _____

_____

23. Vesalius_____

_____

Labeling

1. Using the AST logo (Figure 1-1) as a visual aid to represent an actual operating room (OR), label each surgical team member with an appropriate title and identify whether or not each is a sterile team member.

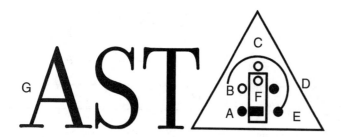

Completion

Mark each job duty with an N if it is performed by a "non-sterile" surgical team member or an S if it is performed by a "sterile" surgical team member.

1. _____ Conducts the preoperative patient interview.

2. _____ Provides additional items to the sterile field during the surgical procedure.

3. _____ Performs a hand scrub and dons a gown and gloves.

4. _____ Maintains the patient's operative record.

5. _____ Organizes the Mayo stand and back table for use during the procedure.

6. _____ Applies sterile dressings to the wound.

Short Answer Discussion

1. Analyze your current lifestyle and compare it to your future lifestyle as a surgical technologist. What differences might there be in your life based on the working conditions and personal characteristics required to be a Certified Surgical Technologist (CST)?

_____

_____

_____

2. List three ways to demonstrate professionalism. Do you think that professionalism is important to a career in surgical technology? Why?

_____

_____

_____

3. What are some benefits of belonging to a professional organization? What is the professional organization dedicated to surgical technology?

_____

_____

_____

4. Define the term "surgical conscience." Do you feel that it is something that is learned or something that you are born with?

_____

_____

_____

5. List three examples of positive nonverbal communication. Why do you feel that nonverbal communication is important in the operating room and in health care in general?

_____

_____

_____

Interactive Learning

1. Trace the history of the profession of surgical technology by drawing a timeline that marks key events that offered advancements to the profession. Share your timeline with other class members.

2. Write a communication scenario to illustrate the differences among social relationships, therapeutic relationships, and professional relationships. Act out your scenario with a class member. Include appropriate subject matter, appropriate dialogue, and the components of effective communication related to each varying relationship.

3. Visit the websites of key organizations related to hospitals, health care organizations, and surgical services. Print out items of interest and share with other class members.

4. Rent the 1991 movie *The Doctor* starring William Hurt and observe the way the film director utilized positive and negative body language to tell the doctor's story. While watching, take notes regarding the nonverbal communication in the movie.

Case Studies

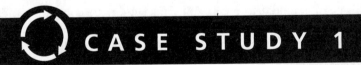

CASE STUDY 1

Rodrigo is a 57-year-old man who was admitted to the emergency department (ED) following a motor vehicle accident. Rodrigo was driving a delivery van that was struck head-on by another vehicle. Rodrigo has severe injuries to both lower extremities: (1) closed femur fracture of the left leg and (2) open fracture of the right tibia and fibula with near amputation. A chest tube was inserted upon arrival in the ED. Rodrigo is neurologically intact. He is now scheduled for surgery on his legs.

(continues)

CASE STUDY 1 *(continued)*

1. This case represents what category of surgical intervention?

_____
_____
_____
_____

2. What is the difference between emergent and urgent surgical intervention?

_____
_____
_____
_____

3. What is elective surgery?

_____
_____
_____
_____

4. Consult with your instructor: Is elective surgical intervention the same as "minor" surgery?

_____
_____
_____
_____

CASE STUDY 2

Kathleen is a 15-year-old female who has been admitted to the hospital for surgery to correct a condition called scoliosis, an abnormal lateral curvature of the spine. This surgical intervention requires a lengthy incision and dissection of spinal muscles. It runs the risk of considerable blood loss and damage to spinal nerves. Distraction rods are placed to help straighten the spine, and bone grafting is required. Match one of the following health careers to each situation described below: orthopedic technologist, physician assistant, orthopedic nurse, EMG technologist or physician, physical therapist, cell saver technologist or perfusionist, diagnostic imaging technologist or radiology technician, and medical laboratory technologist.

1. Intraoperative X-rays are required. Who would perform these, and what department of the hospital would employ this person?

_____
_____

(continues)

⟳ CASE STUDY 2 *(continued)*

_____

_____

2. Blood loss may be countered by filtering the patient's blood and returning it to her. Who would perform this activity?

_____

_____

_____

_____

3. The patient has been admitted to the hospital before. Which department is contacted for the old records?

_____

_____

_____

_____

4. To whom would blood samples be taken to check the hematocrit and hemoglobin levels during the operative procedure?

_____

_____

_____

_____

5. After surgery, Kathleen may need some rehabilitation in working with her muscles. Which allied health unit may assist with ambulation postop?

_____

_____

_____

_____

⟳ CASE STUDY 3

You are a student attending your first clinical rotation in a large hospital. You have been assigned a preceptor with whom you are having trouble working. She will not let you do anything except observe, and, therefore, you are not learning much or logging the cases that you will need to graduate. You know that something has to be done to improve the situation, but what?

1. Apply the principles of communication. How might you effectively communicate with your preceptor while explaining the problem?

_____

(continues)

CASE STUDY 3 *(continued)*

_____

_____

_____

2. What if she does not respond? What will your next step be?

_____

_____

_____

_____

3. You know that communicating and working as a team is essential in the OR. What can you do to work well with someone after there has been a conflict and/or confrontation?

_____

_____

_____

_____

_____

Lab 1: Orientation to Surgical Technology

Introduction

The orientation to surgical technology will help the student better understand the thinking behind and the process that happens with surgery. During the orientation there is very little hands-on experience, but the orientation stresses who, what, where, when, and why for surgery. This lab is set up so that the learner is able to look at the bigger picture and is able to start making critical thinking a part of their learning process.

Game 1: Who Gets Surgery First?

Time involved: One week for setup

Supplies: Paper and pencil, note cards

Instructors: Make a list of surgeries that fall into the different categories including emergent, urgent, elective, and optional. Utilizing either teams or individuals, pair one surgery and another from a different category and ask the learner, "Who gets surgery first?" You can also group surgeries from the same category and see what the student's reaction and thinking is for each. This will help build critical thinking skills.

Students: Study the categories of how surgeries can be grouped. These include emergent, urgent, elective, and optional. Learn where to place each surgery in accordance with the needs of the patient. Making note cards can be a big help but thinking through the patients' needs will also give you better options regarding "Who gets surgery first?"

Game 2: Name That Specialty

Time involved: One week for setup

Supplies: Paper and pencil, note cards

Instructors: Make a listing of all specialties on one side of a note card; on the other side list what areas of the body are worked on in that specialty and some surgeries that correlate to that specialty. Ask the students questions from either side of the note card. Keep in mind that some surgeries can fall into more than one specialty. You should also be prepared to ask the students why they think their answer is correct to get the thinking behind their answer.

Students: On one side of a note card make a list of all the specialties, and on the other side list what areas of the body and different surgeries are performed under that specialty. Study these to help you better understand which doctor is doing which surgery.

Game 3: Name That Role

Time involved: One week for setup

Supplies: Paper and pencil, note cards

Instructors: The roles that the different team members play in surgery can vary widely or can actually be the same depending on their jobs and training. When the learner is better able to distinguish their role and the expectations of the surgical team member, they are better able to focus on the learning. Make a list of job responsibilities on one side of a note card; on the other side of the card, list who would do these jobs including the surgical technologist in the scrub role (STSR), circulator, anesthesia provider, surgeon, first assistant, and also if that person is sterile or nonsterile when they do these jobs. The jobs can be anything from pulling supplies to handing instruments, cleaning the room, and any other role that may come into play with the patient at any time.

Students: Learning the role that you will play in surgery can be a very difficult task. Depending on the hospital and the state you are in, you could play the role of the person that transports the patient, helps in the ED or OR, or handles instruments. It is very crucial that you understand each role so that the patient has the best care that can possibly be provided. Take note cards and list different jobs that will take place as the patient moves along the path of the hospital. You should then list who can do those jobs. Take the time to think about each job and what each person does to make sure things run smoothly for the patient.

Game 4: Telegraph Wire

Time involved: One week for setup

Supplies: Standard OR personal protective equipment including gowns, gloves, masks, hair covers, and eye protection; a radio or other device to make noise

Instructors: Communication is a very large part of what we do. Being able to speak quickly and clearly with a lot of distraction around us will keep our patients safe. Also important is being able to read what is not said but delivered through emotion. Utilizing the distractions that are all around us in the OR is how we play this game. Make a list of statements and emotions that you would have the learner convey to another. These can either be verbal statements or just an emotion without words. Have the learners put on surgical attire including gloves, gowns, masks, eye protection, and hair covers. Then string the students around the room. Starting with the first person on the line, give them either a statement or an emotion. Have them convey this to the next person in line, the next person will then receive the message and pass it along to the next, until it goes from the front of the line to the back. While this is going on feel free to play the radio loud, have other conversations going on, or just create general distractions. When the information has reached the back of the line, ask the students to repeat what was said or what they perceived the emotion to be.

Students: Communication is the key to all that we do to help our patients. Being able to listen with a lot of distractions can be difficult but can be learned. You also need to learn how to understand emotions. This can be a challenge when all that is available is a person's body language or their eyes. Work on verbal and nonverbal communication skills and then play this learning game.

Standards of Conduct

OBJECTIVES

After studying this chapter, the reader should be able to:

C 1. Analyze major concepts inherent in professional practice law.

2. Interpret the legal responsibilities of the surgical technologist and other surgical team members.

3. Analyze the American Hospital Association's Patient Care Partnership.

4. Describe the need for professional liability insurance policies.

A 5. Analyze the key elements related to developing a surgical conscience.

R 6. Assess the resources that aid the surgical technologist in interpreting and following professional standards of conduct.

7. Develop an increased sensitivity to the influence of ethics in professional practice.

8. Analyze the role of morality during ethical decision making.

9. Cite examples of ethical situations and problems in the health professions.

10. Analyze scope of practice issues as they relate to surgical technology.

11. Evaluate the role of the risk management department in the health care facility.

E 12. Apply principles of problem solving in ethical decision making.

13. Assess errors that may occur in the operating room and devise a plan for investigation, correction, and notification.

Select Key Terms

Define the following, using your textbook glossary or a medical dictionary if necessary:

1. abandonment _____

_____

2. accreditation _____

_____

3. advance directive _____

_____

4. affidavit _____

_____

5. bioethics _____

_____

6. code of ethics _____

_____

7. credentialing _____

_____

8. deontological approach _____

_____

9. ethics _____

_____

10. formalism _____

_____

11. incident report _____

_____

12. informed consent _____

_____

13. liability _____

_____

14. malpractice _____

_____

15. moral principles _____

_____

16. negligence _____

_____

17. Patient Care Partnership _____

_____

18. Patient's Bill of Rights _____

_____

19. risk management _____

_____

20. Safe Medical Device Act _____

_____

21. scope of practice _____

_____

22. surgical conscience _____

_____

23. tort law _____

_____

24. utilitarianism _____

_____

Matching I

Match each term with the correct definition.

_____ A. Certification

_____ B. Licensure

_____ C. Registration

_____ D. Aeger Primo

_____ E. Doctrine of Borrowed Servant

_____ F. Doctrine of Foreseeability

_____ G. Doctrine of Personal Liability

_____ H. Primum non nocere

_____ I. Res ipsa loquitur

_____ J. HIPAA

1. Motto of AST: "The patient first."

2. "Above all, do no harm."

3. The ability to reasonably anticipate that harm or injury may result because of certain acts or omissions. This doctrine could be applied to not applying a safety strap, or a side rail being left down while transporting a patient.

4. Recognition by an appropriate body that an individual has met a predetermined standard.

5. Federal act that establishes privacy standards to protect patients' medical records and other health-related information.

6. Formal process by which qualified individuals are listed in a registry.

7. "The thing speaks for itself."

8. Legal right granted by a government agency in compliance with a statute that authorizes and oversees the activities of a profession.

9. Each person is responsible for his or her own conduct, even though others may be liable as well. This doctrine could be applied to a surgeon delegating a task outside of your scope of practice. The surgeon is wrong to do this, but if you perform the task, you will be liable.

10. The one controlling or directing the employee has greater responsibility than the one paying the employee. This doctrine could be applied to the surgeon and the "captain of the ship" doctrine.

Matching II

Match each term with the correct definition.

____ A. Tort

____ B. Liability

____ C. Negligence

____ D. Abandonment

____ E. Incident report

____ F. Standard of care

____ G. Ethics

____ H. Malpractice

____ I. Iatrogenic injury

____ J. Slander

11. Lack of skill or care. Departure from the standard of care.

12. Oral statement that damages a person's reputation.

13. A civil wrong that causes injury to another person which may be intentional or unintentional.

14. Adverse outcome that results from the activity of health care professionals.

15. Description of expected conduct for a given circumstance. What a prudent caregiver would do in a similar circumstance.

16. Leaving a patient who needs care and is dependent on their presence as a caregiver.

17. Professional misconduct, lack of judgment or skill that results in harm to another.

18. Report of an irregular or adverse patient occurrence.

19. Legally responsible for damages. An obligation to do or not do something. May be personal or corporate.

20. System of moral principles and rules that become standards for professional conduct.

Short Answer Discussion

1. Explain the difference between general consent and special (informed) consent processes.

_____

_____

_____

2. Define the following terms in your own words.

Law: _____

_____

_____

Ethics: _____

_____

_____

Morals: _____

_____

_____

3. Based on your definitions of law, ethics, and morals, explain the importance of each as related to health care. How are these concepts important in surgery specifically?

_____

_____

_____

SAMPLE

(Name of Facility)   (Patient Identification–Stamp)

Standard Consent to Surgery or Special Procedure

Patient Name _____

Attending Physician _____

Surgeon or Supervising Physician _____

1. (*Name of facility*) maintains personnel and facilities to assist your/the patient's physicians and surgeons in their performance of various surgical or other special diagnostic or therapeutic procedures. These operations and procedures may involve risks of unsuccessful results, complications, injury, or death, from known and/or unforeseen causes, and no warranty or guarantee is made as to results or cure.

   You have the right to be informed of such risks as well as the nature of the operation or procedure; the expected benefits of such; and any available alternatives and their risks and benefits. Except in case of emergency, operations or procedures are not performed until you have had the opportunity to receive this information and have given your consent. You have the right to consent or refuse any proposed operation or procedure any time prior to its performance.

2. Your/the patient's physician/surgeon has recommended the operation or procedure set forth below. Upon your authorization and consent, the operation or procedure set forth below, together with any different or further procedures which in the opinion of the supervising physician/surgeon may be indicated due to an emergency, will be performed on you/the patient. The operation or procedure will be performed by the supervising physician or surgeon named above (or in the event of an emergency causing his/her inability to complete the procedure, a qualified substitute supervising physician or surgeon), together with associates and assistants, including anesthesiologists, pathologists and radiologists from the medical staff of (*name of facility*) to whom the supervising physician or surgeon may assign designated responsibilities. The persons in attendance for the purpose of performing specialized medical services such as anesthesia, radiology or pathology are not agents, servants, or employees of the facility and your/the patient's supervising physician or surgeon, but are independent contractors, and therefore your agents, servants, or employees.

3. The pathologist is hereby authorized to use his/her discretion in disposing any member, organ, or other tissue removed from your/the patient's person during the operation or procedure set forth below.

4. Your signature below constitutes your acknowledgment that: you have read and agree to the foregoing; that the operation or procedure set forth below has been adequately explained to you by the above named physician/surgeon and by your/the patient's anesthesiologist and that you have received all of the information that you desire concerning such operation or procedure; and that you authorize and consent to the performance of the operation or procedure.

Procedure: _____

_____

_____

_____

Signature (Patient/Parent/Conservator/Guardian)   Relationship (if other than patient)

_____

Date   Time   Witness

I have been informed of the risks/benefits and alternatives of blood product infusions. I consent to the use of blood product infusions.

_____

Signature (Patient/Parent/Conservator/Guardian)   Relationship (if other than patient)

_____

Date   Time   Witness

(Name of Facility)   (Patient Identification–Stamp)
(Address of Facility)

4. What is "time-out" and how is it important to the quality patient care provided by the surgical team? List three errors or incidents that could potentially occur if the "time-out" was not performed.

_____

_____

_____

5. In Chapter 1, you were asked to define "surgical conscience" and whether you felt that it is something that you are born with or something learned. Do you still agree with your original answer based on your further study of morals and ethics?

_____

_____

_____

Interactive Learning

1. While working with a partner, complete the sample surgical consent as if you were having elective surgery. Have one person sign as the surgical patient and role-play while your partner presents the consent as a hospital employee.

2. Research a bioethical topic and write a summary that includes the pro-argument and the con-argument, and close your paper with your own feelings regarding the topic you've chosen. Share this research with your class and/or your instructor.

3. Discuss scope of practice as a class and research whether or not there is a scope of practice specific to surgical technologists in your state. Review examples of AST Recommended Standards of Practice and various Guideline Statements and discuss how they could protect you as a professional.

4. Reflect on your own life and past experiences and write about an ethical dilemma that you have encountered. Describe the event, how you felt about it, and how you resolved the issue. This paper can be written for submission or as a journal-style entry for personal use.

Case Studies

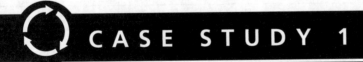

CASE STUDY 1

Mollie is a 9-year-old girl admitted to the hospital following a seizure on the playground at school. She has been diagnosed with a cerebral arteriovenous malformation (AVM). A craniotomy with attendant clipping and removal of the AVM has been proposed. Mollie is in a foster home with a guardian. Her biological parents are both dead.

1. What information is needed for a valid consent for surgery in this case?

_____

_____

(continues)

CASE STUDY 1 *(continued)*

2. Who can give consent in this case?

_____

_____

3. Review the consent form sample. What is the role of the witness regarding the consent form?

_____

_____

CASE STUDY 2

Harold is still a relatively new surgical technologist. Since passing the national certification examination, he has been working in a large teaching hospital. He loves the work and being at a hospital "on the cutting edge." He is surprised to find out that several of the staff members do not think they should be performing some of the procedures they do. They feel that it is experimenting on human beings.

1. Do you believe health care professionals are required to do everything necessary to save and prolong human life?

_____

_____

2. What is more important: quality or quantity of life? How do you know what quality is?

_____

_____

3. Is there such a thing as a "right to die"?

_____

_____

4. Does a health care professional have the right to refuse to participate in approved procedures?

_____

_____

Lab 2: Standards of Conduct

Introduction

The Standards of Conduct portion of this manual will give the student a better understanding of the moral and ethical expectations of being a surgical technologist and a health care worker. When the student knows the expectations and rules before starting a task, they will have a better chance for success in the end. There is very little in the way of practical work here, but when the student starts the practical portion they will understand more fully the expectations placed on them as far as patient care; surgical conscience; and moral, ethical, and legal issues.

Game 1: Legal Term Jeopardy®

Time involved: One week for setup

Supplies: Paper and pencil, note cards, and a display (either whiteboard, blackboard, or computer)

Instructors: Legal Term Jeopardy® can be played several different ways. You can download from a PowerPoint presentation–style game from the Internet; it can be used on a whiteboard or blackboard, or you can work from note cards. Here are a few ways that may work for you. Your categories may include what surgical technologists do, how surgical technologists are used in the OR, or who they protect, and then decide how many answers you will place in each category. Make a list of legal terms that fall into the different categories; then you can use the terms or their meanings for your questions. The what, where, when, why, and how of the legal terms are used to pose the questions; students will give you the "What is _____" answers. You may utilize either teams or individuals. This will help build critical thinking skills.

Students: Study the legal terms, their meanings, and their uses. Making note cards can be a big help. Make as many note cards as you are able and study them each chance you get. If you carry the cards around with you, each time you have a few minutes of free time, pull them out and work on them. This will greatly enhance learning.

Game 2: Moral vs. Ethical

Time involved: One week for setup

Supplies: Your mind

Instructors: Make a listing of ethical and moral situations. Give the students a situation that fits into either or both categories of ethical or moral. Ask the students if the situation fits into a moral or ethical category or both. You should also be prepared to ask the students why they think their answer is correct in order to reveal the thinking behind their answer. Give points for correct answers, and correct thinking.

Students: This game takes on a lot more thinking than memorizing. Understanding the difference between morals and ethics can be difficult. Study the definitions of both and then think about what may fall into either category or both. Understanding the difference between the two will greatly enhance patient care. Make as many note cards as you are able and study them each chance you get. If you carry the cards around with you, each time you have a few minutes of free time, pull them out and work on them. This will greatly enhance learning.

Game 3: Name that Acronym

Time involved: One week for set up

Supplies: Paper and pencil, note cards

Instructors: Make a list of all acronyms that you expect the students to know. Have students write the acronyms on one side of a note card, and on the other side, list what they mean. Ask the students questions from either side of the note card. You should also be prepared to ask the students why the think their answer is correct in order to reveal the thinking behind their answer. Give points for correct answers. You can place students in teams or work as individuals.

Students: Write acronyms on one side of each note card, and on the other side list the definitions for each acronym.

CHAPTER 3

The Surgical Patient

OBJECTIVES

After studying this chapter, the reader should be able to:

C 1. Assess the patient's response to illness and hospitalization.

A 2. Demonstrate awareness that all surgical patients have the right to the highest standards and practices in asepsis.

R 3. Distinguish and assess the physical, spiritual, and psychological needs of a patient.

E 4. Distinguish and assess cultural and religious influences on the surgical patient.

Select Key Terms

Define the following, using your textbook glossary or a medical dictionary if necessary:

1. Maslow's Hierarchy of Needs _____

_____

2. patient _____

_____

3. physical need _____

_____

4. psychological need _____

_____

5. social need _____

_____

6. spiritual need _____

_____

Matching

Match each stage of Maslow's Hierarchy with the correct description.

_____ A. Physiological needs

_____ B. Safety needs

_____ C. Belongingness and love needs

_____ D. Prestige and esteem needs

_____ E. Self-actualization

1. This is the need to fulfill what one believes is one's purpose.

2. This level of need refers to a positive evaluation of oneself and others, a need to be respected and to respect others.

3. These needs refer to the perception on the part of the individual that his or her environment is safe.

4. The most basic needs are biological needs like water, oxygen, food, and temperature regulation.

5. These are basic social needs—to be known and cared for as an individual and to care for another.

Short Answer Discussion

1. Describe what self-actualization means to you. Do you feel that everyone reaches this stage in their life?

_____

_____

2. Some health care professionals have little or no direct contact with patients. Do you feel that a thorough understanding of patient care, patient needs, and therapeutic relationships are necessary to the surgical technologist's role specifically?

_____

_____

3. Imagine yourself as the surgical patient undergoing a body-image changing procedure. What are your physiological needs vs. your emotional needs? How do you feel while being wheeled into the operating room?

_____

_____

4. America is a culturally diverse country. Do you think that understanding cultural and religious beliefs is an integral part of caring for the surgical patient? Provide an example of a culture different from your own and explain how you could make the patient from this culture more comfortable in the operating room.

_____

_____

5. Do you agree with Maslow's theory of a hierarchical progression of developmental stages? Why or why not? Is there another developmental theory with which you agree more?

_____

_____

6. Compare and contrast the three definitions of death. Describe which definition is used when considering the patient a candidate for organ transplantation.

_____

_____

_____

7. Types of surgery: What type of procedure is intended to provide the patient with symptomatic relief? What type of surgery treats or manages a disease?

_____

_____

8. What is the significance of an advance directive? Could an advance directive be considered euthanasia? If so, what type of euthanasia is it?

_____

_____

9. Describe briefly Kubler-Ross's Five Stages of Grief.

_____

_____

10. In some states a death that occurs in the operating room may be considered a coroner's case. When preparing the patient for a coroner's autopsy, all tubes such as the endotracheal tube, IV line, or Foley are left in place. Why do you think that the coroner would want to be notified?

_____

_____

Interactive Learning

1. Reflect on your own life and past experiences. Label Maslow's Hierarchy on Figure 3-1; next to each section of the hierarchy write a sentence or two about a time you could personally relate to that category of needs. Discuss how many of your class members feel that they have reached the top (self-actualization) of the hierarchy in their own lives.

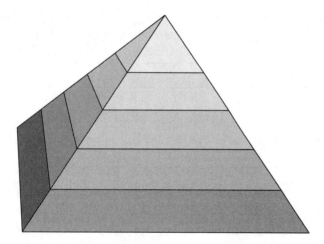

Figure 3-1

Case Study

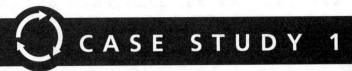

CASE STUDY 1

Myrtle is scheduled for a total hip arthroplasty in about half an hour. She is in the preoperative holding area and has just expressed to her nurse a fear that she will not survive the procedure. Myrtle has asked to speak with the chaplain.

1. What type of need is Myrtle expressing?

_____
_____
_____
_____

2. Should her premonition be taken seriously?

_____
_____
_____
_____

3. With the procedure scheduled to take place shortly, will time allow the chaplain to be called?

_____
_____
_____
_____

CASE STUDY 2

Johanna is a 14-year-old Jehovah's Witness and has just been involved in a car accident while driving with her mother. The trauma team in the ER ordered a CT, which showed that she has internal bleeding and a broken pelvis. She has been rushed to the OR for her life-threatening injuries.

1. What are beliefs regarding blood products amongst the Jehovah's Witness religion?

_____
_____
_____
_____

(continues)

CASE STUDY 2 *(continued)*

2. What decisions will the surgical team and Johanna's family be faced with if it is determined that Johanna needs a blood transfusion to survive surgery? *Note: this may require independent research. Consult with your instructor.*_____

_____

_____

_____

3. Prioritize Johanna's situation as related to Maslow's Hierarchy. Which should take priority, her physiological needs or her spiritual needs? Why?

_____

_____

_____

_____

CASE STUDY 3

Two days ago Carl received the news that he has prostate cancer. Today, Carl has been waiting to see the surgeon for over an hour to discuss possible surgical options that may help his diagnosis. Susan, the receptionist, just received a call that Dr. Thomkins will be delayed another 40 minutes. When she gives Carl this news, he becomes very angry and shouts "It seems like doctors only care about time when they are charging you! I've waited here for over an hour today, maybe I should charge him in 15-minute increments for my time today!" and storms out the door before Susan can even respond.

1. Why do you think Carl may have gotten so upset?

_____

_____

_____

_____

2. What is the Roy Adaptation Model and do you think it applies to Carl? If so, why?

_____

_____

_____

_____

3. List and describe four coping mechanisms that Carl may be working through.

_____

_____

_____

_____

Lab 3: The Surgical Patient

Introduction

The surgical patient portion of this manual will give the student a better understanding of the surgical patient and his or her needs physiologically, sociologically, and psychologically. There is really no practical portion to this lab, but it helps the students to use their thinking and reasoning skills to better benefit patients by meeting their needs while they are under our care.

Game 1: Placing the Need

Time involved: One week for setup

Supplies: Paper and pencil, note cards, and a display (either whiteboard, blackboard, or computer)

Instructors: Placing the needs can be accomplished in several different ways. You will utilize Maslow's Hierarchy of Needs for this game. Using a display, you will make a pyramid. You will then make different note cards with different needs, using the Maslow description, but also the needs themselves. You may have one card that states physiological need and more cards that state needs that fit into this category. The what, where, when, why, and how of the needs are used to fill up the pyramid. The student or team will be given a stack of cards with the needs upside down. Each person will then pull off the top card in order and will be expected to place the card in the correct category. Each right answer is awarded a point; when one is missed, another team can be allowed to steal the point if they get the right answer, and if the steal is wrong the team will lose a point. Set a time limit for each point and each steal. This activity will help build critical thinking skills.

Students: Study Maslow's Hierarchy of Needs. Fit actual attributes into each category on the pyramid. Making note cards can be a big help. Make as many note cards as you are able and study the cards each chance you get. If you carry these around with you, each time you have a few minutes of free time, pull them out and work on them. This will greatly enhance learning.

Game 2: Characteristics

Time involved: One week for setup

Supplies: Paper and pencil, note cards, and your acting skills

Instructors: Make a list of emotions, physical attributes, or other characteristics of patients. This can encompass a patient's age along with a feeling, or a patient's facial expression. Place each on a note card that will be given to the student. The idea is to then have the student act out what is on the note card. Although acting out fear may be easy, what about denial or malaise? Give the students a little time to get into character, and also give them time to ask you questions. You may expect some of these characteristics to be acted out with only facial expressions, whereas others may need the students to ask questions or work within a skit to get the meaning. The student is not permitted to tell their team what their task is, and will be given points when their team gets it right, or else the other team is allowed to guess the correct answer. You can also ask the students how they would handle this situation or patient. Set a time limit. Assign points accordingly.

Students: This game involves a lot more thinking than memorizing. Understanding how the patient thinks is one thing, but being able to convey this to another student is quite different. Understanding how to read different patients will better help you understand how to deal with these situations. Between the two you will greatly enhance patient care.

CHAPTER 4

Special Populations

OBJECTIVES

After studying this chapter, the reader should be able to:

C 1. Compare and contrast the surgical care considerations for pediatric patients and patients who are obese, diabetic, pregnant, immunocompromised, disabled, geriatric, or experiencing trauma.

2. Evaluate the unique physical and psychological needs of each special population.

A 3. Compare and contrast the intraoperative considerations that relate to postoperative wound healing for pediatric patients and patients who are obese, diabetic, immunocompromised, geriatric, or traumatized.

R 4. Evaluate the role of the surgical technologist for the surgical care of each special population.

E 5. Assess the ethical commitment that is required of surgical technologists as it relates to care of special populations.

6. Determine the general needs associated with special populations of surgical patients.

Select Key Terms

Define the following, using your textbook glossary or a medical dictionary if necessary:

1. arterial blood gases (ABGs) _____

_____

2. autoimmune diseases _____

_____

3. central venous catheter _____

_____

4. diabetes mellitus _____

_____

5. enterocolitis _____

_____

6. golden hour _____

_____

7. human immunodeficiency virus (HIV) _____

_____

8. hypothermia _____

_____

9. immunocompetence _____

_____

10. intra-arterial measurement _____

_____

11. Kaposi's sarcoma _____

_____

12. kinematics _____

_____

13. kernicterus _____

_____

14. penetrating trauma _____

_____

15. pneumothorax _____

_____

16. Revised Trauma Score _____

_____

17. septic shock _____

_____

18. splenectomy _____

_____

19. splenomegaly _____

_____

20. torticollis _____

_____

21. urine output _____

_____

22. venous compression device _____

_____

Matching I

Match the age group with its ego quality/tasks. Knowing what is valued or important to the patient can help you relate to the patient.

_____ A. Infancy

_____ B. Toddler

_____ C. Preschool

_____ D. School age

_____ E. Adolescence

_____ F. Young adult

_____ G. Early middle age

_____ H. 50–70 years

_____ I. 70 Years–death

1. Wisdom; learns to accept help and body changes.

2. Fidelity and devotion to others; adjusts to body changes; privacy; peers.

3. Competence; distinguish gender roles; develop skills; increased socialization.

4. Productivity, consideration, charity; adjust to aging parents and children becoming adults.

5. Hope; bond to mother.

6. Direction, purpose, conscience; learn basic right from wrong; identification.

7. Intimate affiliation and love; select partner.

8. Self-control and willpower; parents; autonomy versus shame and doubt.

9. Develops relationships; at the pinnacle of power in career.

Short Answer Discussion

1. List the correct terms to describe pediatric patient ages from birth through 12 years of age.

_____

_____

_____

_____

2. Why is temperature regulation so important in the pediatric patient? Specifically in the infant patient younger than 6 months of age?

_____

_____

_____

_____

3. At what age do the vitals signs of pediatric patients reach adult norms?

_____

_____

_____

_____

4. Research the difference between obese and morbidly obese. How many pounds overweight is someone who is diagnosed as "obese"?

_____

_____

_____

_____

5. Which type of diabetes would a patient be diagnosed with if the patient's pancreas produced little or no insulin and he or she was required to have daily doses of insulin?

_____

_____

_____

_____

6. When placing the pregnant patient in the supine position, care should be taken to position the patient with a rolled towel or sheet under the _____ hip. Why?

_____

_____

_____

_____

7. In relationship to trauma assessment, how is the Glasgow Coma Scale used and what population of patients are typically assessed by using this scale? Independent research may be required; consult with your instructor.

_____

_____

_____

_____

8. Why are kinematics or mechanisms of injury (MOI) important to the health care team in caring for the trauma patient?

_____

_____

_____

_____

9. Why should the health care provider avoid placing a urinary catheter in the neonatal or infant patient? What is a normal urine output for an infant?

_____

_____

_____

_____

10. Review the developmental theories in Table 4-1 of your textbook. Which life stage development theory do you most agree with? Do you find Piaget's or Erikson's theories more applicable?

_____

_____

_____

_____

11. Using what you learned in Chapter 3 about patients and their unique needs, how do you feel the surgical technologist should interact with patients to establish an environment of care and concern?

_____

_____

_____

_____

12. Compare and contrast the physiological and psychological needs of the following special populations:
    - obese (bariatric) patients

    _____

    - diabetic patients

    _____

    - pediatric patients

    _____

    - pregnant patients

    _____

    - immunocompromised patients/isolation patients

    _____

    - disabled patients

    _____

    - geriatric patients

    _____

    - trauma patients

    _____

Interactive Learning

As a group, role-play as special-needs patients and their caregivers. Examples: For a visually impaired patient, smear Vaseline on a pair of old glasses to imitate what it would be like to have cataracts. For a hearing-impaired patient, place cotton balls in your ears and have someone give you instructions in a normal tone of voice. Be creative, and record your observations to share with the class.

Case Studies

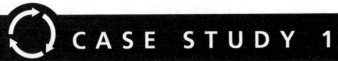

CASE STUDY 1

Seven-year-old Alexandra lost control of her scooter as she was riding down her sloped driveway. She inadvertently rode into the street and was hit by a car. She was not wearing a helmet.

1. What is the first priority of the emergency team that arrives at the scene to assist Alexandra?

   _____

   _____

   _____

   _____

2. The emergency team suspects that Alexandra may have sustained a neck injury during the accident. What should be done to protect the spinal cord?

   _____

   _____

   _____

   _____

3. Alexandra appears to be going into hypovolemic shock. What step(s) should be taken to prevent the hypovolemia from becoming severe?

   _____

   _____

   _____

   _____

CASE STUDY 2

Baby boy Daniels's birth was traumatic. He sustained a bone fracture and the left side of his face appears to droop.

1. What is the most common type of bone fracture that occurs during traumatic birth?

   _____

   _____

   _____

   _____

(continues)

CASE STUDY 2 *(continued)*

2. What is most likely causing the neonate's face to droop?

_____

_____

_____

_____

3. Is the facial droop expected to resolve? If so, how soon?

_____

_____

_____

_____

CASE STUDY 3

The circulator has just come to the preoperative holding area to pick up 18-month-old Henry to take him to the operating room for his ear surgery. Henry took one look at the circulator and began screaming and clinging to his mother.

1. Use the life tasks approach to determine if Henry's behavior is appropriate for his age group.

_____

_____

2. Using what you learned previously about Maslow's Hierarchy of Needs, which of Henry's needs may not be met when he is taken from his mother by the circulator to go to the operating room?

_____

_____

3. What can be done to make the transition from being in his mother's care to being in the care of the circulator a smooth one for Henry?

_____

_____

Lab 4: Special Populations

Introduction

The special populations portion of this manual will give the student a better understanding of surgical patients and their needs, physiologically, sociologically, psychologically, and spiritually. There is really no practical portion to this lab, but it helps students use their thinking and reasoning skills to better benefit patients by meeting their needs while they are under our care.

Game 1: Characteristics

Time involved: One week for setup

Supplies: Paper and pencil, note cards, and your acting skills

Instructors: Make a list of emotions, physical attributes, or other characteristics of the special populations patient. This can encompass a patient's age along with a feeling. Place these on a note card that will be given to the student. The idea is to then have the student act out what the note card says. Although acting out fear may be easy, what about denial or malaise? Give the students a little time to get into character, and also give them time to ask you questions. You may expect some of these characteristics to be acted out with only facial expressions, whereas others may need the students to ask questions or work within a skit to get the meaning. The student is not permitted to tell their team what their task is, and will be given points when their team gets it right, or the other team is allowed to guess the correct answer. You can also ask the students how they would handle this situation or patient. Set a time limit. Assign points accordingly.

Students: This game requires a lot more thinking than memorizing. Understanding how the patient thinks is one thing; being able to convey this to another student is quite different. Understanding how to read different patients will better help you understand how to deal with these situations. Understanding how a patient thinks and how to read different patients will greatly enhance the patient care you give.

Physical Environment and Safety Standards

OBJECTIVES

After studying this chapter, the reader should be able to:

C 1. Recognize the hazards to the patient in the operative environment.

2. Distinguish between support services that work with the operating room (OR) team in the care of the patient.

A 3. Review the type of air-handling system required in the OR and the temperature and humidity required to maintain a sterile field.

4. Indicate cleaning procedures, traffic patterns, and routines required in the operative environment.

R 5. Analyze the role of the surgical technologist in the protection of self, patients, and others from hazards in the operative environment.

E 6. Recognize the design types of the OR.

7. Classify hospital departments that relate to surgical services.

8. Recognize the working environment of the OR.

9. Determine the physical components of the OR.

Select Key Terms

Define the following, using your textbook glossary or a medical dictionary if necessary:

1. airborne bacteria _____

_____

2. back table _____

_____

3. decontamination room _____

_____

4. electrosurgical unit _____

_____

5. hamper_____

_____

6. high-efficiency particulate air (HEPA) filter _____

_____

7. hypothermia _____

_____

8. ionizing radiation _____

_____

9. laminar air flow _____

_____

10. Mayo stand _____

_____

11. polymethyl methacrylate (PMMA) _____

_____

12. Occupational Safety and Health Administration (OSHA) _____

_____

13. pathology department _____

_____

14. perfusionist _____

_____

15. personal protective equipment (PPE) _____

_____

16. plume _____

_____

17. postanesthesia care unit (PACU) _____

_____

18. prophylaxis _____

_____

19. restricted area _____

_____

20. Standard Precautions _____

_____

21. suction outlet _____

_____

22. surgical site infection (SSI) _____

_____

23. triboelectrification _____

_____

Short Answer

1. Which OR design plan features a clean central core surrounded by a series of operating rooms?

   _____

   _____

   _____

2. What are the correct settings for temperature and humidity in the operating room?

   _____

   _____

   _____

3. Describe positive pressure air supply. What is its purpose in the OR?

   _____

   _____

   _____

4. How many air exchanges are required per hour in the OR?

   _____

   _____

   _____

5. At what percentage does humidity become conductive to spark transmission?

   _____

   _____

   _____

6. List three safety precautions that must be followed when a laser is used during a case.

   _____

   _____

   _____

7. Glutaraldehyde is a liquid disinfectant and sterilizing agent. What is the commercial name for glutaraldehyde? What precautions must be taken when working with it?

   _____

   _____

   _____

8. List the three main concerns the surgical technologist should have if a fire occurs in the OR.

   _____

   _____

   _____

9. What does EtO stand for and how is it used? What are the hazards associated with EtO processes?

_____

_____

_____

10. What is formalin used for in the operating room? Which body system is most at risk if handling precautions are not followed?

_____

_____

_____

Short Answer Discussion

1. Discuss common situations that put staff at risk for blood borne exposure and safety strategies that can be implemented to prevent a sharps injury or blood borne exposure in the OR.

_____

_____

_____

2. Discuss symptoms of latex allergies and the risks that health care workers and latex-sensitive patients are faced with. Check your lab to see how many of the supplies that you use are latex-free.

_____

_____

_____

3. *Independent Activity.* Create a color-coded chart that highlights the colors of the tanks and/or hoses for gases used in the operating room. Discuss where they would be shut off in an emergency situation. Consult your instructor for specific information.

_____

_____

_____

Interactive Learning

1. With a group of classmates, design your own OR department. On one side of a poster-board design your entire OR department including the necessary elements discussed in the chapter (e.g., traffic patterns, division of restricted and unrestricted areas, and clean from dirty rooms and hallways). On the back side of the poster, magnify one of your ORs—again being sure to include the necessary elements discussed in the chapter (e.g., room setup, required equipment and furniture, room temperature and humidity, and outlets). Share your design with your class.

2. Visit the Occupational Safety and Health Administration (OSHA) or the Centers for Disease Control and Prevention (CDC) web page and familiarize yourself with how these agencies present their research findings, which dictate our health care guidelines. Print out items of interest to share with other class members.

3. If you are not yet in a clinical rotation, ask your instructor to set up a tour of your local hospital or surgical center. On your tour, visit the OR and Central Sterile Supply and Processing Department to compare what you've read in this chapter to the "real-world." Discuss your findings as a class and ways in which that facility could be made safer.

Case Studies

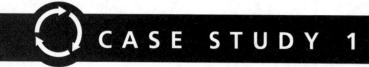

CASE STUDY 1

Eloise is preparing to scrub for an open reduction internal fixation (ORIF) of a tibial plateau fracture. Intraoperative X-rays will be taken with possible cast application.

1. What special communications with other departments/personnel will be necessary prior to this procedure?

_____

_____

_____

_____

2. Will Eloise need to wear any personal protective equipment (PPE) for this procedure?

_____

_____

_____

_____

3. Will the patient require any safety equipment during the procedure?

_____

_____

_____

_____

4. The presence of an X-ray tech (radiology technician) in the room presents a special situation. What responsibility does Eloise have during this time?

_____

_____

_____

_____

⟳ C A S E   S T U D Y   2

Today is Saturday; the staff in the operating room is limited. Marcus has been assigned to a femoropopliteal bypass surgery that could take six to eight hours. During the week, the OR staff can expect to be relieved for lunch, but today Marcus knows that is unlikely to happen.

1. What do you think Marcus must do in advance to physically prepare himself for this lengthy procedure?

   _____

   _____

   _____

   _____

2. Are there any tips that you can give Marcus to reduce the strain on his body while the case is in progress?

   _____

   _____

   _____

   _____

3. What are some of the proper body mechanics that Marcus will want to keep in mind prior to any heavy lifting of patients and/or instrument sets?

   _____

   _____

   _____

   _____

Lab 5: Physical Environment and Safety Standards

Introduction

The Physical Environment and Safety Standards portion of this manual will give the student a better understanding of the environment and the safety that is needed to keep the student and patient safe. Safety should always be the first consideration for surgical technologists. Keeping safe will ensure that the learner's family and the patient will also be safe. The easy thinking is that if it is warm, wet, and not yours, you should be wearing PPE. The more difficult afterthought is that if I do not put myself in jeopardy, my family and my future patients will be kept safe because I did not catch something I could transfer to them now or in the future.

Game 1: Patient Pathway

Time involved: One week for setup

Supplies: Paper and pencil, note cards, and a display (either whiteboard, blackboard, or computer)

Instructors: Draw several different surgery department pathways on a visual display. Have the students place the different departments or rooms within those pathways and indicate the proper attire for each department and what happens in each of those areas. You can either point to an area on the display or pull the names out of a hat and assign each to a team or individual.

Students: This game involves a lot more thinking than memorizing. Understanding the flow of the patient through the hospital and OR gives you a better understanding of what is taking place and why. Work on the different flow charts for the different OR setups to help you with this game.

Game 2: Equipment Jeopardy®

Time involved: One week for setup

Supplies: Paper and pencil, note cards, and a display (either whiteboard, blackboard, or computer)

Instructors: Equipment Jeopardy® can be played several different ways. You can download a PowerPoint presentation–style game from the Internet, you can use a whiteboard or blackboard, or you can work from note cards. Here are a few ways that may work for you. Your categories may include the function of the equipment, what procedures it may be used for, or the name of the equipment; then decide how many answers you will place in each. Make a list of the equipment that fall into the different categories, or use pictures of the equipment, and then you can use these for your questions. The what, where, when, why, and how of the equipment are used to pose the questions; students will give you the "What is _____" answer. You can utilize either teams or individuals. This exercise will help build critical thinking skills.

Students: Study the different pieces of equipment and their uses. Making note cards can be a big help. Make as many note cards as you are able and study them each chance you get. If you carry the cards around with you, each time you have a few minutes of free time, pull them out and work on them. This will greatly enhance learning.

Game 3: Fire Safety, Extinguisher Type

Time involved: One week for setup

Supplies: Paper and pencil, note cards, and a display, (either whiteboard, blackboard, or computer)

Instructors: This is a simple question-and-answer format. You will ask the students for answers to questions that you expect the student to know as part of this area. The questions should relate to fire safety, fire extinguishers, and their classes, types, and uses. It should also include the different types of fires, components needed for a fire, and what to do in case of a fire while at the hospital.

Students: Study the fire safety section. Making note cards can be a big help. Make as many note cards as you are able and study the cards each chance you get. If you carry the cards around with you, each time you have a few minutes of free time, pull them out and work on them. This will greatly enhance learning.

Game 4: Standard Precautions

Time involved: One week for setup

Supplies: Paper and pencil, note cards, and a display (either whiteboard, blackboard, or computer)

Instructors: Make a list of hazards that the learner will encounter at the hospital. These can be things such as blood on the floor, a TB-positive patient, and broken glass. Ask the student how they would handle the situation, but also ask why they would do it that way.

Students: Study standard precautions, hospital policy, and CDC policy on how to handle situations that may arise in the hospital. Making note cards can be a big help. Create as many note cards as you can and study them each chance you get. If you carry the cards around with you, each time you have a few minutes of free time, pull them out and work on them. This will greatly enhance learning.

Game 5: Material Safety Data Sheet (MSDS) Bingo

Time involved: One week for setup

Supplies: Paper and pencil, note cards, and a display (either whiteboard, blackboard, computer)

Instructors: MSDS bingo can be accomplished in several different ways. You can download several different free bingo cards from the Internet. It just takes a little searching to find these items. Either ask your students to identify matching answers on their bingo cards while you provide the questions or have them identify matching questions while you provide the answers. Utilize what is known and must be provided on the MSDS sheets, but also what chemicals they may encounter while working in the hospital setting. You should make a list of chemicals that you are going to ask the students about, so that they can study ahead of time.

Students: Study the list of chemicals that has been provided to you by your instructor; also note the information that should be listed on an MSDS. Look up the MSDS for each of the chemicals. Making note cards can be a big help. Create as many note cards as you can and study them each chance you get. If you carry the cards around with you, each time you have a few minutes of free time, pull them out and work on them. This will greatly enhance learning.

Principles and Practice of Surgical Technology

CHAPTER 6

Biomedical Science

OBJECTIVES

After studying this chapter, the reader should be able to:

C 1. Recognize basic components of a computer system.

2. Apply electrical safety precautions.

3. Interpret terms related to physics.

4. Interpret the basic concepts of robotics.

A 5. (No objectives focused on asepsis in this chapter; however, the practice of sterile technique will be necessary when using related equipment in the OR.)

R 6. Demonstrate basic word processing, Internet, and e-mail functions.

7. Apply computer knowledge to safe patient care.

8. Analyze the geometric concepts of robotics and the mechanisms of the robotic system.

E 9. Cite the basic principles of electricity and their application in the OR.

10. Apply the principles of robotics to safe patient care practices in the OR.

11. Apply the principles of physics to safe patient care practices in the OR.

Select Key Terms

Define the following, using your textbook glossary or a medical dictionary if necessary:

1. active electrode _____

_____

2. Cartesian coordinate geometry _____

_____

3. central processing unit (CPU) _____

_____

4. circuit _____

_____

5. degrees of freedom _____

_____

6. dispersive (inactive) electrode _____

_____

7. electrons _____

_____

8. free electrons _____

_____

9. generator _____

_____

10. ground wire _____

_____

11. infrared waves _____

_____

12. insulator_____

_____

13. load _____

_____

14. mass _____

_____

15. modem _____

_____

16. monitor _____

_____

17. mouse _____

_____

18. neutrons _____

_____

19. periodic table _____

_____

20. plasma _____

_____

21. power _____

_____

22. pressure _____

_____

23. protons _____

_____

24. quarks _____

_____

25. refraction _____

_____

26. resistance _____

_____

27. switch _____

_____

28. volume _____

_____

29. weight _____

_____

30. X-rays _____

_____

Matching: Robotics

Match the robotic term with the appropriate definition:

_____ A. Cartesian geometry

_____ B. Resolution

_____ C. Binaural hearing

_____ D. Degrees of freedom

_____ E. Degrees of rotation

_____ F. Manipulator

_____ G. Telechir

_____ H. Articulation

_____ I. Second generation

_____ J. Third generation

1. Stereo similar to human

2. Remotely controlled robot

3. The angles of a joint that allow movement clockwise or counterclockwise around a joint/axis.

4. Robotic arm

5. Number of dimensions that a manipulator can move (usually 3)

6. Autonomous or insect robot

7. Monitored robot with pressure or tactile sensors and vision or hearing capabilities

8. Ability to differentiate between two objects

9. Joint

10. Mathematical design that allows arm movement in a perpendicular axes along x, y, and z axes (up–down, right–left, and front–back)

Matching: Lasers

Match the laser with the correct description:

_____ A. Argon

_____ B. ND:YAG

_____ C. Holmium

_____ D. Carbon dioxide

_____ E. Laser head

_____ F. Electromagnetic spectrum

_____ G. Energy pump

_____ H. Delivery system

_____ I. Tissue effects

_____ J. Laser beam characteristics

11. Solid crystal invisible beam; useful clear fluid environments; requires cooling system; fiber system delivery with contact or noncontact fibers; tips require careful handling

12. Absorption, reflection, or transmission

13. Blue or green light beam; travels through clear fluid/tissues; useful for ophthalmic or cystoscopy surgery; absorbed by hemoglobin; useful in port wine dermabrasion; 208- or 220-volt service

14. Flexible fiber delivery; 208-volt service; useful arthoscopy/cystosocpy; clear fluid environments

15. Articulated arm, fixed optical array or fiber

16. Monochromatic; collimated; fluence; coherent

17. Most common; least expensive; gas media; invisible beam; articulated mirror/lens delivery system requires care; useful all surgery except clear fluid environments; absorbed by water

18. Contains the media with mirrors at either end

19. Radio waves, microwaves, infrared waves, visible light, ultraviolet light X-ray, and gamma ray

20. Excitation with electrical energy, chemical energy, or flash lamps.

Short Answer

1. Which portable storage device has the largest storage capacity? (Note: Additional options may be available other than those listed in textbook.)

_____

_____

_____

2. What term is used to describe the visual display of shortcuts to available programs from the desktop or home page when using the Internet?

_____

_____

_____

3. What hardware component is considered the "brains" of the computer that processes, manages, and coordinates the operations of the computer?

_____

_____

_____

4. Place the following in ascending order of memory size: terabyte, megabyte, kilobyte, gigabyte, googlebyte.

_____

_____

_____

5. Why might the patient's jewelry be hazardous in the OR?

_____

_____

_____

6. Name the scientific law that mathematically explains the relationship between voltage, current (amps), and resistance as it pertains to electricity.

_____

_____

_____

7. Use Figure 6-1 to label the circuit of an electrosurgical unit (ESU) as related to monopolar usage.

A. _____ B. _____ C. _____ D. _____

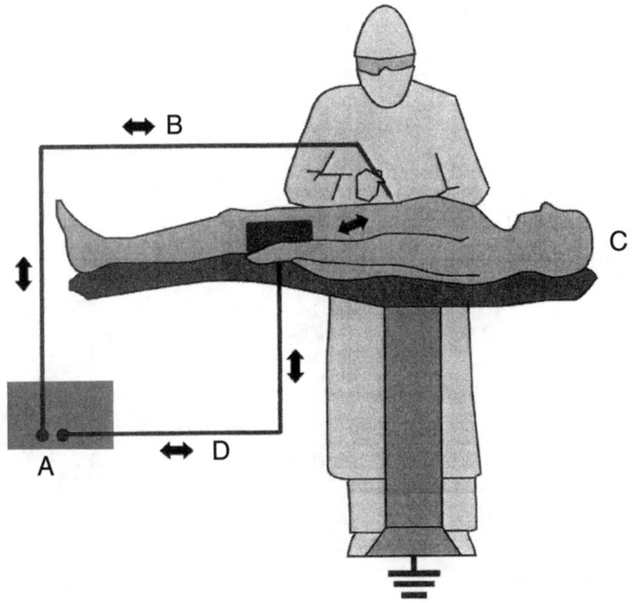

Figure 6-1

8. Compare monopolar and bipolar currents. What are the major differences?

_____

_____

_____

9. Discuss five patient safety precautions to take prior to ESU usage.

_____

_____

_____

10. Define radiofrequency (RF) capacitive coupling. How can it be prevented?

_____

_____

_____

Short Answer Discussion

1. In your opinion, why are the biomedical sciences so important to the surgical technologist? Provide examples of surgical applications related to these sciences.

   _____

   _____

   _____

2. Describe technological advances such as surgical robotics and telesurgery. Compare the pros and cons of surgical robots used in surgery.

   _____

   _____

   _____

Interactive Learning

1. Visit the AST website at: http://www.ast.org and add it to your Favorites function.

2. Create a 10- to 12-slide PowerPoint presentation on a topic related to surgical technology. Slides should include various formatting techniques such as bullets and insertion of graphics. Send a copy to your instructor by attaching the document to an e-mail.

3. Visit the Valleylab website and complete the "Principles of Electrosurgery" online tutorial at: http://www.valleylab.com/education/

4. Review physics and Newton's Laws of Motion with interactive online tutorials like these:

   • http://teachertech.rice.edu
   • http://www.physicsclassroom.com

5. Visit the Intuitive Surgical website and review the development of the da Vinci robot at: http://www.intuitivesurgical.com

---

Case Studies

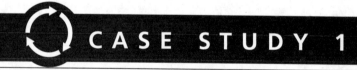

CASE STUDY 1

Norman is a surgical technologist who is circulating during a hip nailing. During the surgical procedure, the surgeon asks to see the patient's X-rays and blood test results, since hepatitis B may be involved. Norman is going to use the computer in the operating room to send an e-mail requesting that the Radiology Department's unit secretary immediately bring over the patient's x-rays. He will send another e-mail to the laboratory technologist requesting that the blood test results be e-mailed to him in the OR.

1. Which icon will Norman use to reply to the e-mail message?

   _____

   _____

   _____

   _____

(continues)

CASE STUDY 1 *(continued)*

2. Norman wants to emphasize the patient's name and facility identification number. Briefly describe two ways to create emphasis using word-processing functions.

_____

_____

_____

_____

3. Norman wants to ensure that the individual at the Surgery Department control desk sees the e-mail (so that he or she will know which OR to deliver the x-rays to when they arrive), but that individual does not need to reply. What function would Norman use?

_____

_____

_____

_____

4. Norman recently visited the Centers for Disease Control and Prevention (CDC) website and noticed an update on hepatitis B. List three ways that he can find that site again.

_____

_____

_____

_____

CASE STUDY 2

A female patient is brought to the operating room for a right oophorectomy. The surgeon is planning to use the AESOP robotic system to perform the surgical procedure. The surgical technologist in the scrub role (STSR) is responsible for setting up the robotic manipulator before the patient enters the OR.

1. Describe how the robotic components are cleaned and sterilized. What is the manipulator?

_____

_____

_____

_____

2. The surgeon will be able to speak commands and the manipulator will adjust. How is this possible?

_____

_____

_____

_____

(continues)

↻ C A S E   S T U D Y   2   (continued)

3. The surgeon requests pitch and then yaw. What is he asking for?

_____

_____

_____

_____

Lab 6: Biomedical Sciences

Introduction

The biomedical sciences portion of this manual will give the student a better understanding of physics, computers, electricity, and robotics. It is through greater need that surgical technologists are learning these pieces. Computers and robots are becoming more and widely used throughout hospitals, and understanding the electrical and physics aspects of their function is becoming more critical.

Game 1: Internet Searches

Time involved: One week for setup

Supplies: Computer

Instructors: Assign the students a topic and have them use different search engines such as Google, Lycos, or others to find the topic and print out the information.

Students: Take the assigned topic and using different search engines, find the topic on the Internet. Print out the material and present it to the instructor.

Game 2: Computer Jeopardy®

Time involved: One week for setup

Supplies: Paper and pencil, note cards, and a display (either whiteboard, blackboard, or computer)

Instructors: Computer Jeopardy® can be played several different ways. You can download from the Internet a PowerPoint presentation–style game and it can be used on a whiteboard or blackboard, or you can work off note cards. Here are a few ways that may work for you. Make some categories about this chapter's topics and what they do, how they are used, or what they are. Make a list of the computer equipment that falls into the different categories, or use pictures, and then you can use these for your questions. The what, where, when, why, and how of the equipment is used to pose the questions; students will give you the "What is _____" answers. You can utilize either teams or individuals. This will help build critical thinking skills.

Students: Study the computer components and their uses. Making note cards can be a big help. Make as many note cards as you can and study them each chance you get. If you carry the cards around with you, each time you have a few minutes of free time, pull them out and work on them. This will greatly enhance learning.

Game 3: e-Mail

Time involved: One week for setup

Supplies: Computer

Instructors: There are three things we are trying to accomplish with this task. Setting up an e-mail account (this may be provided already at your institution), sending and receiving e-mails, and attaching documents to an e-mail. Using either the institution's e-mail system or another free e-mail solution, have the students set up an e-mail account. The student should then send an e-mail to you saying this has been accomplished. You will then respond to their e-mail by assigning them a one-paragraph paper to be completed in a word-processing program of your choosing, such as Microsoft Word or WordPerfect. The student should then attach this paper as a file to the e-mail response to you—not as a cut and paste.

Students: Set up an e-mail account, and follow the instructions provided by your instructor. Learn to send and receive email and attach files to e-mail.

Game 4: Physics Games

Time involved: One week for setup

Supplies: Computer

Instructors: Have your students search for physics games on the Internet. These games should be free to use. Have the students learn to play the physics games and then explain the rules, how they work, and what the student learned from utilizing these tools.

Students: Search the Internet for free physics games. See how they are played and play them. Teach the other students how the game is played and comment on what the game is trying to teach in the way of physics.

Game 5: Robot Parts

Time involved: One week for setup

Supplies: Paper and pencil, note cards, and a display, (either whiteboard, blackboard, or computer)

Instructors: Take pictures of the different robot components. Label them on the back and also write down what they do, where they go, and how they move or function. Show the students the pictures and ask them specific questions about each piece. Go until all the parts are known and can be given the right answer. You should make a list of robot parts that you are going to ask the students about so they can study ahead of time.

Students: Study the list of robot parts that you have been provided by your instructor. Making note cards can be a big help. Make as many note cards as you can and study them each chance you get. If you carry the notes cards around with you, each time you have a few minutes of free time, pull them out and work on them. This will greatly enhance learning.

Game 6: Name That Laser

Time involved: One week for setup

Supplies: Paper and pencil, note cards, and a display (either whiteboard, blackboard, or computer)

Instructors: Using note cards, list each laser on one side; on the other side list the facts about the laser. This should include what it does, where it is used, on what tissue, which surgeries, etc. Ask the students questions either related to the laser or about the laser. You can also add in questions about laser safety.

Students: Study the laser section. Making note cards can be a big help. You can make several different note cards for each laser. Make as many note cards as you can and study them each chance you get. If you carry the cards around with you, each time you have a few minutes of free time, pull them out and work on them. This will greatly enhance learning.

CHAPTER 7

Asepsis and Sterile Technique

OBJECTIVES

After studying this chapter, the reader should be able to:

C 1. Discuss the relationship between the principles of asepsis and practice of sterile technique and surgical patient care.

2. Define and discuss the concept of surgical conscience.

A 3. Discuss the principles of asepsis.

4. Define the terms related to asepsis.

5. Discuss the sterile practices related to the principles of asepsis.

6. Identify the principles and procedures related to disinfection and sterilization.

R 7. Demonstrate competency related to the practice of sterile technique.

8. Demonstrate competency in the procedures related to disinfection and sterilization.

E 9. Discuss the surgical environment and the application of the principles of asepsis to the environment.

Select Key Terms

Define the following, using your textbook glossary or a medical dictionary if necessary:

1. asepsis_____

_____

2. autoclave _____

_____

3. bioburden _____

_____

4. biological indicator _____

_____

5. Bowie-Dick test _____

_____

6. chelation _____

_____

7. chemical indicator _____

_____

8. colonization _____

_____

9. contaminated _____

_____

10. emulsification _____

_____

11. endoscope _____

_____

12. event-related sterility _____

_____

13. flash sterilization _____

_____

14. immersion _____

_____

15. integrity _____

_____

16. intermediate-level disinfection _____

_____

17. Julian date _____

_____

18. Lister _____

_____

19. lumen _____

_____

20. pathogen _____

_____

21. permeability _____

_____

22. sterile field _____

_____

23. sterile technique _____

_____

24. sterilization _____

_____

25. surgical conscience _____

_____

26. surgical site infection (SSI) _____

_____

27. ultrasonic cleaner _____

_____

Matching

Match each term with the correct definition.

____ A. Asepsis	1. Contamination of a person or object by another
____ B. Pathogen	2. "Father of Bacteriology," established the germ theory of disease
____ C. Fomite	3. An inanimate object that harbors microorganisms
____ D. Bioburden	4. Free of all microorganisms, including spores
____ E. Cross-contamination	5. "Father of Antiseptic Surgery," established principles of asepsis including use of carbolic acid as an antiseptic
____ F. Event-related sterility	6. Microbe capable of causing disease
____ G. Sterile	7. Sterility related to handling of an item rather than time elapsed
____ H. Spore	8. Number of microbes or organic debris with which an object is contaminated
____ I. Louis Pasteur	9. Persistent form of certain types of bacteria that allows it to survive in adverse conditions
____ J. Joseph Lister	10. Absence of pathogenic microorganisms

Matching: Microorganisms

Match each microorganism with the correct description.

____ A. Escherica coli	1. Prion transferred via items contaminated with CNS tissue
____ B. Staphylococcus aureus	2. Virus causing chronic disease without jaundice
____ C. Hepatitis C	3. Gram-negative rod that causes ulcers
____ D. Creutzfeldt-Jakob Disease	4. Spore forming anaerobic gram-positive rod, causes gas gangrene
____ E. Streptococcus pyogenes	5. Pathogen outside the intestine; common UTI
____ F. Pseudomonas aeruginosa	6. Gram-positive aerobic cocci causes rheumatic fever

____ G. Clostridium perfringes

____ H. Mycobacterium tuberculosis

____ I. Candida albicans

____ J. Helicobacter pylori

7. Opportunistic fungus that affects the immunocompromised

8. Most common SSI pathogen, found commonly on skin

9. Transmissible airborne nuclei; identified via positive acid-fast stain and culture; maybe MDR

10. Gram-negative rod found commonly in burns

Short Answer

1. Analyze and interpret the chart regarding minimum steam sterilization exposure cycles. What is the minimum steam sterilization exposure cycle time for a wrapped instrument set at 250 degrees?

_____

_____

_____

2. What is the flash sterilization time for a metal instrument containing no lumen?

_____

_____

_____

3. Describe why a towel should be placed between metal basin sets before wrapping the basins for steam sterilization.

_____

_____

_____

4. Summarize the three essential components of monitoring the sterilization process.

_____

_____

_____

5. Differentiate between chemical and biological methods of monitoring the sterilization process.

_____

_____

_____

6. Describe briefly the five General Principles of Packaging.

_____

_____

_____

7. Compare the sterilization times for Cidex and peracetic acid.

_____

_____

_____

8. Compare disinfection, antisepsis, and sterilization.

_____

_____

_____

9. Does terminal cleaning take place at the end of the day or at the end of the case? What is involved in the terminal cleaning process?

_____

_____

_____

10. List the three steps of instrument preparation and explain what happens during each phase.

_____

_____

_____

11. Analyze the process of sterilization and describe the monitoring that is required for all loads containing an implantable.

_____

_____

_____

True or False

_____ 1. The most commonly transmitted pathogen in the operating room is HIV.

_____ 2. Bacterial meningitis may be caused by aerobic gram-negative cocci called *N. meningitides*.

_____ 3. The skin, hair, and nares of operating room personnel are reservoirs of bacteria that may cause an SSI in the surgical patient.

_____ 4. Infection spread by contaminated instruments is an example of direct contact transmission.

_____ 5. Increased age and obesity play a vital role in the risk of the patient contracting an SSI.

_____ 6. Semicritical items must be sterile and free from spores prior to use.

_____ 7. Contact time and the amount of bioburden on an item do not influence the efficiency of disinfectants.

_____ 8. Glutaraldehyde requires a minimum exposure time of 20 minutes to disinfect an item.

_____ 9. Instruments should always be soaked in saline to initiate the cleaning process prior to the end of the case.

_____ 10. The ultrasonic cleaner uses the process of cavitation for cleaning instruments.

Completion

Complete each principle of sterile technique and provide an example of its application.

1. Instruments such as _____ that are used on the skin should not be _____.

   Example: _____

   _____

   _____

2. Contaminated cases require a _____ setup, which should be used only for _____ portions of the case.

   Example: _____

   _____

   _____

   _____

3. The _____ of a sterile, draped table is the _____ portion that is considered sterile.

   Example: _____

   _____

   _____

   _____

4. Once sterile _____ have been applied, they should not be _____.

   Example: _____

   _____

   _____

   _____

5. The _____ of sterile packages must be _____ prior to _____.

   Example: _____

   _____

   _____

   _____

6. The sterile gown is considered sterile from the _____ to the _____ in front and to _____ inches above the _____ on the sleeves.

   Example: _____

   _____

   _____

   _____

7. Members of the surgical team should only _____ when the entire surgical procedure will be performed _____ _____.

   Example: _____

   _____

   _____

   _____

8. If a member of the sterile team must stand on a platform, the platform should be positioned _____ the individual approaches the sterile field.

   Example: _____

   _____

   _____

   _____

9. A nonsterile person must maintain a minimum of _____ inches from any sterile item, area, or field to prevent _____.

Example: _____

_____

_____

_____

10. When in doubt, _____ it _____!

Example: _____

_____

_____

_____

Interactive Learning

Role-play to demonstrate correct and incorrect aseptic technique practices while your classmates critique the incorrect techniques.

Case Studies

CASE STUDY 1

Brittney telephones her physician to report that she is experiencing a fever of 101°F seven days following her laparoscopic tubal ligation. She also states that she is experiencing urinary frequency and burning during urination. The physician suspects that Brittney may have a urinary tract infection because of the catheter that was used to empty her bladder during the surgical procedure. The physician has asked Brittney to schedule an appointment later in the day so that he may examine her and obtain a "clean catch" urine sample.

1. Would Brittney's infection be considered a surgical site infection (SSI)? If not, what type of infection is it?

_____

_____

_____

_____

2. What is the most likely reason that Brittney has an infection?

_____

_____

_____

_____

CASE STUDY 2

Ned is preparing the operating room for an emergency procedure. He is rushing because he knows that the patient will soon be brought into the room and he may not have time to complete his preparations. Ned is opening the final item; just as he is about to place the item on the back table, he notices a small hole in the wrapper.

1. What moral/ethical concept will Ned use to make the "right" decision?

   _____

   _____

   _____

   _____

2. What are Ned's options, and what is the best choice?

   _____

   _____

   _____

   _____

3. If Ned makes the wrong choice, what possible impact could this have on the patient?

   _____

   _____

   _____

   _____

Lab 7: Asepsis and Sterile Technique

Introduction

Asepsis and sterile technique are probably some of the most important things a student will learn in surgical technology. Knowing what is sterile and what is not can save patients' lives and keep everyone healthy. Working with this lab, it is important that the student always practice as if the situation is real. Do not ever treat the situation of aseptic technique lightly. The patient's life depends on this. Although we have games to learn, these do not treat aseptic technique lightly. They are there to help understand different areas, and to help the student see what is all around us in the areas where we live and work.

Game 1: What's on Hand?

Time involved: One week for setup

Supplies: Sterile agar plates or the supplies to make these, at least two for each student

Instructors: This happens to be one of the most fun labs the students can do. The students are going to find out what is either growing on their hands or around the different areas of the institution. You can either purchase commercial agar plates, make your own with recipes found on the Internet, or have the biology labs at your institution make them for you, if this is an option. Have students place their fingers on the agar, swab different areas of the institution such as stair rail, bathroom, or water fountain, and then watch the material grow. Some students may wash their hands, others may not, and still others may use a hand sanitizer. You can also leave some plates open and closed to see what may show up.

Students: Look for different areas around your institution that you think may harbor bacteria and molds. After the plates have been allowed to grow, see what pops up. Know that these things are always a threat to our patient and our own health. This is why we wash our hands and use sanitizers.

Game 2: What is Sterile and What is Not?

Time involved: One week for setup

Supplies: Paper and pencils

Instructors: Identification of sterile versus nonsterile: Set up a sterile field. Have the students identify which objects and team members of the operating room are considered sterile, and those that are not. (Include the people that will be working within those areas, the equipment, the instruments, and the surrounding pieces of furniture.) State the item. Instruct students to indicate on paper the name of the item and if it is sterile or nonsterile. Ask students to observe your movements and to let you know if there is a "break" in the sterile technique. You can show the students how easy it is to contaminate an area just by walking or by turning your back on the field. This can be a learning activity, pop quiz, or game.

Students: Make two lists. On one list you should place sterile areas and supplies and people. On the other list, place nonsterile elements.

Practical

a. Hand washing

b. Package wrapping

    1. Envelope fold

    2. Square fold

    3. Peel pack

    4. Container system

Skill Assessment 7-1

Student Name					
SKILL	**Basic Handwash**				
Instructions	Instructor will demonstrate skill. Practice skill set with your partner. When ready, notify instructor to schedule the check-off. Skills assessment must be completed satisfactorily by _____ (due date).				
Supplies	• Sink with adjustable water faucet • Soap dispenser		• Nail cleaner/brush (as needed) • Towels		

	Practice with Partner Date:		**Skills Testing Date:**		
	PROCEDURAL STEPS				**COMMENTS**
	1. Student is able to state purpose of basic handwash.	Correct	Needs Review		
	2. Student is able to identify circumstances when a handwash should be performed.	Correct	Needs Review		
	3. Student has assembled necessary supplies and/or equipment.	Correct	Needs Review		
	4. Removes any jewelry. Nails are natural, neatly trimmed, and polish-free.	Correct	Needs Review		
	5. Turns on faucet and adjusts the water flow and temperature; inspects the skin integrity of hands and wrists.	Correct	Needs Review		
	6. Wets hands and wrists while keeping fingertips pointed downward and then applies soap from dispenser.	Correct	Needs Review		
	7. Uses moderate friction, circular motions, and interlaces fingers to facilitate adequate cleaning of all areas of hands and wrists, and cleans under the fingernail with a nail brush if necessary.	Correct	Needs Review		
	8. Washes hands for the prescribed amount of time and all surfaces are clean (approximately 15 seconds).	Correct	Needs Review		
	9. Rinses hands from the wrist to fingertips, keeping fingertips pointed downward.	Correct	Needs Review		
	10. Dries hands and wrists with a paper towel, turns off water using paper towel. Discards paper towel appropriately.	Correct	Needs Review		

		Rating
Performance Evaluation Criteria	• Student demonstrated appropriate knowledge of purpose and necessary times for performing a basic handwash. • Student is prepared and performed procedure independently without prompting. • Student performed procedure in accordance with proper aseptic technique.	
	Overall Rating (Satisfactory; Must Redo; Fail):	
Instructor Comments		

Student Signature	*Date*
Instructor Signature	*Date*

Skill Assessment 7-2

Student Name				
SKILL	**Packaging Technique—Wrap (Envelope Fold)**			
Instructions	Instructor will demonstrate skill. Practice skill set with your partner. When ready, notify instructor to schedule the check-off. Skills assessment must be completed satisfactorily by _____ (due date).			
Supplies	• Appropriate size wrappers • Autoclave tape • Labeling materials	• Internal and external indicators • Item to be wrapped		

	Practice with Partner Date:	**Skills Testing Date:**		
	Note: Student must perform skill independently without prompting.			
	PROCEDURAL STEPS			**COMMENTS**
	1. Student is able to state purpose for envelope-style wrap.	Correct	Needs Review	
	2. Student is able to state examples for usage of an envelope-style wrap.	Correct	Needs Review	
	3. Dons appropriate attire and washes hands in accordance with Standard Precautions.	Correct	Needs Review	
	4. Assembles necessary supplies and equipment.	Correct	Needs Review	
	5. Orients the wrap material diagonally on a flat surface.	Correct	Needs Review	
	6. Places item to be wrapped on the wrapper.	Correct	Needs Review	
	7. Inserts internal sterilization indicator.	Correct	Needs Review	
	8. Folds first flap. Ensures top of item is covered completely.	Correct	Needs Review	
	9. Folds second (left) flap.	Correct	Needs Review	
	10. Folds third (right) flap.	Correct	Needs Review	
	11. Folds fourth flap.	Correct	Needs Review	
	12. Applies second wrapper if necessary and secures final flap.	Correct	Needs Review	
	13. If multiple items or free items (screws) are possible, apply a third wrapper in sequential fashion.	Correct	Needs Review	
	14. Properly labels item for processing, places external indicator, and places in designated area.	Correct	Needs Review	

		Rating
Performance Evaluation Criteria	• Student is able to state the purpose and necessary times for performing an envelope-style wrap.	
	• Student is prepared and performed procedure independently without prompting.	
	• Student performed procedure in accordance with the principles of aseptic technique.	
	Overall Rating (Satisfactory; Must Redo; Fail):	
Instructor Comments		

Student Signature	*Date*
Instructor Signature	*Date*

Skill Assessment 7-3

Student Name	
SKILL	**Packaging Technique—Wrap (Square Fold)**
Instructions	Instructor will demonstrate skill. Practice skill set with your partner. When ready, notify instructor to schedule the check-off. Skills assessment must be completed satisfactorily by _____ (due date).
Supplies	• Appropriate size wrappers • Internal and external indicators • Autoclave tape • Labeling materials • Item to be wrapped

Practice with Partner Date:		**Skills Testing Date:**		
Note: Student must perform skill independently without prompting.				
PROCEDURAL STEPS				**COMMENTS**
1. Student is able to state purpose for square fold wrap.	Correct	Needs Review		
2. Student is able to state examples for usage of a square fold wrap.	Correct	Needs Review		
3. Dons appropriate attire and washes hands in accordance with Standard Precautions.	Correct	Needs Review		
4. Assembles necessary supplies and equipment.	Correct	Needs Review		
5. Orients the wrap material squarely on a flat surface.	Correct	Needs Review		
6. Places item to be wrapped on wrapper.	Correct	Needs Review		
7. Inserts internal sterilization indicator.	Correct	Needs Review		
8. Folds first flap, ensuring top of item is covered completely.	Correct	Needs Review		
9. Folds second flap.	Correct	Needs Review		
10. Folds third flap.	Correct	Needs Review		
11. Folds fourth flap.	Correct	Needs Review		
12. Applies second wrapper in sequential fashion if necessary and secures final flap.	Correct	Needs Review		
13. Properly labels item for processing, applies external indicator, and places in designated area.	Correct	Needs Review		

	Rating
Performance Evaluation Criteria • Student is able to state the purpose and necessary times for using square fold to wrap an item. • Student is prepared and performed procedure independently without prompting. • Student performed procedure in accordance with the principles of aseptic technique.	
Overall Rating (Satisfactory; Must Redo; Fail):	

Instructor Comments	

Student Signature	*Date*	
Instructor Signature	*Date*	

Skill Assessment 7-4

Student Name	
SKILL	**Packaging Technique—Peel Pack**
Instructions	Instructor will demonstrate skill. Practice skill set with your partner. When ready, notify instructor to schedule the check-off. Skills assessment must be completed satisfactorily by _____ (due date).
Supplies	• Appropriate size peel packs • Internal and/or external indicators • Labeling materials • Item(s) to be wrapped

Practice with Partner Date:	Skills Testing Date:

Note: Student must perform skill independently without prompting.

PROCEDURAL STEPS			COMMENTS
1. Student is able to state purpose for using a peel pack–style package.	Correct	Needs Review	
2. Student is able to state examples for usage of a peel pack.	Correct	Needs Review	
3. Dons appropriate attire and washes hands in accordance with Standard Precautions.	Correct	Needs Review	
4. Assembles necessary supplies and equipment.	Correct	Needs Review	
5. Places item(s) to be wrapped in peel-pack pouch.	Correct	Needs Review	
6. Inserts internal sterilization indicator. Seals package ensuring there are no gaps or creases.	Correct	Needs Review	
7. Applies second pouch if necessary and secures package, ensuring there are no gaps or creases.	Correct	Needs Review	
8. Properly labels item(s) for processing and places in designated area.	Correct	Needs Review	

Performance Evaluation Criteria		Rating
	• Student is able to state the purpose and necessary times for using a peel pack to package an item.	
	• Student is prepared and performed procedure independently without prompting.	
	• Student performed procedure in accordance with the principles of aseptic technique.	
	Overall Rating (Satisfactory; Must Redo; Fail):	

Instructor Comments	

Student Signature	*Date*
Instructor Signature	*Date*

Skill Assessment 7-5

Student Name				
SKILL		**Packaging Technique—Container System**		
Instructions		Instructor will demonstrate skill. Practice skill set with your partner. When ready, notify instructor to schedule the check-off. Skills assessment must be completed satisfactorily by _____ (due date).		
Supplies		• Rigid instrument container • Locking device • Labeling materials	• Internal and external indicators • Item(s) to be sterilized/processed	

Practice with Partner Date:	**Skills Testing Date:**

Note: Student must perform skill independently without prompting.

PROCEDURAL STEPS			COMMENTS
1. Student is able to state purpose for using a container system.	Correct	Needs Review	
2. Student is able to state examples for usage of a container system.	Correct	Needs Review	
3. Dons appropriate attire and washes hands in accordance with Standard Precautions.	Correct	Needs Review	
4. Assembles necessary supplies and equipment.	Correct	Needs Review	
5. Prepares container system, secures filter(s).	Correct	Needs Review	
6. Places item(s) to be processed into container.	Correct	Needs Review	
7. Inserts internal sterilization indicator.	Correct	Needs Review	
8. Applies lid and seals container with appropriate security device.	Correct	Needs Review	
9. Properly labels item for processing, ensures external indicator in place, and places in designated area.	Correct	Needs Review	

Performance Evaluation Criteria	• Student is able to state the purpose and necessary times for using a rigid container system to process an item. • Student is prepared and performed procedure independently without prompting. • Student performed procedure in accordance with the principles of aseptic technique.	**Rating**
	Overall Rating (Satisfactory; Must Redo; Fail):	
Instructor Comments		

Student Signature	*Date*
Instructor Signature	*Date*

Skill Assessment 7-6

Student Name	
SKILL	**Use of Sterilizer (Flash Autoclave)**
Instructions	Instructor will demonstrate skill. Practice skill set with your partner. When ready, notify instructor to schedule the check-off. Skills assessment must be completed satisfactorily by _____ (due date).
Supplies	• Perforated instrument tray / • Internal and external indicators • Item(s) to be sterilized/processed

Practice with Partner Date:	**Skills Testing Date:**

Note: Student must perform skill independently without prompting.

PROCEDURAL STEPS			COMMENTS
1. Student is able to state purpose and acceptable situations for using a flash autoclave.	Correct	Needs Review	
2. Student is able to state the difference between a gravity and prevacuum autoclave.	Correct	Needs Review	
3. Dons appropriate attire and washes hands in accordance with Standard Precautions.	Correct	Needs Review	
4. Assembles necessary supplies and equipment.	Correct	Needs Review	
5. Prepares container with appropriate items for flash sterilization.	Correct	Needs Review	
6. Places internal indicator.	Correct	Needs Review	
7. Opens autoclave according to manufacturer's recommendations. Checks the drain valve to be sure it is open with no previous indicators or trash.	Correct	Needs Review	
8. Secures autoclave door. Selects cycle and time appropriately for situation given. Adds a biological monitor if an implant is required.	Correct	Needs Review	
9. Properly documents item being processed in the flash autoclave log book.	Correct	Needs Review	
10. Checks mechanical and internal indicators and documents results. Removes item appropriately following manufacturer's recommendations and transfers items in a manner that maintains sterility of the item.	Correct	Needs Review	

	Rating
Performance Evaluation Criteria • Student is able to state the purpose and necessary times for using a flash autoclave system to process an item. • Student is prepared and performed procedure independently without prompting. • Student performed procedure in accordance with the principles of aseptic technique.	
Overall Rating (Satisfactory; Must Redo; Fail):	

Instructor Comments	

Student Signature	*Date*
Instructor Signature	*Date*

Skill Assessment 7-7

Student Name				
SKILL	**Use of Sterilizer (Steris Unit for Heat-Sensitive Items)**			
Instructions	Instructor will demonstrate skill. Practice skill set with your partner. When ready, notify instructor to schedule the check-off. Skills assessment must be completed satisfactorily by _____ (due date).			
Supplies	Just in Time sterilization unit (peracetic acid) Supplies for unit	• Internal indicators • Item(s) to be sterilized/processed If necessary, supplies for leak test		

	Practice with Partner Date:		**Skills Testing Date:**	
	Note: Student must perform skill independently without prompting.			
	PROCEDURAL STEPS			**COMMENTS**
	1. Student is able to state purpose and acceptable situations for using a Just in Time sterilization unit.	Correct	Needs Review	
	2. Student is able to state the hazards of the peracetic acid in concentrated form and how to store and properly dispose of spills.	Correct	Needs Review	
	3. Dons appropriate attire and washes hands in accordance with Standard Precautions.	Correct	Needs Review	
	4. Assembles necessary supplies and equipment for the item to be sterilized.	Correct	Needs Review	
	5. Prepares container appropriately ensuring that all connections are lined up correctly.	Correct	Needs Review	
	6. Places internal indicator.	Correct	Needs Review	
	7. Places the peracetic sterilant cup in place gently. Ensures there are no kinks in tubing.	Correct	Needs Review	
	8. Secures lid ensuring item is not damaged.	Correct	Needs Review	
	9. Properly documents item being processed in the autoclave log book.	Correct	Needs Review	
	10. Checks mechanical and internal indicators and documents results. Removes item appropriately following manufacturer's recommendations and transfers items in a manner that maintains sterility of the item.	Correct	Needs Review	

		Rating
Performance Evaluation Criteria	• Student is able to state the purpose and necessary times for using a peracetic acid (Steris) to process an item. • Student is prepared and performed procedure independently without prompting. • Student performed procedure in accordance with the principles of aseptic technique.	
	Overall Rating (Satisfactory; Must Redo; Fail):	
Instructor Comments		

Student Signature	*Date*
Instructor Signature	*Date*

Skill Assessment 7-8

Student Name	
SKILL	**Use of Sterilizer (Sterrad Unit for Heat-Sensitive Items)**
Instructions	Instructor will demonstrate skill. Practice skill set with your partner. When ready, notify instructor to schedule the check-off. Skills assessment must be completed satisfactorily by _____ (due date).
Supplies	Sterrad unit (hydrogen peroxide sterilization unit) Packaging supplies for unit • Internal and external indicators • Item(s) to be sterilized/processed

Practice with Partner Date:	**Skills Testing Date:**

Note: Student must perform skill independently without prompting.

PROCEDURAL STEPS			COMMENTS
1. Student is able to state purpose and acceptable situations for using a Sterrad sterilization unit.	Correct	Needs Review	
2. Student is able to state the hazards of the unit and how to properly utilize the unit.	Correct	Needs Review	
3. Dons appropriate attire and washes hands in accordance with Standard Precautions.	Correct	Needs Review	
4. Assembles necessary supplies and equipment for the item to be sterilized.	Correct	Needs Review	
5. Prepares item in package appropriately ensuring internal indication is correctly placed.	Correct	Needs Review	
6. Places external indicator.	Correct	Needs Review	
7. Places the package in the unit. Ensures manufacturer's recommendations are followed.	Correct	Needs Review	
8. Secures door and initiates cycle.	Correct	Needs Review	
9. Properly documents item being processed in the autoclave log book.	Correct	Needs Review	
10. Checks mechanical and chemical indicators; documents results. Removes item appropriately following manufacturer's recommendations and transfers items in a manner that maintains sterility of the item.	Correct	Needs Review	

		Rating
Performance Evaluation Criteria	• Student is able to state the purpose and necessary times for using a Sterrad unit to process an item.	
	• Student is prepared and performed procedure independently without prompting.	
	• Student performed procedure in accordance with the principles of aseptic technique.	
	Overall Rating (Satisfactory; Must Redo; Fail):	

Instructor Comments	

Student Signature	*Date*
Instructor Signature	*Date*

Skill Assessment 7-9

Student Name	
SKILL	**Use of Glutaraldehyde (Cidex) for High-Level Disinfection**
Instructions	Instructor will demonstrate skill. Practice skill set with your partner. When ready, notify instructor to schedule the check-off. Skills assessment must be completed satisfactorily by _____ (due date).
Supplies	• Glutaraldehyde • Container for glutaraldehyde • Gloves and eyewear for placement • Sterile gloves, mask, and eyewear for removal • Glutaraldehyde monitor strip • Item(s) to be sterilized/processed • Sterile basin with sterile water for rinsing

Practice with Partner Date:	**Skills Testing Date:**

Note: Student must perform skill independently without prompting.

PROCEDURAL STEPS			COMMENTS
1. Student is able to state purpose and acceptable situations for using glutaraldehyde.	Correct	Needs Review	
2. Student is able to state the hazards of the glutaraldehyde, how to mix, how to store and how to properly dispose of spills.	Correct	Needs Review	
3. Dons appropriate attire and washes hands in accordance with Standard Precautions.	Correct	Needs Review	
4. Assembles necessary supplies and equipment for the item to be disinfected. Mixes glutaraldehyde appropriately or checks expiration date and solution strength using monitor strip.	Correct	Needs Review	
5. Prepares container appropriately ensuring that the lid is in place when items are not being placed or retrieved from the solution.	Correct	Needs Review	
6. Dons appropriate PPE, places dry item in the glutaraldehyde ensuring all lumens are filled or submerged.	Correct	Needs Review	
7. Maintains the item submerged for the appropriate length of time according to the manufacturer's recommendation.	Correct	Needs Review	
8. Prepares sterile rinse basin and sterile area to receive the item.	Correct	Needs Review	
9. Dons appropriate PPE, removes glutaraldehyde lid, dons sterile gloves, and removes item. Rinses item in water and then transfers the item in a manner that maintains status of item.	Correct	Needs Review	
10. Properly documents item being processed in the glutaraldehyde log book.	Correct	Needs Review	

Performance Evaluation Criteria	• Student is able to state the purpose and necessary times for using a peracetic acid (Steris) to process an item. • Student is prepared and performed procedure independently without prompting. • Student performed procedure in accordance with the principles of aseptic technique.	**Rating**
	Overall Rating (Satisfactory; Must Redo; Fail):	

Skill Assessment 7-9 (*continued*)

Instructor Comments	
Student Signature	*Date*
Instructor Signature	*Date*

CHAPTER 8

Hemostasis and Emergency Situations

OBJECTIVES

After studying this chapter, the reader should be able to:

1. Compare and contrast methods of hemostasis and blood replacement and demonstrate the preparation and use of appropriate agents or devices.

2. Recognize developing emergency situations, initiate appropriate action, and assist in treatment of the patient.

3. Apply knowledge of radiological and chemical injuries and biological warfare to the treatment of the patient.

Select Key Terms

Define the following, using your textbook glossary or a medical dictionary if necessary:

1. autologous _____

_____

2. cardiac dysrhythmia _____

_____

3. CPR (cardiopulmonary resuscitation) _____

_____

4. hemolysis _____

_____

5. hemostasis _____

_____

6. hemostat _____

_____

7. homologous _____

_____

8. Rh factor _____

_____

9. suction _____

_____

Short Answer

1. A visual representation of clotting can help you see the flow of the clot. Fill in the chart in Figure 8-1 with a description of each step that occurs when a blood vessel is injured.

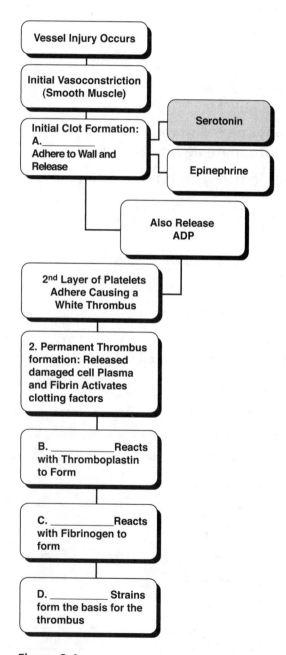

Figure 8-1

2. Describe why aspirin is discontinued one week prior to surgery.

_____

_____

_____

3. Identify at least four conditions or hemostatic defects that can affect coagulation.

_____

_____

_____

4. Analyze each type of hemostatic device and identify which method of achieving hemostasis it uses: Mechanical (M), Chemical (C), or Thermal (T).

_____ A. Silver nitrate   _____ K. Pledget

_____ B. Ligating clips   _____ L. Avitene

_____ C. Cryotherapy   _____ M. Bipolar

_____ D. Suture   _____ N. Hemostat

_____ E. Electrosurgery   _____ O. Harmonic scalpel

_____ F. Epinephrine   _____ P. Gelfoam

_____ G. Stick tie   _____ Q. Tourniquet

_____ H. Bone wax   _____ R. Surgi-cel

_____ I. Thrombin   _____ S. LASER

_____ J. Sponge stick/pressure   _____ T. DeBakey vascular clamp

5. Second Assistant Function of Cutting Suture:

A. When cutting suture for the surgeon who is using monofilament suture, leave a tail of approximately how long?

_____

B. What is the purpose of leaving the tail?

_____

_____

6. What types of material are ligating clips made of?

_____

_____

_____

7. What are kitners and peanuts used primarily for?

_____

_____

_____

8. Pledget use:

A. What is a pledget made of?

_____

_____

B. Describe the purpose of a pledget.

_____

_____

_____

C. Describe how the pledget is used.

_____

_____

_____

9. Bone wax use:

A. What is bone wax made of?

_____

_____

B. Describe the purpose of bone wax.

_____

_____

_____

C. Describe how to prepare bone wax for use.

_____

_____

_____

D. Why is bone wax used in a limited fashion?

_____

_____

_____

E. Describe where bone wax is commonly used.

_____

_____

_____

10. What is suction used for during surgery?

_____

_____

_____

Matching I

Match the drain with the use:

_____ A. Penrose

_____ B. Jackson Pratt

_____ C. Hemovac

_____ D. Sump

_____ E. Water seal

_____ F. T-tube

1. Passive drain placed in CBD

2. Active closed round collection device

3. Gravity drain uses capillary action

4. Chest tube device

5. Active closed drainage "grenade"

6. Utilizes air to displace fluid

Short Answer

1. Describe the purpose of sequential stockings.

_____

_____

_____

2. Tourniquet use:

   A. Describe the purpose of the tourniquet.

   _____

   _____

   _____

   B. When using a tourniquet the surgeon must be notified of what?

   _____

   _____

   _____

   C. What is the maximum time for tourniquet use?

   _____

   _____

   _____

   D. What happens if the surgery lasts longer than the maximum time recommended?

   _____

   _____

   _____

3. Thermal hemostasis:

   A. What is the most commonly used thermal device?

   _____

   _____

   _____

B. How does it provide hemostasis?

_____

_____

_____

C. When the ESU (Bovie) pencil is not in use, what is done with it?

_____

_____

_____

D. What type of energy does the LASER use?

_____

_____

_____

E. Compare LASER and ESU utilization. What is the benefit of using the LASER?

_____

_____

_____

F. What type of energy does the harmonic scalpel use?

_____

_____

_____

G. What are the advantages of the harmonic scalpel?

_____

_____

_____

Matching II: Chemical Hemostasis/Pharmacological Agents

Match the agent with the appropriate description.

_____ A. Avitene

_____ B. Epinephrine

_____ C. Gelfoam

_____ D. Silver nitrate

_____ E. Surgicel or Nu-Knit

_____ F. Thrombin

1. Gelatin powder or pad deposits fibrin

2. Collagen kept dry prior to placement

3. Oxidized cellulose removed from vessels/nerves prior to closure

4. Bovine enzyme applied directly to site, never injected IV

5. Vasoconstrictor mixed with Gelfoam or soaked sponges

6. Caustic pencil for cervical or nasal bleeding

Short Answer

Blood Loss and Blood Replacement

1. When utilizing suction canisters from the field to monitor blood loss, what important information must be monitored and reported by the surgical technician in the scrub role (STSR)? Why?

_____

_____

_____

_____

2. Describe how blood loss is calculated when using sponges.

_____

_____

_____

_____

3. At the end of the case when the closed wound collection device is applied to the drain, what should be monitored or conveyed to the surgeon?

_____

_____

_____

_____

4. Who is responsible for monitoring and reporting estimated blood loss (EBL)?

_____

_____

_____

_____

5. Describe four types of blood replacements given.

_____

_____

_____

_____

6. Describe why blood products may be given.

_____

_____

_____

_____

Matching III: Blood Products

Match types of blood products with the appropriate description:

____ A. A, B, AB, O

____ B. Autologous

____ C. Hemolysis

____ D. Homologous

____ E. Rh factor

____ F. Transfusion reaction

____ G. Type AB

____ H. Type O

1. From patient either stored or cell saver autotransfusion

2. Donated from another; requires type and cross match

3. Four main blood type groups

4. Universal donor

5. Universal recipient

6. Occurs when mismatched blood is given (mild to anaphylactic shock)

7. Antigen found in RBCs of most people

8. Specific type of reaction occurs with Rh mismatch

Short Answer

1. Blood replacement:

   A. What parameters are required for blood that is stored in the OR prior to use?

   _____

   _____

   _____

   _____

   B. Describe how blood is recovered from the sterile field using suction or sponges.

   _____

   _____

   _____

   _____

   C. Describe situations in which lost blood cannot be given back to the patient.

   _____

   _____

   _____

   _____

   D. If you do not have a cell saver machine, describe two ways that you can still recover the patient's own blood.

   _____

   _____

   _____

   _____

2. Transfusion reaction:

   A. Describe typical signs and symptoms of a transfusion reaction.

   _____

   _____

   _____

   _____

   B. What signs and symptoms may you see with a patient under general anesthesia?

   _____

   _____

   _____

   C. What actions are taken if a transfusion reaction is suspected?

   _____

   _____

_____

_____

Emergency Situations

3. Anticipation is important. Describe at least four indicators that indicate an emergency may occur.

_____

_____

_____

_____

4. Many things may occur all at once. If there is a situation in which all of these occur at once, describe how you would anticipate what instruments, equipment, or actions are needed next.

_____

_____

_____

_____

5. Prioritize the conditions in the best order of treatment from 1 to 10.

_____ A. Chest Injuries   _____ F. Shock; fallen blood pressure

_____ B. Breathing   _____ G. Comfort for patient

_____ C. Fractures   _____ H. Circulation; pulse

_____ D. Hemostasis maintained for severe   _____ I. Wound protection/closure
       blood loss

_____ E. Patent Airway

6. What is a designated trauma center?

_____

_____

_____

_____

7. When a sudden cardiac arrest (SCA) occurs, how long before permanent brain damage occurs?

_____

_____

_____

_____

8. What are some warning signs of impending cardiac arrest?

_____

_____

_____

_____

9. What is the first priority of CPR for an adult after establishing unresponsiveness for an adult?

_____

_____

_____

_____

10. Describe the best technique for opening the airway in an injured patient.

_____

_____

_____

_____

11. What is the ratio of compressions to breathing for CPR for one- or two-person adult CPR?

_____

_____

_____

_____

12. When providing CPR for unresponsive infants and children, when do you call 911?

_____

_____

_____

_____

13. What is the ratio of compressions to breathing for two-person CPR in a child?

_____

_____

_____

_____

14. AED:

A. What does AED stand for?

_____

B. What age groups are appropriate for the use of an AED?

_____

C. What is the adult initial setting for defibrillation?

_____

15. What is the primary role of the STSR during CPR in the OR setting?

_____

_____

_____

16. Malignant hyperthermia (MH):

    A. Describe the symptoms of MH.

    _____

    _____

    _____

    B. What are the first symptoms to develop?

    _____

    _____

    _____

    C. What is one of the last symptoms to develop?

    _____

    _____

    _____

17. What triggers an MH episode?

    _____

    _____

    _____

18. How is a predisposition or MH trait diagnosed?

    _____

    _____

    _____

19. What is the drug used to treat an MH crisis?

    _____

    _____

20. A 46-year-old male demonstrates masseter rigidity (tightness). Describe the priorities of treatment.

    _____

    _____

    _____

21. Disseminated intravascular coagulation (DIC):

    A. Describe what occurs with DIC.

    _____

    _____

    _____

    B. What blood replacements or intravenous therapy may be used to treat DIC?

    _____

    _____

    _____

C. Describe the prognosis for patients who develop DIC.

_____

_____

_____

Matching IV: Emergency Conditions

Match the emergency condition with the appropriate description:

_____ A. Syncope

_____ B. Bradycardia

_____ C. Asystole

_____ D. Seizure

_____ E. Grand mal

_____ F. Petit mal

_____ G. Anaphylactic shock

_____ H. Dirty radiological bomb

_____ I. Nerve agent

_____ J. Mustard gas (vesicant)

_____ K. Phosgene (choking agent)

_____ L. Anthrax

_____ M. Botulism

_____ N. Smallpox

_____ O. Most likely bioweapons

1. Neuroparalysis (nausea and vomiting); blurred vision; slurred speech; dysphagia)

2. Treated with epinephrine for extreme cases

3. Skin blisters, burns; dyspnea; conjunctivitis

4. Smallpox and anthrax

5. Thermal burns; flash blindness; poor immune response

6. Skin lesions; flu-like symptoms; dyspnea; high fever; shock

7. Pulmonary edema

8. Loss of consciousness with convulsive body movement

9. Sudden loss of consciousness

10. Rhinorrhea, dyspnea; seizure; paralysis

11. Pulse less than 60 and symptomatic

12. Occurs without warning; very short in duration; stare into space

13. No pulse; start CPR

14. Abnormal brain electrical activity (focal, grand mal, petit mal)

15. Fever; aches; pain; malaise; painful vesicular/pustular skin rash

True or False

_____ 1. Patients exposed to a "dirty bomb" may have blast injuries only and do not need any decontamination.

_____ 2. Decontamination by clothing removal, bathing, and wound irrigation with normal saline is important to reduce radioactive exposure.

_____ 3. Chemical injury may present a vapor exposure hazard for health care personnel.

_____ 4. With mustard gas or other chemical exposure decontamination includes clothing removal and irrigation with household bleach (1 to 10 parts) to decontaminate all areas exposed to the chemical.

_____ 5. Chemical exposure protocol recommends a no-touch technique during decontamination and debridement while wearing double gloves with frequent glove changes.

_____ 6. Specimens (excised tissue) from chemical exposure are placed in formalin.

_____ 7. Instruments used on chemical exposure patients must be discarded after use.

_____ 8. The most common method of biological transmission is through direct person-to-person contact.

_____ 9. Biological warfare agents are chosen because of their potential for low mortality rates, which cause panic and disrupt social structures.

_____ 10. Anthrax patients may experience appendicitis necessitating surgery, but otherwise most patients exposed to biologicals will not be treated in surgery unless they received direct injuries from the blast exposure.

____ 11. Anthrax and botulism are treated using standard precautions because person-to-person transmission does not occur.

____ 12. Smallpox treatment includes vaccination and patient isolation precautions to prevent transmission.

____ 13. The first indication of a biological attack is when a large number of patients arrive with the same set of signs and symptoms of a disease that are not endemic to an area.

____ 14. Bioterrorism readiness plans (BRPs) should include annual disaster drills to test and refine the plan.

____ 15. Linen for a patient with smallpox lesions must be autoclaved and then laundered with bleach and water.

Case Studies

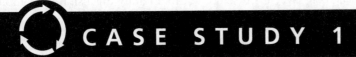

CASE STUDY 1

You are on call and have been alerted by the media of a shopping mall bombing involving multiple injuries. The hospital has more than 40 injured in the emergency room. Viorel is a 10-year-old boy with multiple trauma due to a dirty bomb in the shopping mall. He is scheduled for an emergency exploratory laparotomy. His blood pressure is low and his pulse rate is dropping.

1. What is your first reaction to the media announcement?

_____

_____

_____

_____

2. You have arrived in the OR; how do you prepare to receive casualties from a "dirty bomb"?

_____

_____

_____

_____

3. Viorel has multiple open wounds and is still wearing his clothes. What are the first priorities of treatment?

_____

_____

_____

_____

4. Viorel is hemorrhaging; what means of treatment will you most likely have available?

Chemical: _____

Mechanical: _____

Thermal: _____

(continues)

CASE STUDY 1 (continued)

5. Because this is an emergency and the patient has not been typed and cross matched, what blood replacement (type of blood) will be given if necessary and why?

_____

_____

_____

_____

6. Once the abdomen is entered it is discovered that that the patient has a liver laceration and that piece of shrapnel has penetrated his ileum. The cell saver is on standby; can an autotransfusion be completed? Why?

_____

_____

_____

_____

CASE STUDY 2

Virginia-May is scheduled for hemicolectomy because of carcinoma of the transverse colon. Virginia-May is 67 years old and an incidental splenorrhaphy is completed during the surgery. She receives a blood transfusion during the surgical procedure.

1. As the STSR, you notice blood pooling in the abdomen during the transverse colectomy. You notify the surgeon of your observation but do not ask for the cell saver/perfusionist. Why?

_____

_____

_____

2. Anesthesia asks the circulator how much blood is in the suction canister. What information does the STSR need to give to the team to help determine the amount of blood loss? Why?

_____

_____

_____

_____

3. The circulator weighs the sponges. How is blood loss calculated from weighing the used sponges?

_____

_____

(continues)

CASE STUDY 2 *(continued)*

_____

_____

4. The patient's blood type is B negative. What does this mean?

_____

_____

_____

_____

5. Blood is brought to the OR. How is the blood product verified prior to administration?

_____

_____

_____

_____

6. After the blood is started, the patient's blood oxygen level (pulse oximeter reading) drops to 85%. What should be done?

_____

_____

_____

_____

Lab 8: Hemostasis and Emergency Situations

Introduction

Hemostasis and emergency situations deal with just that. How do we keep bleeding under control and what do we do during different situations? Working with the different options for hemostatic agents and with the different emergencies, we can better understand how we should react under the different situations.

Game 1: Radiological, Chemical, or Biological?

Time involved: One week for setup

Supplies: Pen and paper

Instructors: List common terms related to different aspects of radiological, biological, and chemical areas. Have the students decide which term best fits each area.

Students: Categorize the terms of radiological, biological, and chemical areas. List each on a note card.

Skill Assessment 8-1

Student Name	
SKILL	**Hemostatic Devices Used During Surgery**
Instructions	Instructor will demonstrate skill. Practice skill set with your partner. When ready, notify instructor to schedule check off. Skills assessment must be completed satisfactorily by _____ (due date).
Supplies	• If available—any hemostatic supplies as described below.

	Practice with Partner Date:		Skills Testing Date:		
	PROCEDURAL STEPS				**COMMENTS**

	1. Describe appropriate care of thermal units:
	  A. ESU (holder when not in use; Bovie scraper to clean tip)
	  B. Laser unit (moist towels around site, special wrapped ETT for oral procedures, special eyewear, sign on door, pretest unit)
	  C. Harmonic scalpel (correct assembly of tips)
		Correct	Needs Review		

	2. Describes appropriate preparation and use of chemical hemostatic agents:
	  A. Gelfoam—gelatin that may be in foam pads, which may be cut or compressed and soaked in thrombin or epinephrine
	  B. Avitene—collagen that may be in sheets or powder and must be passed dry
	  C. Surgicel or Oxycel is compressed cellulose that is usually used dry and is removed from around vessels or nerves prior to closure to prevent stricture formation
	  D. Epinephrine—label appropriately; be alert to strength of solutions; is never injected into digits, penis, earlobes, or tip of nose
	  E. Thrombin—mixed just prior to use; never injected IV; stored in refrigerator; possible Bovine allergies
		Correct	Needs Review		

Skill Assessment 8-2

Student Name	
SKILL	**Emergency Skills**
Instructions	Instructor will demonstrate skill. Practice skill set with your partner. When ready, notify instructor to schedule the check-off. Skills assessment must be completed satisfactorily by _____ (due date).
Supplies	• Mock paper vials/AED/defibrillator cards labeled defibrillation 360 joules; defibrillation 200 joules; atropine; lidocaine; Benadryl; epinephrine; IV fluids; Trendelenburg • Mannequin—able to complete jaw thrust and compressions • PPE—gloves, gowns, eyewear, shoe covers

Note: Student must perform skill independently without prompting.

Practice with Partner Date:		**Skills Testing Date:**		
PROCEDURAL STEPS				**COMMENTS**
1. Washes hands.	Correct	Needs Review		
2. Assembles supplies and equipment.	Correct	Needs Review		
3. Describes appropriate treatment for asystole.	Correct	Needs Review		
4. Describes CPR administration for adult patient correctly (30 compressions to two breaths). Demonstrates appropriate compression technique.	Correct	Needs Review		
5. Describes priorities of the STSR during a cardiac arrest during surgery.	Correct	Needs Review		
6. Describes appropriate treatment for ventricular fibrillation.	Correct	Needs Review		
7. Describes appropriate treatment for symptomatic bradycardia (infant with HR of 60 or adult with HR <60 and dropping blood pressure or change in LOC).	Correct	Needs Review		
8. Demonstrates how to open airway for potential cervical spine injury (jaw thrust method).	Correct	Needs Review		
9. Describes how the STSR can assist with controlling the temperature during an MH crisis (ice packs, chilled irrigation fluids; swift anticipation of surgeon's needs to close as quickly as possible).	Correct	Needs Review		
10. Describes the priorities of care during a seizure (protection from injury, description of seizure activity).	Correct	Needs Review		
11. Describes the significance of a latex or contrast media allergy. Identifies signs and symptoms of an allergic reaction (itching, swelling, hives, dyspnea, bronchospasm, laryngeal edema, hypotension, tachycardia, oliguria [shock], and cardiac arrest). Identifies drug treatment that may be used (Benadryl for mild reactions and epinephrine for anaphylactic reactions; IV fluids and Trendelenburg for shock).	Correct	Needs Review		

Skill Assessment 8-2 (*continued*)

	12. Demonstrates/properly identifies PPE for the following: A. radiological "dirty bomb" exposure B. chemical agents (double glove/change gloves frequently) C. anthrax exposure (Standard Precautions) D. smallpox (vaccination, Standard Precautions, and isolation) E. botulism (Standard Precautions)	Correct	Needs Review	
	13. Describes how to decontaminate wound from radiological "dirty bomb."	Correct	Needs Review	
	14. Describes how to decontaminate a wound, specimens, instruments, and linen from chemical agents (mustard gas or phosgene or nerve agents). (Steps 1-10 part 5% sodium hypochlorite (bleach); Specimens placed in 5% sodium hypochlorite; instruments soaked in bleach 10 minutes; linen soaked in bleach.	Correct	Needs Review	

		Rating
Performance Evaluation Criteria	• Demonstrated initiative. Assembled all supplies and equipment needed.	
	• Demonstrated infection control measures correctly. Identified and demonstrated appropriate PPE equipment for the situation given. Decontaminated equipment prior to use; protected mannequin prior to use; cleaned equipment after use.	
	• Demonstrated knowledge of emergency conditions and appropriate treatment. Demonstrated CPR correctly including opening of airway and compressions, and identified appropriate treatment for the emergency condition including asystole, bradycardia, ventricular fibrillation, and cervical injury.	
	• Demonstrated knowledge of appropriate patient care in the event of an MH crisis, seizure, or allergic reaction.	
	• Demonstrated knowledge of radiological or chemical injury management during chemical or nuclear warfare.	
	• Student prepared and responded independently without hesitation to the situation given.	
	Overall Rating (Satisfactory; Must Redo; Fail):	
Instructor Comments		

	Student Signature	*Date*	
	Instructor Signature	*Date*	

CHAPTER 9

Surgical Pharmacology and Anesthesia

OBJECTIVES

After studying this chapter, the reader should be able to:

C 1. Recognize general terminology and abbreviations associated with pharmacology and anesthesia.

2. Assess the action, uses, and modes of administration of drugs and anesthetic agents used in the care of the surgical patient.

3. Recognize the side effects and contraindications for use of drugs and anesthetic agents.

4. Interpret the factors that influence anesthesia selection for individual patients.

A 5. Demonstrate safe practice in transferring drugs and solutions from the nonsterile area to the sterile field.

6. Demonstrate the procedure for identifying a drug or solution on the sterile field.

7. Analyze how sterile technique is used in relation to certain anesthesia procedures.

R 8. Convert equivalents from one system to another and accurately identify, mix, and measure drugs for patient use.

9. Compare and contrast the roles of the STSR and circulator during the administration of anesthesia.

E 10. Demonstrate the precautions in identifying drugs and solutions in the OR.

11. List the equipment used as an adjunct to anesthesia.

Select Key Terms

Define the following, using your textbook glossary or a medical dictionary if necessary:

1. agonist _____

_____

2. amnesia _____

_____

3. anaphylaxis _____

_____

4. anesthesia _____

_____

5. antagonist _____

_____

6. antimuscarinic _____

_____

7. aspiration _____

_____

8. biotechnology _____

_____

9. buccal _____

_____

10. capnography_____

_____

11. contraindication_____

_____

12. Doppler _____

_____

13. drug _____

_____

14. generic _____

_____

15. homeostasis_____

_____

16. hypnosis _____

_____

17. indication_____

_____

18. induction _____

_____

19. intra-articular _____

_____

20. laryngospasm _____

_____

21. NPO _____

_____

22. PACU _____

_____

23. parenteral _____

_____

24. pharmacodynamics _____

_____

25. pharmacokinetics _____

_____

26. pharmacology _____

_____

27. prophylaxis _____

_____

28. topical _____

_____

29. volatile agents _____

_____

Conversions

Perform the following computations and exercises. Refer to a medical dictionary or the textbook if necessary. Identify the following abbreviations.

1. C _____

2. m _____

3. kg _____

4. L _____

5. mL _____

6. F _____

7. mm _____

8. mg _____

9. g _____

10. ung _____

11. lb _____

12. sc _____

13. oz   _____

14. cm   _____

15. gtt   _____

16. DEA   _____

17. mEq   _____

18. IV   _____

19. PO   _____

20. IM   _____

21. DVT   _____

22. UTI   _____

23. PONV   _____

24. GERD   _____

25. ARDS   _____

26. LMA   _____

27. ETT   _____

28. SARA   _____

29. ABG   _____

30. PT or PTT _____

31. CSF   _____

32. CNS   _____

33. USP   _____

34. FDA   _____

35. BIS   _____

Calculate the following weight conversions.

36. 1.5 g =   _____ mg

37. 52 lb =   _____ kg

38. 46 kg =   _____ lb

39. 78 kg =   _____ lb

40. 500 mg = _____ g

41. 4000 g = _____ kg

42. 5 g =   _____ mg

43. 240 lb = _____ kg

44. 300 mg = _____ g

45. 2 g =   _____ mg

46. 220 kg = _____ lb

47. 175 lb = _____ kg

Calculate the following length conversions.

48. 1 m = _____ inches

49. 1 inch = _____ cm

50. 4 cm = _____ inches

51. 10 cm = _____ inches

52. 12 inches = _____ cm

53. 30 cm = _____ inches

54. 6 inches = _____ cm

55. 1 yard = _____ inches

Calculate the following volume conversions.

56. 1 mL = _____ mL

57. 4 cc = _____ mL

58. 2 oz = _____ mL

59. 5 L= _____ mL

60. 1.5 L = _____ mL

61. 0.5 oz = _____ mL

62. 500 cc = _____ L

63. 0.75 L = _____ mL

64. 1 gallon = _____ mL

65. 12 mL = _____ oz

66. 15 gtt or minims = _____ mL

Calculate the following temperature conversions.

67. 36°C = _____ F

68. 32°F = _____ C

69. 98.6°F = _____ C

70. 100°C = _____ F

71. 18°C = _____ F

72. 101°F = _____ C

73. 104°F = _____ C

74. 212°F = _____ C

75. 37.7°C = _____ F

76. 91.4°F = _____ C

Match the following basic conversions:

____ 1. 1 g a. 30 cc

____ 2. 1 kg b. 14–15 minims

____ 3. 1 cc c. 1000 cm

____ 4. 1 L   d. 37°C

____ 5. boiling point 212°F   e. 1000 mg

____ 6. 1 minim   f. 100 cc

____ 7. 1 oz   g. 1 gtt

____ 8. 98.6°F   h. 1000 cc

____ 9. 100 mL   i. 100°C

____ 10. 1 m   j. 2.2 lb

Classifications

Match the classification with the definition.

____ 1. Analgesic   a. Blocks parasympathetic impulses

____ 2. Anesthetic   b. Colors or marks tissue

____ 3. Antibiotic   c. Constricts pupil

____ 4. Anticholinergic or antimuscarinic   d. Drugs with potential for addiction

____ 5. Anticoagulant   e. Prevents clot or thrombus formation

____ 6. Antiemetic   f. Paralyzes the ciliary muscle of eye

____ 7. Anti-inflammatory   g. Appears radiopaque on x-ray

____ 8. Antipyretic   h. Prevents or treats nausea and vomiting

____ 9. Controlled substance   i. Relieves fever

____ 10. Contrast media   j. Secretion of endocrine gland

____ 11. Cycloplegic   k. Relieves pain

____ 12. Diuretic   l. Prevents or treats infections

____ 13. Dye   m. Dilates pupil

____ 14. Fibrinolytic   n. Increases blood pressure

____ 15. Hemostatic   o. Dissolves clots or thrombus—enzyme

____ 16. Hormone   p. Reduces mental anxiety and promotes sleep

____ 17. Miotic   q. Increases urine output or treat edema

____ 18. Mydriatic   r. Prevents or treats pain, redness, swelling, or heat

____ 19. Sedative   s. Produces partial or complete loss of sensation

____ 20. Vasoconstrictor   t. Enhances formation of clot or thrombus

Match the drug with the description.

____ 1. Lidocaine   a. Hormone vasoconstrictor

____ 2. Dantrolene   b. Gas anesthetic may increase ear pressure

____ 3. Epinephrine   c. Antiarrhythmia and anesthetic

____ 4. Benzodiazepines   d. Anticoagulant use for vascular cases

____ 5. Atropine   e. Osmotic diuretic

____ 6. Nitrous oxide

____ 7. Heparin

____ 8. Thrombin

____ 9. Mannitol

____ 10. Bacitracin

f. Hemostatic agent never given via IV

g. Antibiotic

h. Preoperative sedative

i. Treatment for malignant hyperthermia

j. Anticholinergic or antimuscarinic—decrease mucous secretions or treat bradycardia

Identification

1. The names for several commonly used medications are listed in the left column. Provide the generic name and classification for each one. Note: Medications may have more than one classification.

Common (Trade) Name	Generic Name	Classification
Adrenalin		
Ancef		
Anectine		
Benadryl		
Coumadin		
Dantrium		
Decadron		
Demerol		
Flagyl		
Gelfoam		
Heparin		
Humulin		
Kantrex		
Lasix		
Marcaine		
Narcan		
Papaverine		
Pentothal Sodium		
Pitocin		
Renografin		
Silvadene		
Solu-Cortef		
Sublimaze		
Surgicel or Oxycel		
Tagamet		
Toradol		
Tracrium		
Valium		

Versed		
Wydase		
Xylocaine hydrochloride		

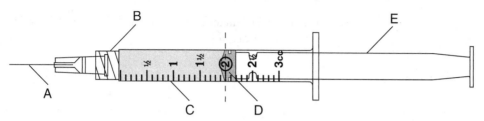

Figure 9-1

2. Identify the components of the syringe shown in Figure 9-1.

A. _____   D. _____

B. _____   E. _____

C. _____

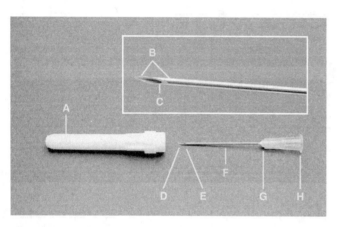

Figure 9-2

3. Identify the components of the needle shown in Figure 9-2.

A. _____   E. _____

B. _____   F. _____

C. _____   G. _____

D. _____   H. _____

See package insert for complete product information.
Store at controlled room temperature 20° to 25°C (68° to 77°F) [see USP].
Each mL contains: heparin sodium, 1,000 USP Units. Also, sodium chloride, 9 mg; benzyl alcohol, 9.45 mg added as preservative.
811 317 804
Pharmacia & Upjohn Company
Kalamazoo, MI 49001, USA

NDC 0009-0268-01   10 mL
**Heparin Sodium
Injection, USP**
from beef lung
1,000 Units/mL
For subcutaneous or intravenous use

See package insert for complete product information.
Store at controlled room temperature 20° to 25° C (68° to 77° F) [see USP].
Each mL contains: Heparin sodium, 5,000 USP Units. Also, sodium chloride, 9 mg; benzyl alcohol, 9.45 mg added as preservative.
Pharmacia & Upjohn Company
Kalamazoo, MI 49001, USA

NDC 0009-0291-01
10 mL
**Heparin Sodium
Injection, USP**
from beef lung
5,000 Units/mL
For subcutaneous or intravenous use

Figure 9-3

4. The physician has ordered 5000 units of Heparin. What volume of Heparin will be needed? Use the medication labels pictured in Figure 9-3 to determine your answer.

5. From which source is Heparin derived?

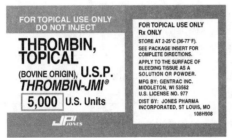

Figure 9-4

6. The surgeon preference card calls for topical thrombin. Where will the STSR initially locate the medication?

7. In which drug form is topical thrombin manufactured?

8. What must be done to prepare the medication for use?

9. What unit of measure is used to determine the dose of topical thrombin? Use the medication label pictured in Figure 9-4 to determine your answer.

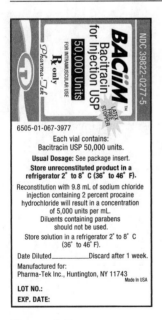

Figure 9-5

10. The physician has ordered 100,000 units of Bacitracin, diluted in 1000 cc of saline, for irrigation of the abdominal cavity. How many vials of Bacitracin will be needed? Use the medication label pictured in Figure 9-5 to determine your answer.

_____

11. In which drug form is Bacitracin manufactured?

_____

12. What must be done to prepare Bacitracin for use?

_____

13. How will the Bacitracin/saline solution be introduced into the abdominal cavity? What supplies will be necessary?

_____

14. Cocaine HCL 4% has been ordered as a local anesthetic for a patient having nasal surgery. How is the cocaine administered?

_____

15. What is the drug classification for cocaine?

_____

16. If any cocaine remains at the end of the procedure, what procedure is necessary to ensure proper disposal of this drug? Why?

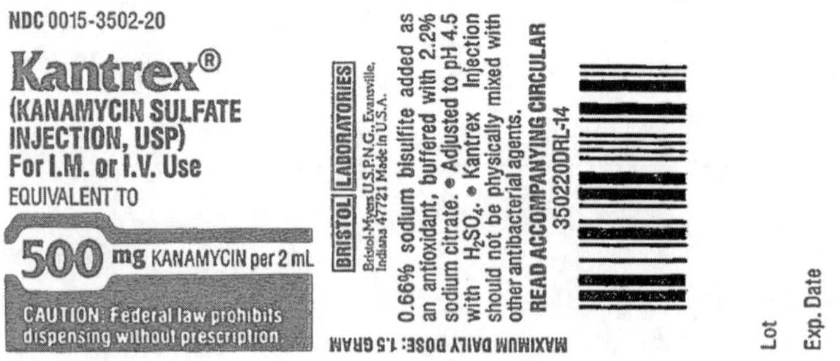

_____

NDC 0015-3502-20

Kantrex®
(KANAMYCIN SULFATE INJECTION, USP)
For I.M. or I.V. Use
EQUIVALENT TO

500 mg KANAMYCIN per 2 mL

CAUTION: Federal law prohibits dispensing without prescription.

BRISTOL LABORATORIES
Bristol-Myers U.S.P.N.G., Evansville, Indiana 47721 Made in U.S.A.

0.66% sodium bisulfite added as an antioxidant, buffered with 2.2% sodium citrate. • Adjusted to pH 4.5 with H₂SO₄. • Kantrex Injection should not be physically mixed with other antibacterial agents.
READ ACCOMPANYING CIRCULAR
350220DRL-14

MAXIMUM DAILY DOSE: 1.5 GRAM

Lot
Exp. Date

Figure 9-6

17. The physician preference card calls for 1 g of kanamycin sulfate. How many vials of kanamycin will be needed? Use the medication label in Figure 9-6 to determine your answer.

_____

18. What is the drug classification for kanamycin?

_____

19. For what purpose would kanamycin be ordered?

_____

20. What is the drug classification for oxytocin?

_____

21. In what situation(s) in the operating room is the use of oxytocin indicated?

_____

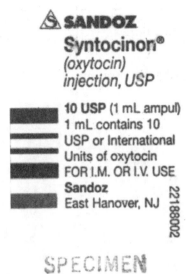

△ SANDOZ
Syntocinon®
(oxytocin)
injection, USP

10 USP (1 mL ampul)
1 mL contains 10
USP or International
Units of oxytocin
FOR I.M. OR I.V. USE
Sandoz
East Hanover, NJ

SPECIMEN

Figure 9-7

22. The surgeon has requested that the STSR have 20 units of oxytocin available on the sterile field. How many vials will be necessary? Use the medication label in Figure 9-7 to determine your answer.

_____

23. Via which route(s) is oxytocin administered?

_____

Interactive Learning

1. Using the sample medication file card, choose one of the following medications that are frequently found on the STSR's back table from the list below and complete a sample card. Attach a copy of the research material to the card you completed.

Heparin

Bacitracin

Xylocaine

Xylocaine with epinephrine

Bupivacaine

Bupivacaine with epinephrine

Renografin

Methylene blue

Thrombin

Sample:

front

Drug Name: _____ Drug Classification: _____

Drug Action: _____ Route(s) of Administration: _____

_____

_____

_____

_____

_____

Possible Iatrogenic, Adverse, or Idiosyncratic Reactions: _____

_____

Contraindications: _____

Sample:

back

Antagonist: _____ Special Administration and Storage Instructions: _____

Usual Dosages: _____ Onset: _____

Peak Effect: _____

Preoperatively: _____ Duration Time: _____

Pain Management: _____

Drug Interactions: _____

MAO Inhibitors: _____

Overdose Symptoms: _____

Overdose Management: _____

2. Identify two websites that provide information including potential side effects and maximum doses.

_____

_____

Case Studies

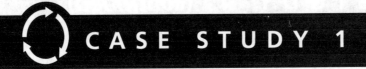

CASE STUDY 1

Amanda, a 22-month-old female, is scheduled to have a tympanoplasty under general anesthesia at 7:30 am. Her mother states that she has been NPO (not eating or drinking) since last evening when she drank a bottle of 2% milk at about 8:00 PM.

1. Amanda will be having a general anesthetic. Describe the stages of general anesthesia.

   _____

   _____

   _____

2. As Amanda undergoes general anesthesia, what precautions are taken during induction and extubation? Why (what are you trying to prevent)?

   _____

   _____

   _____

3. If Ketamine is used as an induction agent, what side effect may occur for Amanda?

   _____

   _____

   _____

4. Her anesthesiologist will not use nitrous oxide for maintenance of the anesthesia. Why not?

   _____

   _____

   _____

5. Has Amanda been NPO for an adequate amount of time? How much time is considered adequate?

   _____

   _____

   _____

6. Why is it important for Amanda to be NPO?

   _____

   _____

   _____

7. As a child, Amanda is highly susceptible to hypothermia. What devices can be used to prevent hypothermia?

   _____

   _____

   _____

(continues)

C A S E   S T U D Y   1   *(continued)*

8. What monitoring anesthesia equipment will be needed to care for Amanda?

_____

_____

C A S E   S T U D Y   2

Tony, an 86-year-old man weighing 140 lbs, is scheduled for a repair of an abdominal aortic aneurysm with general anesthesia. His mother died of an elevated temperature above 106°F during a routine hysterectomy when he was six years old. He had fluids for lunch less than four hours ago. The surgeon orders Cefotan IV 30 minutes prior to the incision.

1. What position(s) will be necessary for Tony's surgery? After anesthesia is administered, will it be necessary for the circulator to position the patient?

_____

_____

_____

2. A gas inhalation drug may be used to maintain anesthesia. The anesthesiologist usually uses Forane, but not today. Why?

_____

_____

_____

3. During intubation, the circulator is asked to provide pressure on the cricoid ring. What is this called and why is it done?

_____

_____

_____

4. Since this is a vascular procedure, what medication will be added to the irrigation solution for this case? Why?

_____

_____

_____

(continues)

CASE STUDY 2 (continued)

5. Why is the Cefotan given as a one-time dose prior to the incision? What is the drug classification?

_____

_____

_____

6. Why is timing important in the administration of the Cefotan? Relate timing to the process of pharmacokinetics and peak effect.

_____

_____

_____

CASE STUDY 3

Danny, a 56-year-old male weighing 185 lbs, is scheduled for a ventral herniorrhaphy. The surgeon routinely injects the site with lidocaine 1% during the procedure.

1. During the procedure, describe how the STSR receives the drug lidocaine onto the field.

_____

_____

_____

2. Describe the procedure for passing the medication to the surgeon.

_____

_____

_____

3. What is the purpose of a neutral zone? Describe how the neutral zone is achieved.

_____

_____

_____

4. Tony received over 600 mg of the amino amide. What is the maximum dose? Is this dose appropriate? If not, what can happen?

_____

_____

_____

Lab 9: Surgical Pharmacology and Anesthesia

Introduction

Medications are a part of any surgical technologist's job. It is our responsibility to make sure the right medication and dosage (expiration date checked) are found and followed to secure patient safety. We as surgical technologists need to know what the medication is and what it does to make sure our patient is safe. There are two pieces of this lab that can help accomplish this. The first part comes as a learning exercise "game," and the second part encompasses some practical exercises for hands-on training.

Game 1: Name That Med

Time involved: Two to three weeks setup

Instructors: Make a list of medications that you expect students to know. Divide this list among the students, giving each student an equal portion of the list. Give the students some specifics of what you expect them to know about the medications such as:

1. common (trade) name

2. generic name

3. classification of medications (i.e., analgesics, narcotics, sedative)

4. maximum dose

5. administration route

6. duration of action

7. indications for use

8. etc.

Students: Take your list of medications and make cards (flash cards) for each of the medications that you have been assigned. Once you have made the cards, make copies of each of the cards for your fellow students to study, and give a copy to your instructor. The cards could include some of the following information, but ask your instructor for specifics.

1. trade (common) name

2. generic name

3. classification of medications (i.e., analgesic, narcotic, sedative)

4. maximum dose

5. administration route

6. duration of action

7. indications

Supplies: Paper, writing utensils, a copy machine or printer, source for information (book, computer)

How the Game Is Played

After each student has been given time to find the material, make copies, and study the content, the game can begin. Teams can be either individuals or groups. Have the instructor give a piece of the information gained from the research, and then ask the students by team to give the correct answer back. (Example: This drug has the generic name of diphenhydramine; what is the brand name? Answer: Benadryl). Do this in a set order, and allow teams to "steal points" if another team gives the wrong answer. Go through each of the cards and ask different questions about different aspects from each card. The team with the most points wins.

Practical

a. Sellick's maneuver

b. Draw up medication in a syringe (off the sterile field)

c. Draw up medication in a syringe (into the sterile field)

d. Accept medication into the sterile field (into a container)

Skill Assessment 9-1

Student Name	
SKILL	**Sellick's Maneuver**
Objective	Student will demonstrate knowledge and application of Sellick's maneuver.
Instructions	Instructor will demonstrate maneuver. Practice Sellick's maneuver with your partner. When ready, notify instructor and schedule the check-off. Skills Assessment check-off must be completed satisfactorily by _____ (due date).
Supplies	• None • Mannequin

Note: Student must perform skill independently without prompting.

Practice with Partner Date:		Skills Testing Date:		
PROCEDURAL STEPS				**COMMENTS**
1. Defines Sellick's maneuver.		Correct	Needs Review	
2. States purpose of Sellick's maneuver.		Correct	Needs Review	
3. Gives two examples in which Sellick's maneuver may be indicated.		Correct	Needs Review	
4. Positions self at patient's right side.		Correct	Needs Review	
5. Identifies correct anatomy. Uses self to demonstrate how to find anatomical structures.		Correct	Needs Review	
6. Positions hand properly.		Correct	Needs Review	
7. Applies adequate pressure.		Correct	Needs Review	
8. Maintains cricoid pressure until asked to release by instructor (anesthesia).		Correct	Needs Review	

Performance Evaluation Criteria

RATING

- Assembled necessary supplies and equipment
- Described Sellick's maneuver correctly as the application of cricoid pressure to reduce the risk of aspiration by closing the esophagus. Examples: Emergency surgery when patient has eaten recently, NPO status cannot be verified, or patient is experiencing GI bleeding. May be used during CPR as needed.
- Student prepared and performed procedure independently.
- Performed each step in appropriate sequence.
- Demonstrated correct technique—firm pressure with the thumb and index finger forming a V on the cricoid cartilage. States cricoid pressure is applied prior to induction of anesthesia as instructed by anesthesia personnel until endotracheal tube is placed, placement verified, cuff inflated, and waits for instruction to release by anesthesia personnel.

Overall Rating (Satisfactory; Must Redo; Fail):

Instructor Comments	
Student Signature	*Date*
Instructor Signature	*Date*

Skill Assessment 9-2

Student Name	
SKILL	**Draw Up Medication in a Syringe (Off the Sterile Field)**
Objective	Student will demonstrate knowledge and application of drawing up medication in a syringe (off the sterile field).
Instructions	Instructor will demonstrate maneuver. Practice skill with your partner. When ready, notify instructor and schedule skills check-off. Skills assessment must be completed satisfactorily by _____ (due date).
Supplies	• Medication bottle • Label and skin marker • Syringe × 2 • Withdrawal needle (18 gauge) × 2 • Injection needle (22–25 gauge) × 2 • Ampule—labeled for medication • Vial—labeled for medication • Mannequin with armband • Preference card with medication listed • Chart with allergies noted • Potential medications as assigned by instructor—know medication classification and any precautions for _____.

Note: Student must perform skill independently without prompting.

Practice with Partner Date:		Skills Testing Date:	
PROCEDURAL STEPS			**COMMENTS**
1. Identifies medication correctly.	Correct	Needs Review	
2. Assembles all necessary supplies.	Correct	Needs Review	
3. Demonstrates application of the "Six Rights."	Correct	Needs Review	
4. Verifies allergies of patient and that patient is not allergic to drug.	Correct	Needs Review	
5. Prepares medication container for withdrawal of medication.	Correct	Needs Review	
6. Withdraws medication correctly for container (ampule and vial).	Correct	Needs Review	
7. Needle for injection is applied to syringe.	Correct	Needs Review	
8. Medication label is rechecked for accuracy. States vial/ampule is kept in room until end of case.	Correct	Needs Review	
9. Medication is labeled correctly according to local policy.	Correct	Needs Review	

| **Performance Evaluation Criteria** | • Assembled necessary supplies and equipment.
• Described medication appropriately. Possible medications: Lidocaine—local anesthetic or antiarrhythmia medication; monitor for lidocaine toxicity; lidocaine with epinephrine is never injected into digits. Heparin—anticoagulant for irrigation; reversal agent protamine sulfate. Bacitracin—antibiotic; stored in refrigerator; check for allergies. And/or medication as assigned by instructor
• Demonstrated application of "Six Rights." Ensures right patient, right drug, right dose, right route of administration, right time, and right label/documentation. Uses preference card to identify right drug, right dose, right route of administration, right time, and right label/documentation. Identifies right patient and verification of allergies using simulated chart and patient ID band.
• Student prepared and performed procedure independently.
• Performed each step in appropriate sequence. | **RATING** |

Skill Assessment 9-2 (*continued*)

	• Demonstrated correct technique with no contamination. Ampule—opens correctly; inserts 18-gauge needle, bevel down; withdraws. Vial—cleans top/alcohol, injects equal amount of air, inverts and withdraws appropriate amount of solution. Labels correctly according to local policy.	
	Overall Rating (Satisfactory; Must Redo; Fail):	
Instructor Comments		
	Student Signature	**Date**
	Instructor Signature	**Date**

Skill Assessment 9-3

Student Name	
SKILL	**Draw Up Medication in a Syringe (Onto the Sterile Field)**
Objective	Student will demonstrate knowledge and application of drawing up medication in a syringe (onto the sterile field).
Instructions	Instructor will demonstrate. Practice skill with your partner. When ready, notify instructor to schedule the check-off. Skills assessment must be completed satisfactorily by _____ (due date).
Supplies	• Medication bottle: Ampule—labeled and/or vial—labeled*** • "Sterile" half-sheet • "Sterile" gown/glove setup • "Sterile" pack (three wrappers) • Mannequin with armband • Preference card - medication listed • Chart with allergies noted • Circulator—(second student who follows directions of STSR) • Potential medications as assigned by instructor—know medication classification and any precautions for _____ ○ Label(s) and skin marker ○ Syringe × 2 ○ Withdrawal needle (18 gauge) × 2 ○ Injection needle (22–25 gauge) × 2 ○ Container(s) ○ Hemostat × 1–2

Note: Student must perform skill independently without prompting.

Practice with Partner Date:		Skills Testing Date:		
PROCEDURAL STEPS				**COMMENTS**
1. Identifies medication correctly.	Correct	Needs Review	
2. Assembles all necessary supplies.	Correct	Needs Review	
3. Opens sterile supplies without contamination.	Correct	Needs Review	
4. Scrubs in correctly; dons sterile gown/gloves.	Correct	Needs Review	
5. Demonstrates application of the "Six Rights." Identifies total amount of medication given at end.	Correct	Needs Review	
6. Verifies allergies of patient and that patient is not allergic to drug.	Correct	Needs Review	
7. Circulator is instructed by STSR and prepares for withdrawal of medication correctly.	Correct	Needs Review	
8. STSR and circulator verify visually and verbally identification of medication.	Correct	Needs Review	
9. STSR withdraws medication correctly for container (ampule and/or vial). States vial/ampule is kept in room until end of case.	Correct	Needs Review	
10. Needle for injection is applied to syringe.	Correct	Needs Review	
11. Medication is labeled correctly according to local policy.	Correct	Needs Review	
12. Medications passed to surgeon/instructor as requested. STSR identifies medication.	Correct	Needs Review	

Skill Assessment 9-3 (*continued*)

		RATING
Performance Evaluation Criteria	• Assembled necessary supplies and equipment • Identifies medication information (classification, dose, strengths, administration precautions, etc.) correctly. Medication(s) as assigned by instructor: _____	
	• Demonstrates application of "Six Rights." Ensures right patient, right drug, right dose, right route of administration, right time, and right label/documentation. Uses preference card to identify right drug, right dose, right route of administration, right time, and right label/documentation. Identifies right patient and verification of allergies using simulated chart and patient ID band. Identifies for documentation the total amount of medication administered at end of "case." • Student prepared and performed procedure independently. • Performed each step in appropriate sequence. • Demonstrated correct sterile technique. Guards sterile field. Sterile items transferred correctly. • Demonstrated correct technique with no contamination: Ampule—opens correctly; inserts 18-gauge needle, bevel down; withdraws. Vial—circulator cleans top/alcohol, STSR injects equal amount of air into inverted container and withdraws correctly. Labels correctly according to local policy.	
	Overall Rating (Satisfactory; Must Redo; Fail):	
Instructor Comments		

Student Signature	Date
Instructor Signature	Date

Skill Assessment 9-4

Student Name	
SKILL	**Accept Medication into the Sterile Field (Into a Container)**
Objective	Student will demonstrate knowledge and application of accepting medication into the sterile field (into a container).
Instructions	Instructor will demonstrate maneuver. Practice skill with your partner. When ready, notify instructor and schedule the check-off. Skills assessment must be completed satisfactorily by _____ (due date).

Supplies	• Medication bottle: vial/container, labeled
	• "Sterile" half sheet
	• "Sterile" gown/glove setup
	• "Sterile" pack (three wrappers)
	• Mannequin with armband
	• Preference card—medication listed
	• Chart with allergies noted
	• Circulator—(second student who follows directions of STSR)
	
	• Potential medications as assigned by instructor, know medication classification and any precautions for_____
	  ○ Label(s) and skin marker
	  ○ Syringe × 2
	  ○ Withdrawal needle (18 gauge) × 2
	  ○ Injection needle (22–25 gauge) × 2
	  ○ Container(s)
	  ○ Hemostat × 1–2

Note: Student must perform skill independently without prompting.

Practice with Partner Date:		Skills Testing Date:	
PROCEDURAL STEPS			**COMMENTS**
1. Identifies medication correctly.	Correct	Needs Review	
2. Assembles all necessary supplies.	Correct	Needs Review	
3. Opens sterile supplies without contamination.	Correct	Needs Review	
4. Scrubs in correctly; dons sterile gown/glove.	Correct	Needs Review	
5. Demonstrates application of the "Six Rights." Identifies total amount given at end of case.	Correct	Needs Review	
6. Verifies patient is not allergic to drug.	Correct	Needs Review	
7. Circulator is instructed by STSR and prepares medication for transfer to sterile field.	Correct	Needs Review	
8. STSR and circulator verify visually and verbally identification of medication.	Correct	Needs Review	
9. STSR presents or places container at edge of sterile field correctly to receive medication. States container kept in room for referral as needed.	Correct	Needs Review	
10. Medication is transferred to sterile field.	Correct	Needs Review	
11. Medication is correctly identified visually and verbally. Container is labeled correctly.	Correct	Needs Review	
12. Medication is prepared for administration. Drawn up and diluted prn correctly.	Correct	Needs Review	
13. Medication labeled according to local policy.	Correct	Needs Review	
14. Medications passed to surgeon/instructor as requested. STSR identifies medication.	Correct	Needs Review	
15. At end of exercise, STSR identifies correct amount administered during exercise.	Correct	Needs Review	

Skill Assessment 9-4 (*continued*)

		RATING
Performance Evaluation Criteria	• Assembled necessary supplies and equipment	
	• Describes medication (classification, strength, dose, administration, etc.) appropriately. Medication as assigned by instructor: _____	
	• Demonstrates application of "Six Rights." Ensures right patient, right drug, right dose, right route of administration, right time, and right label/documentation. Uses preference card to identify right drug, right dose, right route of administration, right time, and right label/documentation. Identifies right patient and verification of allergies using simulated chart and patient ID band. Identifies for documentation the total amount used at end of "case."	
	• Student prepared and performed procedure independently.	
	• Performed each step in appropriate sequence.	
	• Demonstrated correct sterile technique. Guards sterile field. Sterile items transferred correctly.	
	• Demonstrated correct technique with no contamination: Ampule—opens correctly; inserts 18-gauge needle, bevel down; withdraws. Vial—circulator cleans top/alcohol, STSR injects equal amount of air into inverted container and withdraws correctly. Labels correctly according to local policy.	
	Overall Rating (Satisfactory; Must Redo; Fail):	
Instructor Comments		

Student Signature	*Date*	
Instructor Signature	*Date*	

Skill Assessment 9-5

Student Name				
SKILL	**Correctly Identify Medication Dosage**			
Objective	To correctly read and calculate medication amounts administered by syringe with 100% accuracy.			
Instructions	Instructor will demonstrate testing station. Practice skill with your partner. When ready, notify instructor and schedule the check-off. Skills assessment must be completed satisfactorily by _____ (due date).			
Supplies	• TB syringe X 2 • Insulin syringe • 3-cc or 5-cc syringe(s) as used by local facilities • 10-cc syringe • Larger syringes as used by local facilities • Instructor/student fills syringes with different amounts of solutions			

Note: Student must perform skill independently without prompting.

Practice with Partner Date:

Skills Testing Date:

PROCEDURAL STEPS			COMMENTS
1. Correctly identifies amount drawn up into a TB and/or insulin syringe correct. Correctly identifies each mark.	Correct	Needs Review	
2. Correctly identifies how much has been administered if syringe was full at start of case..	Correct	Needs Review	
3. Correctly identifies amount drawn up into each 3-cc and/or 5-cc syringe. Correctly identifies each mark.	Correct	Needs Review	
4. Correctly identifies how much has been administered if syringe was full at start of case.	Correct	Needs Review	
5. Correctly identifies amount drawn up into each 10-cc syringe. Correctly identifies each mark.	Correct	Needs Review	
6. Correctly identifies how much has been administered if syringe was full at start of case.	Correct	Needs Review	
7. Correctly identifies amount drawn up into each large syringe. Correctly identifies each mark.	Correct	Needs Review	
8. Correctly identifies how much has been administered if syringe was full at start of case.	Correct	Needs Review	

Performance Evaluation Criteria	• Identifies each type of syringe and amount left in syringe. • Demonstrates correct calculation of amount administered from a full syringe. • Student prepared and performed procedure independently.	RATING
	Overall Rating (Satisfactory; Must Redo; Fail):	
Instructor Comments		

Student Signature	*Date*
Instructor Signature	*Date*

CHAPTER 10

Instrumentation, Equipment, and Supplies

OBJECTIVES

After studying this chapter, the reader should be able to:

C 1. Associate the relationship between instrumentation, equipment, and supplies and quality patient care in the OR.

A 2. Indicate items that require sterilization prior to use in the sterile field.

R 3. Recognize basic instruments by type, function, and name.

4. Demonstrate proper care, handling, and assembly of instruments.

5. Differentiate the types of special equipment utilized in OR practice and demonstrate proper care, handling techniques, and safety precautions.

6. Cite the names and describe the functions of accessory equipment and demonstrate proper care, handling, and assembly.

7. Collect and prepare supplies used in the OR.

E 8. Associate the relationship between instruments, equipment, and supplies and the OR environment with safety concepts.

Select Key Terms

Define the following, using your textbook glossary or a medical dictionary if necessary:

1. aperture _____

_____

2. bipolar electrosurgery _____

_____

3. capillary action _____

_____

4. catheter _____

_____

5. cottonoid _____

_____

6. cryo- _____

_____

7. drain _____

_____

8. fenestration _____

_____

9. insufflation _____

_____

10. irrigation _____

_____

11. magnification _____

_____

12. monopolar cautery _____

_____

13. pneumatic _____

_____

14. resistance _____

_____

15. retract _____

_____

16. scalpel _____

_____

17. serrations _____

_____

18. stainless steel _____

_____

19. teeth _____

_____

20. ureteral _____

_____

21. urethral _____

_____

Identification

1. Identify the components of the instrument shown in Figure 10-1.

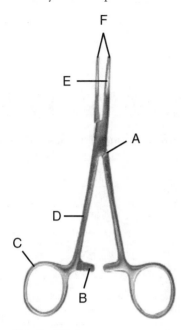

Figure 10-1

A. _____   D. _____

B. _____   E. _____

C. _____   F. _____

2. Classify the instruments listed using the following designations:

Accessory	Probing
Clamping/occluding	Retracting
Cutting	Suctioning
Dilating	Suturing
Grasping/holding	

A. #3 Knife handle   _____

B. Allis   _____

C. Babcock   _____

D. Crile   _____

E. Deaver   _____

F. DeBakey tissue forceps   _____

G. Kocher   _____

H. Metzenbaum   _____

I. Mosquito   _____

J. Needle holder   _____

K. Poole   _____

L. Richardson   _____

M. Towel clamp   _____

N. Yankauer   _____

O. Westcott   _____

P. Frazier   _____

Q. Adson   _____

R. Lowman   _____

S. Kelly   _____

T. Grooved director   _____

3. Using the numbers 1, 2, 3, and 4, organize the following instruments by size from shortest/smallest to longest/largest.

   A. _____ Crile

   B. _____ Mosquito

   C. _____ Pean

   D. _____ Schnidt

4. What does tagging mean?

   _____

   _____

5. Scalpel handles

   A. A #20 knife blade fits on a # _____ knife handle.

   B. A #15 knife blade fits on a # _____ knife handle.

6. Identify each cutting instrument and the type of tissue on which it is usually used. Use Figure 10-2.

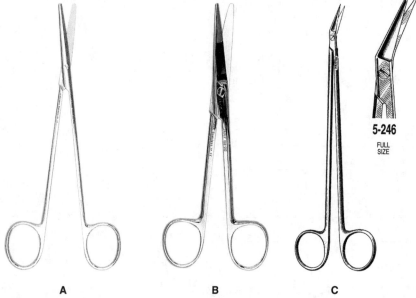

5-246

FULL SIZE

A   B   C

Figure 10-2

A. _____   _____

B. _____   _____

C. _____   _____

7. Identify each instrument and what it might be used for. Use Figure 10-3.

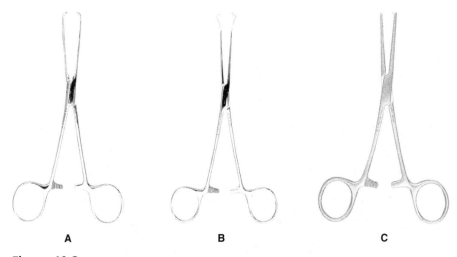

A   B   C

Figure 10-3

A. _____

B. _____

C. _____

8. Identify three atraumatic vascular instruments that may be used on vascular tissue.

_____

_____

9. Identify each retracting instrument and identify if it is self-retaining or hand-held. Use Figure 10-4.

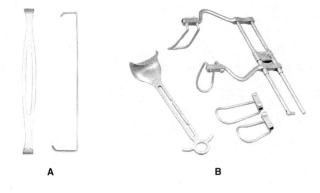

A   B

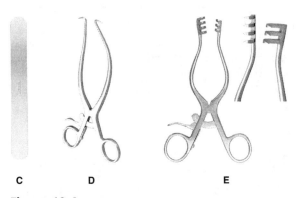

C   D   E

Figure 10-4

A. _____   D. _____

B. _____   E. _____

C. _____

10. Describe how you would choose the appropriate needle holder for the case.

_____

_____

11. Identify the suction that matches the description:

A. Suction with a removable guard used to aspirate abdominal fluids. Why is the guard adjustable or removable?

_____

B. Suction that has a tip that screws on and off; used for tonsillectomy or abdominal cases:

_____

C. Suction used by neurosurgeons that is angled and has variable suction.

_____

D. Suction that resembles a bent hypodermic needle and may be used for ear surgery.

_____

E. Unit used to drain sinuses or gallbladders.

_____

12. How is suction maintained patent during the procedure?

_____

13. Why is a suction tip wrapped with a sponge or applied over cottonoids for use?

_____

14. Describe three reasons that you use an instrument for the intended purpose only.

_____

15. Instrument count sheets:

A. Describe the purpose of using an instrument count sheet when assembling instrument sets.

_____

B. Why should the instrument count sheet be signed after assembly?

_____

C. In an emergency, what is the instrument count sheet used for?

_____

Matching

Match the scope used for viewing to the correct area of the body.

_____ A. Proctoscope   1. Common bile duct

_____ B. Hysteroscope   2. Joint

_____ C. Mediastinoscope   3. Large intestine

_____ D. Ventriculoscope   4. Uterus

_____ E. Fetoscope   5. Rectum

_____ F. Choledochoscope   6. Ear

_____ G. Gastroduodenoscope   7. Abdomen

_____ H. Laparoscope   8. Middle thoracic cavity

_____ I. Arthroscope   9. Cranial cavity

_____ J. Colonoscope   10. Pregnant uterus

_____ K. Otoscope   11. Stomach and duodenum

Short Answer

1. Identify the three possible power sources for power tools used in the OR.

   _____

2. What type of power source uses a pressure gauge on a regulator?

   A. _____

Complete the Sentences:

   B. Internal pressure for the tank must be at least _____psi.

   C. The operating pressure is usually set between _____ and _____psi.

3. Identify the types of motion:

   A. An oscillating saw uses a(n) _____ motion.

   B. A reciprocating saw uses a(n) _____ motion.

   C. A drill, driver, or reamer uses a(n) _____ motion.

4. Microscope (fill in the blanks/complete the sentences):

   A. The objective lens and eyepieces are called _____ and range from _____ to _____ mm.

   B. The distance of the lens from the target tissue is referred to as the _____.

   C. Focusing is controlled by _____.

   D. Two possible attachments to the microscope include _____.

   E. To match the original field of view seen by the surgeon, a camera or second set of binoculars requires a _____.

5. How is a video camera usually sterilized?

   _____

   _____

6. When using an irrigation/aspiration unit, what protection must the surgical team use?

   _____

   _____

7. What type of energy is used by a phaco-emulsifier?

   _____

   _____

8. What three sources are used to generate the cold temperature in a cryotherapy unit?

_____

_____

9. What is the normal laparoscopy intraoperative pressure setting for the insufflator?

_____

_____

10. Insufflators:

    A. What kind of gas does the laparoscopic insufflator use?

    _____

    B. How is the gas introduced?

    _____

11. Identify the nerves that can be identified using a nerve simulator during surgery.

    _____

    _____

12. How is suction tubing secured to the drape?

    _____

    _____

13. Operating room lights:

    A. At what depth of focus should OR lights be set?

    _____

    _____

    B. Describe how to turn OR lights on and off.

    _____

    _____

    C. Why is it important to be careful when turning OR lights on and off?

    _____

    _____

14. Tourniquets

    A. When using a tourniquet what item(s) may be used to exsanguinate the arm?

    _____

    _____

    B. What is the appropriate tourniquet pressure setting?

    _____

    _____

    C. What are the potential complications of tourniquet use?

    _____

    _____

D. Identify the maximum time recommended for tourniquet inflation. What should be done if the surgery exceeds the time limit?

_____

_____

15. What do the sequential compression devices on a patient's legs prevent?

_____

_____

Drapes

1. What is the goal of draping?

_____

_____

2. Describe the following properties of drapes and relate why each is important to the patient.

A. Lint free: _____

_____

B. Fluid resistant: _____

_____

C. Porous: _____

_____

D. Flame retardant: _____

_____

3. Identify one advantage and one disadvantage of each type of fabric.

A. Nonwoven fabrics: _____

_____

B. Woven fabrics: _____

_____

4. Describe each the following types of drapes.

A. Incise drape: _____

_____

B. Aperture drape: _____

_____

C. Isolation drape: _____

_____

D. Fenestrated drape: _____

_____

E. Split sheet: _____

_____

F. Stockinette:_____

_____

5. You are setting up your case and notice the circulator adding an extension onto the table. She states the patient is more than seven feet tall. What concerns do you have about the drape and how can you correct it, if necessary?

_____

_____

Surgical Sponges

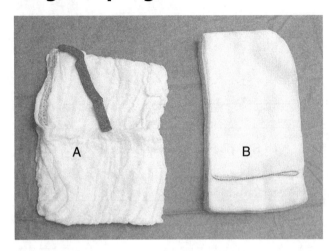

Figure 10-5

1. Identify the types of sponges in Figure 10-5, usual number in a pack, and indicate where they are typically used.

    A. Name _____ Number _____

    Used _____

    B. Name _____ Number _____

    Used _____

2. Neurosurgical sponges:

    A. Name of sponge _____

    B. May be moistened with _____

    C. Number in a pack _____

    D. Where are they arranged on field? _____

3. Describe each one and identify the usual number in a package:

    A. Tonsil Sponge:_____

    B. Kitner:_____

    C. Peanut: _____

4. *Critical thinking exercise.* The surgeon is doing a routine hernia surgery with Raytec on the field. He states that the patient has dead bowel in the groin area and that the abdominal cavity will need to be opened to complete a laparotomy for a bowel resection. Describe what to with the Raytecs and why.

_____

_____

_____

Dressings

1. Describe how dressing sponges differ from surgical sponges.

   _____

   _____

   _____

2. Describe how the incision and surrounding area are prepared for the dressing.

   _____

   _____

   _____

3. Identify the type of dressing material:

   A. Op-site _____

   B. Basic dressing used when drainage is anticipated_____

   C. Collodion _____

   D. Foams _____

   E. Dressing used to reduce edema or hematoma _____

   F. Skin closure tapes_____

   G. Aerosol adhesive spray _____

   H. Dressing used to prevent movement _____

   _____

4. Identify the three types of contact layers that could be used in a three-layer dressing. Give an example of each.

   _____

   _____

   _____

5. Identify the proper type of dressing for the situation.

   A. Dressing that prevents unidirectional movement

   _____

   B. Large three-layer dressing with additional absorbent material but no pressure

   _____

   C. Dressing that eliminates dead space

   _____

   D. Dressing layer provides an airtight and watertight seal

   _____

   E. Dressing layer allows passage of air and fluids

   _____

   F. Dressing layer that draws secretions from the wound by wicking action

   _____

6. Match the type of material used with the situation described.

_____ A. Secures dressing for frequent dressing changes or inspections

1. Hydrocolloid dressing

_____ B. Used to secure dressing when a digit is involved

2. Tape (paper, silk, adhesive)

_____ C. Most frequently used to secure dressings

3. Kerlix, Coban, ace wrap

_____ D. Used for intermediate absorbent layer

4. Montgomery straps

_____ E. Secure a splint dressing on an extremity

5. Vaseline gauze or Xeroform gauze

_____ F. Prevents movement by incorporating proximal and distal joint

6. Telfa or Adaptic

_____ G. Occlusive dressing around a chest tube

7. Fiberglass

_____ H. Semipermeable dressing on chronic wounds to debride

8. Tube gauze

_____ I. Example of a complete three-layer dressing

9. ABD pad

_____ J. Nonadherent—painless when removed

10. Band-Aid

7. Describe the following specialty dressings:

A. Bolster or stent dressing _____

_____

B. Wet to dry gauze _____

_____

C. Queen Anne's collar _____

_____

8. Describe four reasons that packing material such as Nu Gauze may be used.

_____

_____

_____

Catheters

1. Identify the catheters pictured in Figure 10-6 and what each is used for.

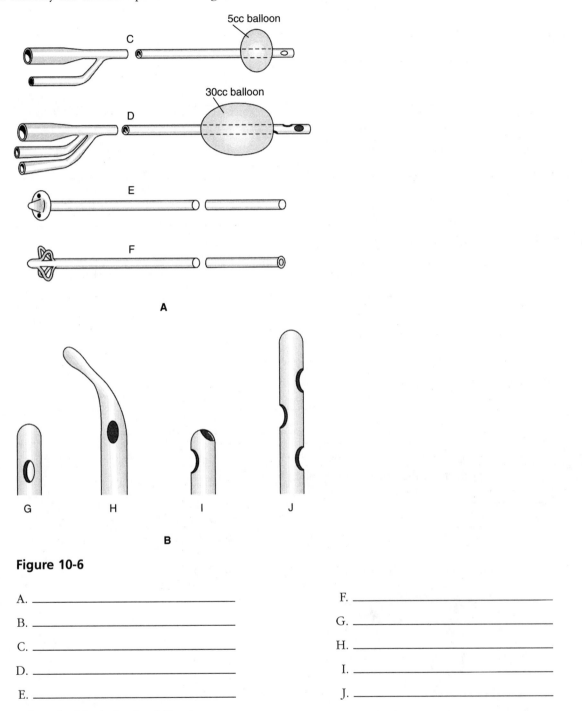

Figure 10-6

A. _____ F. _____

B. _____ G. _____

C. _____ H. _____

D. _____ I. _____

E. _____ J. _____

2. Fill in the blank for the following:

A. Describe how to inflate the Foley catheter balloon in the bladder.

_____

_____

_____

B. Describe how to move a gravity drainage bag.

_____

_____

_____

C. Describe how catheters are sized (measuring unit).

_____

_____

_____

D. Describe the purpose(s) of intravascular catheters.

_____

_____

_____

E. Describe how a Fogarty catheter is used.

_____

_____

_____

Tubes

1. Describe the purpose of the following tubes:

    A. Gastrostomy tube _____

    B. Sump tube _____

    C. ETT _____

2. Identify the three components of the tracheostomy tube.

    A. _____

    B. _____

    C. _____

3. Identify the three components of the chest drainage system in Figure 10-7.

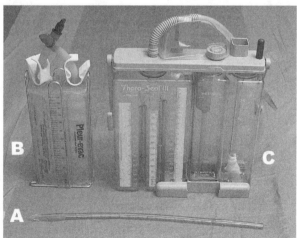

Figure 10-7

A. _____

B. _____

C. _____

4. Answer the following questions related to chest tubes:

A. What is the purpose of a chest tube?

_____

_____

B. If a person has two chest tubes on the same side, what does the chest tube placed in the lower chest evacuate?

_____

_____

C. What does the chest tube placed in the upper chest evacuate?

_____

_____

D. What is the water in the collection unit used for?

_____

_____

E. If the patient has two chest tubes, what can you use to connect them to one drainage system?

_____

_____

Drains

1. Identify the drain/tube/catheter as either passive (P) or active (A).

_____ Penrose   _____ Stryker

_____ Hemovac   _____ Chest tube

_____ T-tube   _____ Gastrostomy tube

_____ Nephrostomy tube   _____ Cystostomy tube

_____ Jackson Pratt

Fill in the blank.

2. Closed wound suction devices connected to active drains utilize _____ to remove fluids and/or air.

3. Passive drains use _____ or absorbent dressings to remove fluids and/or air.

Needles

1. What is the range in length of hypodermic needles?

_____

2. Hypodermic diameter or gauge ranges from 12 to 30.

Place the following sizes in order from smallest to largest.

26, 30, 14, 22, 20, 16

_____

3. Name three biopsy needles commonly used and identify the type of tissue each is used for.

    A. _____

    B. _____

    C. _____

Case Studies

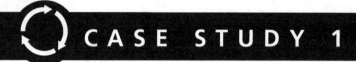

Edward has been assigned to prepare the Cysto Room for a transurethral resection of the prostate (TURP). At the end of the procedure, the physician has ordered a 30-cc three-way 32 Fr Foley inserted and connected to drainage and irrigation.

1. What instrument will be prepared and utilized to visualize the prostate?

    _____

    _____

    _____

    _____

2. The patient is having a three-way Foley inserted at the end of the procedure. What size syringe will you need?

    _____

3. What will you fill the balloon with to hold it in place and why?

    _____

4. When connecting the self-retaining urinary catheter to the drainage bag, what precautions will you take and why?

    _____

    _____

5. Which type of drainage bag is this, passive or active?

    _____

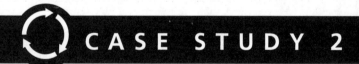

Magdelena is preparing the OR for a neurosurgical procedure (craniotomy). The surgeon needs instrumentation for the case.

1. The surgeon uses a craniotome that is nitrogen powered. What is a craniotome used for?

    _____

    _____

(continues)

CASE STUDY 2 *(continued)*

_____

_____

2. What protects the dura mater?

_____

3. What is the normal operating psi range that should read on the gauge when you test the device prior to use?

_____

4. What type of suction is the surgeon most likely to use?

_____

5. When using this suction, the surgeon will utilize a special sponge called a

_____

6. When packaged, how many of these sponges are bundled together?

_____

7. A microscope with a 400x objective lens is utilized during the procedure. Before bringing the microscope over the sterile field, what will be necessary?

_____

_____

8. During the procedure, what does the surgeon use to increase or decrease the magnification of the microscope?

_____

_____

9. Instrument length is important because of the distance between the lens and target tissue; what is this distance called?

_____

CASE STUDY 3

Tony has fallen and broken his leg and is scheduled for an ORIF (open reduction internal fixation) of his distal tibia. The wound is open and there is a lot of debris in the wound. His blood pressure is 120/76 mm Hg.

1. When pulling supplies and equipment for this case, what will be needed to debride the wound?

_____

_____

2. What will you need to protect the staff from splashing?

_____

_____

(continues)

CASE STUDY 3 *(continued)*

3. What bone holding clamps might be used to hold the bone pieces in place? After the incision is made, the surgeon is given scissors to dissect through the layers of tough connective tissue around the bone. Which scissors will you most likely pass to the surgeon?

_____

_____

4. The surgeon has ordered a tourniquet. List at least two items that will be needed to facilitate the use of the tourniquet.

_____

_____

_____

_____

5. What is the likely pressure setting range that will be used?

_____

_____

6. What should you do if the operating time exceeds the recommended time for tourniquet use?

_____

_____

7. The pack contains the drapes to use. What type of fenestrated drape will most likely be in the pack?

_____

_____

8. Prior to application of the main drape, the surgeon places a drape under the leg. What type of drape will be placed?

_____

_____

9. What can the surgeon use to isolate the foot from the sterile field?

_____

_____

Lab 10: Instrumentation, Equipment, and Supplies

Introduction

The instrumentation, equipment, and supplies portion of this manual will give the student a better understanding of the names classifications, and uses on their setups. The lab practice will allow more hands-on experience with the tools of the trade. This lab should be taught early in the program and continued throughout the core and specialty procedure instruction classes. The student will have to use a lot of memorization skills to learn all the basic and specialty instruments. Introducing small groups of instruments over a longer period will give the students a better chance for success. Add 10 new instruments each week until the students' recall meets the program objectives.

Game 1: Instrument Jeopardy®

Time involved: One week for setup

Supplies: Paper and pencil, note cards, and a display (either whiteboard, blackboard, or computer)

Instructors: Instrument Jeopardy® can be accomplished in several different ways. You can download from the Internet a PowerPoint presentation–style game, you can use on a whiteboard or blackboard, or you can work from note cards. Here are a few ways that may work for you. Make categories that may include what the instruments do, how they are used, or how they look, and then decide how many answers you will place in each category. Make a list of instruments that fall into the different categories; then you can use pictures, descriptions, anatomical areas, and actual instruments. The how, what, where, and when of the instruments are used to pose the questions; students will give the "What is ___" answer. You can have the students respond in teams or as individuals. This will help build critical thinking skills.

Students: Study the categories of how, what, where, and when instruments can be grouped or used. Making note cards can be a big help, but also thinking about the how, where, when, and why an instrument is used will help you to learn to anticipate the surgeon's needs for instruments during surgery.

Practical

A. Assemble an instrument set

B. Instrument handling—load, pass, and unload a scalpel handle

C. Instrument handling—passing various instruments

Skill Assessment 10-1

Student Name	
SKILL	**Assemble an Instrument Set**
Instructions	Instructor will demonstrate assembly. Practice procedure with your partner. When ready, notify instructor to schedule the check-off. Skills assessment must be completed satisfactorily by _____ (due date).
Supplies	• External case or wrapping material—one double-thickness wrap or two wrappers of appropriate material (if no tray top to secure items—three wrappers for inner wrap) • Internal chemical indicator • Outer chemical indicator (sterilization tape or label for case) • Internal protection such as towels, peel packs, or protective tips • Basic instrument count sheet • Tray • Instruments • Inspection supplies to test scissors, gauze • Cleaning supplies/water-soluble lubricant prn

Note: Student must perform skill independently without prompting.

Practice with Partner Date: | **Skills Testing Date:**

PROCEDURAL STEPS			COMMENTS
1. Identifies importance of standardized assembly of sets.	Correct	Needs Review	
2. Demonstrates appropriate attire for instrument processing.	Correct	Needs Review	
3. Demonstrates standard hand washing.	Correct	Needs Review	
4. Assembles equipment and supplies.	Correct	Needs Review	
5. Organizes workspace for most effective ergonomics.	Correct	Needs Review	
6. Utilizes count sheet to assemble correct type and size of instruments.	Correct	Needs Review	
7. Inspects instruments for cleanliness and working condition. Inspects tips, identifies instruments needing sharpening, and replaces defective instruments.	Correct	Needs Review	
8. Assembles tray correctly with lighter instruments on top. All instruments in open position on stringers or disassembled.	Correct	Needs Review	
9. Count sheet/instrument sheet signed.	Correct	Needs Review	
10. Internal indicator placed in tray.	Correct	Needs Review	
11. Contained appropriately for type of packaging material and tray available.	Correct	Needs Review	
12. Outer chemical indicator placed.	Correct	Needs Review	
13. Tray labeled appropriately with name of item, date processed, initials of person preparing set, etc., as per local policy.	Correct	Needs Review	

Skill Assessment 10-1 (*continued*)

		RATING
Performance Evaluation Criteria	• Assembled necessary supplies and equipment.	
	• Discussed importance of standardized sets.	
	• Discussed methods of inspection and testing: tips meet with no crossing, box locks and serrations clean, working action not too loose or too tight; needle holders hold needle, scissors cut appropriately, all parts present, lumens inspected, etc.	
	• Demonstrated correct assembly of tray contents. Lighter objects on top, protective devices as appropriate.	
	• Demonstrated correct preparation of tray for sterilization process including appropriate wrapping, security of item, chemical indicator placement, and labeling.	
	• Student prepared and performed procedure independently.	
	• Performed each step in appropriate sequence.	
	Overall Rating (Satisfactory; Must Redo; Fail):	
Instructor Comments		

Student Signature	*Date*	
Instructor Signature	*Date*	

Skill Assessment 10-2

Student Name	
SKILL	**Basic Passing with Hand Signals**
Instructions	Instructor will demonstrate assembly. Practice procedure with your partner. When ready, notify instructor to schedule check-off. Skills assessment must be completed satisfactorily by _____ (due date).
Supplies	• Towels for setup • Basic instrument tray (various hemostats, scissors, tissue forceps, ringed instruments appropriate to local facility, handheld and self-retaining retractors commonly used, etc.) • Raytec—sponges • Basic instrument count sheet

Note: Student must perform skill independently without prompting.

Practice with Partner Date:		Skills Testing Date:	
PROCEDURAL STEPS			**COMMENTS**
1. Assembles equipment and supplies.	Correct	Needs Review	
2. Organizes workspace for most effective ergonomics. (Prepares towel roll and lays out instruments as a simulated Mayo stand.)	Correct	Needs Review	
3. Identifies all instruments on set correctly.	Correct	Needs Review	
4. Selects correct instrument requested by hand signal or scenario.	Correct	Needs Review	
5. Demonstrates correct passing of unloaded knife handle.	Correct	Needs Review	
6. Demonstrates correct placement and retrieval of sponges. Loads Forester sponge stick correctly.	Correct	Needs Review	
7. Demonstrates safe passing of forceps. Aligns between surgeon's thumb and middle finger (index finger used for stabilization of forceps).	Correct	Needs Review	
8. Demonstrates safe passing of ringed instrument in position to use. Curved instruments are passed with curve aligned with curve of surgeon's hand. Grasps at box locks when possible and does not handle the working tip of the instrument with gloved hand.	Correct	Needs Review	
9. Demonstrates safe passing of ringed instrument with placement designed to elicit the grasp reflex. No student-to-surgeon hand contact—only instrument touches palm.	Correct	Needs Review	
10. Demonstrates safe passing of retractors for type. Chooses retractor correctly and orients tip to tissue depth for scenario given.	Correct	Needs Review	
11. Returns items to storage location on setup. Maintains field in organized manner.	Correct	Needs Review	
12. Breaks down setup and stores appropriately.	Correct	Needs Review	

Skill Assessment 10-2 (*continued*)

		RATING
Performance Evaluation Criteria	• Assembled necessary supplies and equipment.	
	• Demonstrated knowledge of basic instrument set and hand signals. Able to identify 100% correct.	
	• Discussed key principles of passing technique: tips visible; ringed instrument closed on first ratchet, if curved, aligned with curve of surgeon's hand, elicits surgeon's grasp reflex, does not distract surgeon by touching other areas of hand.	
	• Demonstrated safe passing of instruments. If not, area(s) needing improvement: _____	
	• Demonstrated organizational skills. Workspace organized with items placed for safe retrieval. Kept work area organized, immediately retrieved item discarded, and replaced on setup.	
	• Student prepared and performed procedure independently.	
	• Responded appropriately to each hand signal given during session.	
	Overall Rating (Satisfactory; Must Redo; Fail):	
Instructor Comments		

Student Signature	*Date*
Instructor Signature	*Date*

Skill Assessment 10-3

Student Name	
SKILL	**Instrument Sharps Handling—Load, Pass, and Unload Sharps**
Instructions	Instructor will demonstrate assembly. Practice procedure with your partner. When ready, notify instructor to schedule the check-off. Skills assessment must be completed satisfactorily by _____ (due date).
Supplies	• Needle box • Scalpel blade (size[s] to fit scalpel handle[s]) • Suture—small needle (3–0 or 4–0); micro needle (6–0 or 7–0); and large needle (1 or 0) • Basic instrument count sheet • Basic instrument tray (hemostats, needle holders [Crile wood; Mayo Hegar; Haney, and Castroviejo], scalpels, etc.)

Note: Student must perform skill independently without prompting.

Practice with Partner Date:		Skills Testing Date:	
PROCEDURAL STEPS			**COMMENTS**
1. Identifies methods of handling sharps to reduce injury.	Correct	Needs Review	
2. Selects appropriate blade and handle for blade requested.	Correct	Needs Review	
3. Demonstrates safe loading, holding, and storage of blade device (uses hemostat or needle holder on dull side).	Correct	Needs Review	
4. Demonstrates safe holding and passing of scalpel for use.	Correct	Needs Review	
5. Demonstrates safe utilization of neutral zone placement for scalpels and suture passing (may use tray or magnetic pad).	Correct	Needs Review	
6. Demonstrates safe retrieval of scalpel.	Correct	Needs Review	
7. Demonstrates safe removal and disposal of blade.	Correct	Needs Review	
8. Demonstrates correct selection of needle holder for suture requested.	Correct	Needs Review	
9. Demonstrates safe loading of needle holder. No touch technique when possible. (May adjust at curve.)	Correct	Needs Review	
10. Demonstrates correct loading of needle on needle holder for situation (straight or curved Heaney).	Correct	Needs Review	
11. Demonstrates safe passing of needle holder for use. Companion instrument(s) passed with suture as appropriate (pickups or hemostat to first assistant).	Correct	Needs Review	
12. Demonstrates safe handling of suture with control of free end to reduce memory, prevent contamination, or limit the formation of knots. (Places free end near surgeon's hand.)	Correct	Needs Review	
13. Demonstrates safe utilization of neutral zone technique for placement of sutures.	Correct	Needs Review	

Skill Assessment 10-3 (*continued*)

	14. Demonstrates safe retrieval of needle holder. Inspects needle holder to ensure that needle is present and intact. Notifies "surgeon" if needle is not present or intact.	Correct	Needs Review	
	15. Demonstrates safe storage of needle and suture remnant.	Correct	Needs Review	
	16. Breaks down setup and stores appropriately.	Correct	Needs Review	

		RATING
Performance Evaluation Criteria	• Assembled necessary supplies and equipment. • Discussed correct methods of handling sharps including exchange of needles, inspection for completeness, neutral zone guidelines, needle box or sharps containers utilization, counts, utilization of magnetic pads (lateral), and placement on Mayo or back table so that there is no danger of injury or compromise of sterile field. • Demonstrated correct loading of scalpel and needle holder (not less than one-third or greater than one-half of needle length from suture or two-thirds from tip—stated swag section is weak). Selected correct needle holder for each needle size. • Demonstrated correct method of passing sharps or utilization of neutral zone placement for no pass facilities. Needle tip up or blade down. Positioned hand during passing and retrieval to limit chance of injury. (Blades: Usually #10 blade like a steak knife; #15 blade pencil style to use belly of needle.) Controls free end of suture. • Student prepared and performed procedure independently. • Performed each step in appropriate sequence.	
	Overall Rating (Satisfactory; Must Redo; Fail):	
Instructor Comments		

Student Signature	**Date**	
Instructor Signature	**Date**	

Skill Assessment 10-4A

Name	
SKILL	**Instrument Preparation, Handling, and Passing**
Instructions	Instructor will demonstrate assembly. Practice procedure with your partner. When ready, notify instructor to schedule the check-off. Skills assessment must be completed satisfactorily by _____ (due date).
Supplies	• Mayo stand and back table • Back table drape (individual items may be wrapped in drape or wrapped for individual transfer) • Mayo cover • Towels for setup • Sponges or other testing material for scissors • Gown/glove setup × 2 (self and "surgeon") • Draped mannequin/setup to pull up to for setup and passing practice • Basic instrument count sheet • Basic instrument tray (various hemostats, scissors, tissue forceps, ringed instruments appropriate to local facility, handheld and self-retaining retractors commonly used, etc.) • Wrap or instrument case setup for tray

Note: Student must perform skill independently without prompting.

Practice with Partner Date:	Skills Testing Date:		
PROCEDURAL STEPS			**COMMENTS**
1. Assembles and prepares supplies and lab for practice.	Correct	Needs Review	
2. Demonstrates appropriate infection control practices. Washes hands and dons appropriate OR attire.	Correct	Needs Review	
3. Demonstrates correct application of sterile technique principles during exercise. Prepared instruments and tray as "sterilized" appropriately for use in the sterile field.	Correct	Needs Review	
4. Demonstrates correct gown/closed glove technique.	Correct	Needs Review	
5. Demonstrates correct draping of Mayo cover. Creates and places towel roll for effective use. Checks internal indicator when accepting instrument tray.	Correct	Needs Review	
6. Demonstrates preparation of back table and Mayo setup as previously instructed.	Correct	Needs Review	
7. Prepares instruments for use. Assembles, inspects, and tests instruments for working order. (Tips meet, clean, acceptable working action.) Closes instruments on first ratchet.	Correct	Needs Review	
8. Selects correct instrument requested (verbal or hand signal). Identifies all instruments correctly.	Correct	Needs Review	

Skill Assessment 10-4 (*continued*)

	9. Demonstrates safe passing of instrument with placement designed to elicit the grasp reflex without hand contact with surgeon. Utilizes box locks when possible and does not handle working tip of the instrument with gloved hand.	Correct	Needs Review	
	10. Demonstrates safe passing of instrument in position to use. Curved instruments are passed with curve aligned with curve of surgeon's hand. Tissue forceps aligned with surgeon's middle/fore finger and thumb.	Correct	Needs Review	
	11. Returns items to storage location on setup. Maintains field in organized manner.	Correct	Needs Review	
	12. Breaks down setup and stores appropriately.	Correct	Needs Review	
Performance Evaluation Criteria	• Assembled necessary supplies and equipment. • Discussed each type of instrument and identified name and function of each instrument in basic instrument set. • Discussed correct methods of inspection, testing, and preparation of instruments while setting up Mayo. • Demonstrated correct application of sterile technique principles. Complete tasks with no contaminations, breaks in sterile technique, or identified and corrected contaminations appropriately. • Demonstrated safe passing of instrument which safely elicited grasp reflex for "surgeon." Follows *sharps* rules. • Demonstrated attention to detail—setup is completed as instructed and maintained in an organized, clean, and safe manner. If not, needs improvement with: _____ • Student prepared and performed procedure independently. • Performed each step in appropriate sequence. Handled sharps safely.	**RATING**		
	Overall Rating (Satisfactory; Must Redo; Fail):			
Instructor Comments				
	Student Signature	***Date***		
	Instructor Signature	***Date***		

Skill Assessment 10-4B

Name	
SKILL	**Instrument Preparation: Loading and Passing a Needle Holder**
Instructions	Instructor will demonstrate assembly. Practice procedure with your partner. When ready, notify instructor to schedule the check-off. Skills assessment must be completed satisfactorily by _____ (due date).
Supplies	• Draped mannequin/setup to pull up to for setup and passing practice • Gown/gloves as appropriate. • Needle Holders: Crile-Wood, Mayo-Hegar, Castroviejo • Forceps: Rat tooth/tissue or adsons with teeth • Suture: 3-0 or 4-0, 2-0 or 0, 6-0 or 7-0 • Needle box

Note: Student must perform skill independently without prompting.

Practice with Partner Date:	Skills Testing Date:		
PROCEDURAL STEPS			**COMMENTS**
13. Assembles and prepares supplies and lab for practice.	Correct	Needs Review	
14. Demonstrates appropriate infection control practices. Washes hands and dons appropriate OR attire.	Correct	Needs Review	
15. Prepares instruments for use. Assembles, inspects, and tests instruments for working order. (Tips meet, clean, acceptable working action.) Closes instruments on first ratchet.	Correct	Needs Review	
16. Selects correct instrument for suturing choice (verbal or hand signal). Identifies all instruments correctly.	Correct	Needs Review	
17. Loads needle on needle holder correctly (between 1/3 and 1/2 of the length of needle from swaged end).	Correct	Needs Review	
18. Passes needle holder so that the needle tip is pointed up and on the surgeon's thumb side; places end of suture near the surgical site.	Correct	Needs Review	
19. Receives needle holder back correctly (may use neutral zone). Accounts for all pieces, places in needle box correctly.	Correct	Needs Review	
20. Repeats process for Castroviejo needle holder, placing the needle holder along the axis of the index finger.	Correct	Needs Review	

Skill Assessment 10-4B (*continued*)

	21. Demonstrates safe passing of instrument with placement designed to elicit the grasp reflex without hand contact with surgeon. Utilizes box locks when possible and does not handle working tip of the instrument with gloved hand.	Correct	Needs Review	
	22. Demonstrates safe passing of instrument in position to use. Passes tissue forceps aligned with surgeon's middle/fore finger and thumb to the other hand.	Correct	Needs Review	
	23. Returns items to storage location on setup. Maintains field in organized manner.	Correct	Needs Review	
	24. Breaks down setup and stores appropriately.	Correct	Needs Review	
Performance Evaluation Criteria	• Assembled necessary supplies and equipment. • Discussed each type of instrument and identified name and function of each needle holder matching size of suture needle and tissue forceps. • Discussed correct methods of inspection, testing, and preparation of instruments. • Demonstrated correct application of sterile technique principles. Completed tasks with no contaminations, breaks in sterile technique, or identified and corrected contaminations appropriately. • Demonstrated safe passing of instrument which safely elicited grasp reflex for "surgeon." Follows *sharps* rules. • Demonstrated attention to detail—setup is completed as instructed and maintained in an organized, clean, and safe manner. If not, needs improvement with: _____ • Student prepared and performed procedure independently. • Performed each step in appropriate sequence. Handled sharps safely.		**RATING**	
	Overall Rating (Satisfactory; Must Redo; Fail):			
Instructor Comments				
	Student Signature		**Date**	
	Instructor Signature		**Date**	

Skill Assessment 10-4C

Name	
SKILL	**Instrument Preparation: Loading and Passing a Needle Holder Using Free Needles**
Instructions	Instructor will demonstrate assembly. Practice procedure with your partner. When ready, notify instructor to schedule the check-off. Skills assessment must be completed satisfactorily by _____ (due date).
Supplies	• Draped mannequin/setup to pull up to for setup and passing practice • Gown/gloves as appropriate. • Needle holders: Crile-Wood, Mayo-Hegar • Free needles • Suture: As appropriate to size of free needle • Needle box

Note: Student must perform skill independently without prompting.				
Practice with Partner Date:		**Skills Testing Date:**		
PROCEDURAL STEPS				**COMMENTS**
25. Assembles and prepares supplies and lab for practice.		Correct	Needs Review	
26. Demonstrates appropriate infection control practices. Washes hands and dons appropriate OR attire.		Correct	Needs Review	
27. Prepares instruments for use. Assembles, inspects, & tests instruments for working order. (Tips meet, clean, acceptable working action.) Closes instruments on first ratchet.		Correct	Needs Review	
28 Selects correct instrument for suturing choice (verbal or hand signal). Identifies all instruments correctly.		Correct	Needs Review	
29. Loads suture in needle and needle on needle holder correctly (between 1/3 and 1/2 of the length of needle from swaged end).		Correct	Needs Review	
30. Passes needle holder so that the needle tip is pointed up and on the surgeon's thumb side; places end of suture near the surgical site.		Correct	Needs Review	
31. Receives needle holder back correctly (may use neutral zone). Accounts for all pieces, places in needle box correctly.		Correct	Needs Review	
32. Demonstrates safe passing of instrument with placement designed to elicit the grasp reflex without hand contact with surgeon. Utilizes box locks when possible and does not handle working tip of the instrument with gloved hand.		Correct	Needs Review	
33. Returns items to storage location on setup. Maintains field in organized manner.		Correct	Needs Review	
34. Breaks down setup and stores appropriately.		Correct	Needs Review	

Skill Assessment 10-4C (*continued*)

		RATING
Performance Evaluation Criteria	• Assembled necessary supplies and equipment.	
	• Demonstrated correct loading and preparation of the needle and needle holder.	
	• Demonstrated correct and safe passing of instrument which safely elicited grasp reflex for "surgeon."	
	• Follows sharps rules. Demonstrated attention to detail. If not, needs improvement with: _____	
	• Student prepared and performed procedure independently.	
	• Performed each step in appropriate sequence. Handled sharps safely.	
	Overall Rating (Satisfactory; Must Redo; Fail):	
Instructor Comments		
	Student Signature	
	Instructor Signature	

Skill Assessment 10-4D

Name	
SKILL	**Instrument Preparation: Passing Free Ties, Reels, and Tie on Passer**
Instructions	Instructor will demonstrate assembly. Practice procedure with your partner. When ready, notify instructor to schedule the check-off. Skills assessment must be completed satisfactorily by _____ (due date).
Supplies	• Draped mannequin/setup to pull up to for setup and passing practice • Gown/gloves as appropriate. • Instrument: right angle, tonsil hemostat (Schnidt or Adson) • Free suture ties, reels

Note: Student must perform skill independently without prompting.

Practice with Partner Date:	**Skills Testing Date:**		
PROCEDURAL STEPS			**COMMENTS**
35. Assembles and prepares supplies and lab for practice.	Correct	Needs Review	
36. Demonstrates appropriate infection control practices. Washes hands and dons appropriate OR attire.	Correct	Needs Review	
37. Prepares instruments for use. Assembles, inspects, & tests instruments for working order. (Tips meet, clean, acceptable working action.) Closes instruments on first ratchet.	Correct	Needs Review	
38. Selects correct instrument for free tie (verbal or hand signal).	Correct	Needs Review	
39. Loads free tie in the tips of instrument for passing.	Correct	Needs Review	
40. Prepares reel and passes reel with free end on surgeon's thumb side.	Correct	Needs Review	
41. Passes a free tie into surgeon's outstretched hand using sufficient pressure to elicit the grasp reflex.	Correct	Needs Review	
42. Returns items to storage location on setup. Maintains field in organized manner.	Correct	Needs Review	
43. Breaks down setup and stores appropriately.	Correct	Needs Review	

Skill Assessment 10-4D (*continued*)

		RATING
Performance Evaluation Criteria	• Assembled necessary supplies and equipment. • Demonstrated correct loading and preparation of the tie and instrument. Passes correctly. • Demonstrated correct and safe passing of a free tie to elicit the grasp reflex for "surgeon." • Demonstrated correct passing of the reel ready for immediate use. • Demonstrated attention to detail. If not, needs improvement with: _____ • Student prepared and performed procedure independently. • Performed each step in appropriate sequence. Handled sharps safely.	
	Overall Rating (Satisfactory; Must Redo; Fail):	
Instructor Comments		
	Student Signature	*Date*
	Instructor Signature	*Date*

Skill Assessment 10-4E

Student Name	
SKILL	**Advanced Instrument Techniques**
Instructions	Instructor will demonstrate assembly. Practice procedure with your partner. When ready, notify instructor to schedule the check-off. Skills assessment must be completed satisfactorily by _____ (due date).
Supplies	• Sponges, kitners (peanut or cherry), and cottonoids (type used locally) • Suture with needle and ties • Irrigation bowl with solution and Asepto syringe • Active electrode and safety holder • Material for suturing (sticky towels cut, left folded, and facing each other with outer edges taped down can be used, suturing simulator, pig's feet, etc.) to practice cutting suture • Vessel occlusion simulation— (rubber bands or vessel loops secured between two structures with small hinge clips or pieces of suture knotted on both ends on towels or other simulation setup) • Basic instrument count sheet • Basic instrument tray (various hemostats, scissors, tissue forceps, ringed instruments appropriate to local facility, handheld and self-retaining retractors commonly used, etc.)

Note: Student must perform skill independently for each scenario without prompting.

Practice with Partner Date:			
Skills Testing Date:			

PROCEDURAL STEPS			COMMENTS
1. Assembles and prepares supplies and lab for practice.	Correct	Needs Review	
2. Selects instrument requested correctly.	Correct	Needs Review	
3. Demonstrates safe and effective passing of instrument.	Correct	Needs Review	
4. Demonstrates safe preparation, handling, and passing of specialty sponges: sponge stick (load on Forester), kitner dissectors (loaded on Rochester pean/Kelly), and cottonoids (pickups passed with cottonoid offered on back of hand).	Correct	Needs Review	
5. Demonstrates correct sequence of instrument passing for vessel occlusion. Clamp, clamp, cut, tie, suture, scissors.	Correct	Needs Review	
6. Demonstrates preparation and passing of Asepto syringe.	Correct	Needs Review	
7. Demonstrates correctly cutting of suture as on the knot or 3–4 mm or 1/4 inch for skin; slightly shorter for inside 1/8 inch (place blade of scissor on suture, slide scissors down to knot or area above knot, rotate scissor slightly to see knot and amount of tail, and then cut either flush on the knot or slightly above knot leaving tail of appropriate length).	Correct	Needs Review	

Skill Assessment 10-4E (*continued*)

	8. Demonstrates correct passing of active electrode (in holder when not in use) and "buzzing" of hemostat. (Places Bovie tip flat, activates cutting close to tip or holds hemostat with large amount of gloved surface, does not put self in circuit/does not touch patient.) Note: Buzzing of hemostat is not recommended, but if necessary safety precautions are taken to prevent dielectric breakdown of glove/burns.	Correct	Needs Review	
	9. Breaks down setup and stores appropriately.	Correct	Needs Review	

		RATING
Performance Evaluation Criteria	• Assembled necessary supplies and equipment.	
	• Identified and safely passed each instrument/Asepto, which elicited grasp reflex for "surgeon."	
	• Demonstrated safe passing techniques for specialized sponges. Identified handling techniques when counting item (kitners back to holder; cottonoids back table—never kick bucket; sponges opened and dropped into kick bucket).	
	• Anticipated sequence of vessel occlusion correctly. Passed hemostat, hemostat, Metzenbaum scissor, tie, and then suture scissor. Able to manipulate hemostat correctly for "surgeon" to tie.	
	• Demonstrated cutting of suture appropriately for situation given (on skin, flush on knot, and inside tag).	
	• Demonstrates passing pencil-style active electrode and buzzing technique safely.	
	• Demonstrated attention to detail—work area is completed as instructed and maintained in an organized, clean, and safe manner. If not, needs improvement with: _____	
	• Student prepared and performed procedure independently.	
	• Performed each step in appropriate sequence for scenario given.	
	Overall Rating (Satisfactory; Must Redo; Fail):	
Instructor Comments		
	Student Signature	*Date*
	Instructor Signature	*Date*

CHAPTER 11

Wound Healing, Sutures, Needles, and Stapling Devices

OBJECTIVES

After studying this chapter, the reader should be able to:

C
1. Indicate terms relevant to wound healing.

2. Summarize the possible complications of wound healing.

A
3. Recognize the classifications of surgical wounds.

4. Indicate and give examples of types of traumatic wounds.

5. Analyze the factors that influence healing and recognize the manner in which they affect the healing process.

R
6. Recognize the characteristics of inflammation.

7. Cite and interpret common suture terms.

8. Classify and differentiate suture materials and stapling devices and their usage.

9. Recognize the types, characteristics, and uses of natural and synthetic absorbable suture materials.

10. Compare and recognize the common natural and synthetic nonabsorbable sutures, stating their sources, common trade names, and uses.

11. Demonstrate application of recommended preparation and handling techniques for suturing and stapling devices and provide rationale for choice.

12. Cite and interpret common suture techniques.

13. Summarize the basic uses and advantages of stapling instruments.

14. Distinguish, describe the use of, and demonstrate proper handling of the various types of surgical needles.

E
15. Assess the types of injury that cause damage to tissues.

16. Recognize the characteristics of the types of healing.

17. Recognize the stages/phases of wound healing.

Select Key Terms

Define the following, using your textbook glossary or a medical dictionary if needed:

1. adhesion _____

   _____

2. anastomosis _____

   _____

3. approximated _____

   _____

4. chromic gut _____

   _____

5. chronic wound _____

   _____

6. cicatrix _____

   _____

7. dead space _____

   _____

8. debridement _____

   _____

9. dehiscence _____

   _____

10. evisceration _____

    _____

11. first intention _____

    _____

12. French-eyed needle _____

    _____

13. friable _____

    _____

14. herniation _____

    _____

15. immunosuppressed patient _____

    _____

16. inflammation _____

    _____

17. laceration _____

    _____

18. ligated _____

_____

19. monofilament _____

_____

20. packing _____

_____

21. primary suture line _____

_____

22. PTFE _____

_____

23. second intention _____

_____

24. secondary suture line _____

_____

25. swaged _____

_____

26. tensile strength _____

_____

27. third intention _____

_____

28. vessel loop _____

_____

Classify the Surgical Wound

1. When is the wound classification recorded on the intra-operative record?

_____

_____

2. True or False: When reviewing a chart, the wound classification tells us the degree of microbial contamination that was present or occurred during the operation. This information can indicate the likelihood of the patient developing or having a postoperative infection.

_____

_____

3. Identify the wound classification for each instance listed.

Surgical Wound	Wound Classification
Breast biopsy, frozen section indicates cancer	
Laparoscopic cholecystectomy; gallbladder removed with endobag	
Cystoscopy with retrograde pyelogram (RPG); no stones found	
Scheduled bowel resection; scrub observes bloody hole in glove; regloved	
Emergency bowel resection; feces noted during anastomosis	
Laparoscopic-assisted vaginal hysterectomy; purulent left ovary	
Hernia repair; mesh utilized	
Open reduction internal fixation (ORIF) (<4 h) open fracture	
Incision and drainage of groin. STAT gram stain indicates gram-negative rods.	
Gunshot wound to abdomen; bowel resection and liver laceration repaired	

Wound Healing

Match the wound with the appropriate condition description.

_____ 1. Abrasion

_____ 2. Laceration

_____ 3. Contusion

_____ 4. Chronic wound

_____ 5. Puncture

_____ 6. Clean wound

_____ 7. Complicated wound

_____ 8. Contaminated wound

_____ 9. Thermal wound

_____ 10. Closed wound

a. Persists for an extended period

b. Penetrating wound

c. Dirty object damages skin

d. Tissue is lost/destroyed or contains a foreign body

e. Scrape

f. Bruise

g. Cut or tear

h. Occurs by heat or cold

i. Skin intact with damage to underlying tissue

j. Incision made, sutured, heals first intention

Short Answer

11. What is released from the damaged cells to cause the inflammatory response?

_____

_____

12. Normal healing of wounds occurs from _____ to _____ across the wound not from the inside out.

13. Describe the five signs of the inflammatory process.

_____

_____

_____

14. Identify the three phases of normal (primary intention) wound healing. What is the normal length of time for each?

    Phase 1: _____

    _____

    _____

    Phase 2: _____

    _____

    _____

    Phase 3: _____

    _____

    _____

15. Indicate the correct type of wound healing for the description. Indicate if it is first, second, or third intention healing.

Description	Wound Healing Type
Granulation tissue occurs from inside out or bottom upward	
Incision opened under ideal conditions; minimal scar	
Delayed closure	
Produces a weak union with a wide irregular scar	
Wound debrided then closed 4–6 days later to heal	
Used for dirty wounds, produces intermediate scar/tensile strength	
Incision made with rapid wound healing to 70–80% original strength	
Routine negative breast biopsy closure (mammogram mass)	
Which type of healing is most likely used for a decubitus ulcer?	
Which type of healing is most likely to be used initially for a ruptured appendix?	

16. Identify the order in which normal primary intention healing occurs. Place the events in the order of occurrence using the numbers 1–9. There are three primary phases of normal healing. Use the written description and Figure 11-1 in the textbook for reference.

    A. _____ Cicatrix appears, slow increase in tensile strength until 70–80% returns

    B. _____ Fibroblasts secrete collagen; capillary networks form up to 20 days

    C. _____ Scab forms with a weak sealing of wound

    D. _____ Wound contraction occurs as fibroblasts cause the scar to pale

    E. _____ Proliferation phase begins on third to fifth postoperative day

    F. _____ Maturation or remodeling phase begins 14–21 days post injury

    G. _____ Lag phase: Inflammation occurs, with heat, swelling, pain, redness, loss of function

    H _____ May last up to 12 months or longer

    J. _____ 25–30% tensile strength returns at the end of this phase

17. Use additional information derived from an Internet search on the topic of wound healing for each of the issues listed below. Analyze your research and describe how each of the following affects wound healing.

Age: _____

_____

Nutrition: _____

_____

Disease (e.g., diabetes, obesity): _____

_____

Radiation exposure: _____

_____

Smoking: _____

_____

Immunocompromised because of steroid therapy or chemotherapy:

_____

_____

18. Describe the appropriate tissue handling techniques that should be utilized during any case.

_____

_____

_____

Complications

Match the complication with the appropriate description.

_____ 1. Adhesion   A. Microbial contamination occurs

_____ 2. Dehiscence   B. Splitting of suture material

_____ 3. Evisceration   C. Partial or total separation of layer(s)

_____ 4. Fistula   D. Tract between two surfaces open at both ends

_____ 5. Hemorrhage   E. Hypertrophic scar formation

_____ 6. Herniation   F. Abnormal attachment between two surfaces

_____ 7. Infection   G. Exposure of viscera (organs)

_____ 8. Keloid   H. Excessive blood loss

_____ 9. Sinus tract   I. Results from wound dehiscence; found 2–3 months postoperatively

_____ 10. Suture complication   J. Tract between two surfaces open at one end

11. Describe five possible causes of wound dehiscence.

_____

_____

_____

_____

12. Distinguish the difference between dehiscence and evisceration.

_____

_____

13. Which incision is most likely to be a factor in the cause of dehiscence?

_____

14. Analyze the factors leading to wound infection and dehiscence and identify measures that the STSR can take to prevent wound infections and dehiscence.

_____

_____

_____

_____

_____

_____

Suture Material

True or False

_____ 1. 3-0 and 4-0 sutures are most commonly used for subcuticular skin closure.

_____ 2. 6-0 and 7-0 sutures are typically used for very large vessel closure.

_____ 3. 8-0 and 11-0 sutures are typically used for microsurgery such as ophthalmic.

_____ 4. The Brown and Sharpe (B&S) sizing is used for stainless steel wire gauges.

_____ 5. Nonabsorbable suture should be used when continued support is not needed.

_____ 6. Silk suture is common for ligating blood vessels.

_____ 7. GI tissue is weak, but heals quickly and should use absorbable suture for inner layers.

_____ 8. Monofilament rather than multifilament sutures should be used in the presence of infection.

_____ 9. Multifilament suture may be more pliable allowing knots to hold more easily.

_____ 10. Absorbable sutures inhibit tissue reaction such as hydrolysis or digestion.

Ordering

Place the USP sizes in order from smallest to largest. Place the numbers 1–10 next to each size, with 1 being the smallest and 10 the very largest.

11. 0 _____

12. 4-0 _____

13. 11-0 _____

14. 8-0 _____

15. 1 _____

16. 5 _____

17. 3-0 _____

18. 6-0 _____

19. 2-0 _____

20. 2 _____

21. Classify the following suture types according to their characteristics:

Suture Generic Name	Trade Name(s)	Absorbable or Nonabsorbable	Monofilament or Multifilament	Type: Natural or Synthetic	Common Usage	Color Package	Tensile Strength
Plain gut collagen (intestine of sheep or cows)	Plain Gut						
Chromic gut collagen (intestine of sheep or cows treated with salts)	Chromic Gut						
Polyglactin 910 or polyglycolic acid	Vicryl Dexon						
Polydioxanone	PDS II Ethicon						
Stainless steel	Stainless steel						
Polypropylene	Prolene or surgilene						
Nylon	Ethilon Dermalon Nurolon Surgilon						
Silk	Surgical silk						
Cotton	Surgical cotton						

Fill in the Blank: Ligatures

22. When cutting suture for the surgeon on a monofilament suture for skin closure with a "tag," you would typically cut the suture approximately _____ from the knot.

23. When cutting suture for the surgeon on a multifilament suture inside the wound with a "tag," you would typically cut the suture approximately _____ from the knot.

24. Large vessels are typically occluded with suture ligatures or _____ to prevent hemorrhage.

25. The most common sizes of suture ligatures are _____ and _____ and are made of _____ suture material.

26. When passing ligature reels, check the size by the number of holes on the side of the reel and always pull the strand approximately _____ inch(es) away from the reel.

27. The needle should be clamped approximately _____ of the distance from the swaged end of the needle. If tough tissue is anticipated, the needle should be clamped at the _____ mark of the needle.

28. Always wet _____ sutures prior to passing to the surgeon.

29. If a muscle has been transversely incised and must be approximated, you would be prepared to supply the surgeon with a (n) _____ suture.

30. The skin is usually closed with an interrupted or continuous _____ suture on a _____ needle.

31. The preferred method of skin closure is _____ suture line to prevent bacteria and tissue from traveling the length of the wound.

True or False

_____ 32. Ligature reels are a counted item because they can be easily lost in the wound.

_____ 33. Free ties should be placed on the Mayo stand for easy access.

_____ 34. If used, ties-on-passes should be prepared ahead of time to prevent delay.

_____ 35. In delicate tissue, clamp the needle on the swaged segment to allow the surgeon greater depth.

_____ 36. Silk suture should be passed to the surgeon after being moistened.

_____ 37. Memory (bends in the suture) may be removed with a gentle pull from monofilament suture. Be careful not to pull against the swaged end.

_____ 38. Surgical gut should be soaked in normal saline.

_____ 39. The peritoneum is usually closed with a nonabsorbable suture.

_____ 40. Stainless steel staples result in less tissue reaction.

_____ 41. The continuous suture is more likely to result in dehiscence if it fails.

Matching

Match the suture technique or accessory device with the usage.

_____ 42. Reinforces subcuticular stitch—skin must be dry   A. Traction suture

_____ 43. Approximation with noncrushing B-shaped steel   B. Pursestring suture

_____ 44. Nonabsorbable suture placed into a structure to retract   C. Retention

_____ 45. Device prevents pressure from secondary suture line loop   D. Preknotted

_____ 46. Circular stitch placed to close an opening or invert tissue   E. Button

_____ 47. Used for isolation, retraction, temporary occlusion of vessels   F. Bridge or bolsters

_____ 48. Premoistened and loaded onto hemostat   G. Umbilical tape

_____ 49. Secondary suture line to prevent tension   H. Vessel loops

_____ 50. Device used for tendon repair   I. Stapler

_____ 51. Endoscopic suturing   J. Skin closure tapes

Short Answer

Compare sutures regarding the following characteristics.

52. Describe tensile strength and identify what factors affect the tensile strength of the suture.

_____

_____

53. Identify one suture with very strong tensile strength.

_____

_____

54. Describe pliability.

_____

_____

55. Describe how to remove memory.

_____

_____

56. Identify one suture with memory.

_____

_____

Staple Devices and Needles

Short Answer—Staplers and Needles

1. The type of stapler that delivers two double staple lines and contains a knife to transect tissue is called a

_____.

2. A device used to anastomose tubular structures such as the colon is called a(n)

_____.

3. Synthetic material used for fascia defects as a reinforcement or bridge between structures is called

_____.

4. When using a _____ eyed needle, pull the suture into a V-shaped area; however, there is more tissue damage than with use of a swaged needle.

5. A suture with a needle on each end of the suture strand is called

_____.

6. A suture designed to be removed with a quick pull is called a

_____.

7. When using a needle on the skin, you would typically use a _____ needle.

8. When using a needle on delicate gastrointestinal tissue, you would typically use a _____ needle.

9. When using a needle on friable tissue such as the liver or kidney, you could use a _____ needle.

10. The most commonly used body shape is the _____ circle and the most commonly used body shape for skin closure is the _____ circle.

Case Studies

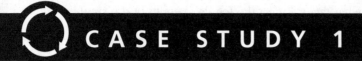
CASE STUDY 1

James, a 12-year-old male, lost control of his trail bike while riding on a course that he and some friends constructed in a vacant lot. He flew over the handlebars into the dirt onto his left arm. His arm is broken, and the bone is sticking out through the skin. It is 10:00 AM.

1. James has sustained a traumatic injury to his left arm. What classification(s) does his wound fall into?

   _____

   _____

   _____

   _____

2. James was immediately taken to the Urgent Care Center. It is determined that James will need surgical treatment and will be transferred by ambulance to the nearest hospital, which is 150 miles away. The surgery is scheduled for 4:00 PM. How will the surgical wound be classified? Why?

   _____

   _____

   _____

   _____

3. Is James at risk for surgical site infection (SSI)? Why? What steps can be taken to minimize the risk of SSI?

   _____

   _____

   _____

CASE STUDY 2

Dorothea just had her ruptured appendix removed. The skin and subcutaneous layers of her wound have been left open. Her surgeon told her that if her wound showed no signs of infection in five days he would finish the closure.

1. During the surgical procedure, the surgeon grasps the appendix for removal. Once he grasps the appendix, he asks for a suture. Why would he use a pursestring stitch at the base of the appendix?

   _____

   _____

   _____

   _____

(continues)

CASE STUDY 2 *(continued)*

2. Why did the surgeon leave the wound partially open? In its present condition, by what method is the wound expected to heal?

   _____

   _____

   _____

   _____

3. When will the surgeon possibly close the wound? How will the surgeon determine if Dorothea's wound may be closed in five days?

   _____

   _____

   _____

   _____

4. If the wound can be closed in five days, what type of healing will then be expected? What is the expected amount of tensile strength that can be regained?

   _____

   _____

   _____

   _____

Lab 11: Wound Healing, Sutures, Needles, and Stapling Devices
Introduction

The Wound Healing, Sutures, Needles, and Stapling Devices portions of this lab will give the student a better understanding of the sutures or stapling devices used. The suture or stapling device needed varies according to the situation such as the location, type of tissue, or mechanisms of healing such as the length of time or tensile strength needed. This lab should be introduced early in the program and continued with the core and specialty procedures. The student will have to memorize the characteristics of basic sutures and specialty sutures, and correctly identify how to handle and use each one. Introducing a few at a time over a longer period will give the students a better chance for success. Add a new suture and/or accessory component each week until students can recall all of the important characteristics.

Game 1: Wound Healing Jeopardy®

Time involved: One week for setup

Supplies: Paper and pencil, note cards, and a display (whiteboard, blackboard, or computer)

Instructors: Wound Healing Jeopardy® can be accomplished in several ways. You can download from the Internet a PowerPoint presentation–style game, it can be used on a whiteboard or blackboard, or you can work from note cards. Here are a few ways that may work for you. Make your categories that may include what the sutures do, how they are used, or how they look, or how long until they break down. Then decide how many answers you will place in each category. Make a list of sutures that fall into the different categories; then you can use pictures, descriptions, anatomical areas, actual sutures. The what, where, and when of the sutures are used to pose the questions; students will give the "What is ___" answers. You can utilize either teams or individuals. This will help build critical thinking skills.

Students: Study the categories of how, what, where and when sutures can be grouped or used. Making note cards can be a big help, but also thinking about the how, where, when, and why a suture is used, will give you the skills to anticipate the surgeon's needs for sutures during surgery.

Practical

a.   Suture/needle/staple handling—Load, pass, and unload a needle holder

b.   Suture/needle/staple handling—Load a non-swaged needle

c.   Suture/needle/staple handling—Pass ties

d.   Suture/needle/staple handling—Load, unload, pass stapling devices

Skill Assessment 11-1

Student Name	
SKILL	**Suture and Tie Passing Techniques**
Instructions	Instructor will demonstrate assembly. Practice procedure with your partner. When ready, notify instructor to schedule the check-off. Skills assessment must be completed satisfactorily by _____ (due date).
Supplies	• Setup with various ties used locally [reels, free ties (2–3 sizes), and "stick ties" suture]. • Towel or tie preparation device as used locally for multiple ties. • Needle box • Vessel occlusion simulation (rubber bands or vessel loops secured between two structures with small hinge clips or pieces of suture knotted on both ends on towels or other simulation setup) • Basic instrument count sheet • Basic instrument tray (various hemostats, scissors, tissue forceps, ringed instruments appropriate to local facility, handheld and self-retaining retractors commonly used, etc.)

Note: Student must perform skill independently without prompting.

Practice with Partner Date:		Skills Testing Date:	
PROCEDURAL STEPS			**COMMENTS**
1. Assembles and prepares supplies and lab for practice.	Correct	Needs Review	
2. Selects instrument requested correctly.	Correct	Needs Review	
3. Demonstrates safe and effective preparation of Mayo setup. Prepares free ties so that multiple sizes are distinguishable from each other in towel setup/tie setup device.	Correct	Needs Review	
4. Demonstrates safe preparation, handling, and passing of reel or free ties. Placement in palm of surgeon's hand with shorter end of tie on surgeon's thumb side.	Correct	Needs Review	
5. Demonstrates correct loading and passing of "tie on a passer." Controls free end of tie; places end of suture on field. Passes companion instrument such as pickups or hemostat to nondominant hand or first assistant.	Correct	Needs Review	
6. Demonstrates safe loading of suture (stick tie). Opens suture packet, applies needle holder. No-touch technique (may adjust angle at curve of needle if necessary).	Correct	Needs Review	
7. Passes suture correctly for right and left hand dominance. Controls free end of suture; places free end on sterile field near surgeon's hand. Passes companion instrument (pickups or hemostat).	Correct	Needs Review	
8. Demonstrates anticipation. Prepares to pass suture scissors without prompting after passing tie or suture.	Correct	Needs Review	
9. Demonstrates correct sequence of instrument passing for vessel occlusion. Clamp, clamp, cut, tie, suture scissors.	Correct	Needs Review	

Skill Assessment 11-1 (*continued*)

	10. Maintains work area neat and organized. Immediately retrieves free ends of suture and disposes in "trash bag."	Correct	Needs Review	
	11. Breaks down setup and stores appropriately.	Correct	Needs Review	

		Rating
Performance Evaluation Criteria	• Assembled necessary supplies and equipment.	
	• Identified and safely passed each instrument/Asepto correctly, elicited the grasp reflex for "surgeon."	
	• Demonstrated safe passing techniques for reel or tie on a passer. Identified handling techniques of suture to prevent fraying, kinks, or knots (controls suture to prevent contamination).	
	• Demonstrated safe passing techniques for "stick tie" suture. (Loaded needle holder correctly—not less than one-third or greater than one-half of needle length from suture or two-thirds from tip—stated swag section is weak.) Selected correct needle holder for needle size.	
	• Anticipated correctly for suture scissors or sequence of vessel occlusion. Passed hemostat, hemostat, Metzenbaum scissor, tie, and then suture scissor. Able to manipulate hemostat correctly for "surgeon" to tie.	
	• Demonstrated attention to detail—work area is completed as instructed and maintained in an organized, clean, and safe manner. If not, needs improvement with: _____	
	• Student prepared and performed procedure independently.	
	• Performed each step in appropriate sequence.	
Instructor Comments	**Overall Rating (Satisfactory; Must Redo; Fail):**	

Student Signature	***Date***	
Instructor Signature	***Date***	

Skill Assessment 11-2

Student Name	
SKILL	**Staple Handling Techniques**
Instructions	Instructor will demonstrate assembly. Practice procedure with your partner. When ready notify instructor to schedule skills check-off. Skills assessment must be completed satisfactorily by _____ (due date).
Supplies	• Setup with various stapling devices used locally (skin staples, linear stapler, intraluminal stapler, other stapling devices as available or demonstrated by sales representative) • Lap sponge • Setup trash bag • Emesis basin or "dirty setup" tray or other mechanism utilized for separation of clean and dirty • Skin closure simulation setup (may use towels) • Basic instrument count sheet • Basic instrument tray (various hemostats, scissors, tissue forceps, ringed instruments appropriate to local facility)

Note: Student must perform skill independently without prompting.

Practice with Partner Date:		Skills Testing Date:	
PROCEDURAL STEPS			**COMMENTS**
1. Assembles and prepares supplies and lab for practice.	Correct	Needs Review	
2. Identifies routine staplers utilized. Selects stapler requested correctly.	Correct	Needs Review	
3. Demonstrates safe preparation, handling, and passing of skin stapler. Offers two Adson forceps with teeth and one skin stapler. Assists with skin closure correctly.	Correct	Needs Review	
4. Demonstrates ability to remove skin staples using a staple remover or hemostat.	Correct	Needs Review	
5. Discusses the difference of a linear stapler with knife or without knife. Stapler without knife may need scalpel or Metzenbaum to separate.	Correct	Needs Review	
6. Discusses or prepares stapler for use. (Removes any protective inserts, opens jaws, and passes item.)	Correct	Needs Review	
7. Discusses or demonstrates safe reloading of inserts. States that stapler inserts utilized on bowel may be contaminated after use and must be removed with an instrument. Free staples must be removed from upper jaws of stapler with folded lap sponge and discarded from field. (Identifies need for separation of clean and dirty; uses technique utilized locally.)	Correct	Needs Review	
8. Discusses or prepares intraluminal circular stapler for use. Identifies the importance of the donut inspection after use.	Correct	Needs Review	
9. Maintains work area neat and organized. Immediately retrieves free ends of suture and disposes in "trash bag."	Correct	Needs Review	
10. Breaks down setup and stores appropriately.	Correct	Needs Review	

Skill Assessment 11-2 (*continued*)

		Rating
Performance Evaluation Criteria	• Assembled necessary supplies and equipment. • Identified and safely passed each instrument/Asepto correctly, which elicited the grasp reflex for the "surgeon." • Demonstrated safe passing techniques for stapler. Identified handling techniques of suture to prevent contamination. • Demonstrated safe reloading techniques for linear stapler. • Demonstrated knowledge of staplers and identified types correctly. Identified precautions regarding use of each type. • Demonstrated attention to detail—work area is completed as instructed and maintained in an organized, clean, and safe manner. If not, needs improvement with: _____ • Student prepared and performed procedure independently. • Performed each step in appropriate sequence.	
Instructor Comments	**Overall Rating (Satisfactory; Must Redo; Fail):**	

Student Signature	*Date*
Instructor Signature	*Date*

CHAPTER 12

Surgical Case Management

OBJECTIVES

After studying this chapter, the reader should be able to:

C 1. Analyze the role of the STSR in caring for the surgical patient.

2. Verify the preoperative routines that must be completed.

3. Demonstrate the transportation of the surgical patient.

4. Apply the principles of surgical positioning.

A 5. Demonstrate techniques of opening and preparing supplies and instruments needed for any operative procedure with the maintenance of sterile technique at all times.

6. Summarize the methods of preparation of the operative site for surgery.

7. Demonstrate the application of thermoregulatory devices.

R 8. Interpret the principles and demonstrate the taking and recording of vital signs.

9. Interpret the principles of urinary catheterization and demonstrate the procedure.

10. Analyze how the principles of operative site preparation and urinary catheterization are related both to patient care and to the principles of asepsis.

E 11. Demonstrate the proper techniques for the surgical hand scrub, gowning, gloving, and assisting of team members.

12. Demonstrate the proper technique for preparing supplies and instruments on a sterile field.

13. Demonstrate and explain in detail the procedure for counting instruments, sponges, needles, and other items on the sterile field.

14. Demonstrate the initial steps for starting a procedure.

15. Demonstrate intraoperative handling of sterile equipment and supplies.

16. Summarize and demonstrate postoperative routines.

Select Key Terms

Define the following, using your textbook glossary or a medical dictionary if needed:

1. adhesive _____

    _____

2. anticipate _____

    _____

3. antimicrobial _____

    _____

4. apical pulse _____

    _____

5. biohazard _____

    _____

6. catheterization _____

    _____

7. circumferentially _____

    _____

8. count _____

    _____

9. craniotomy _____

    _____

10. cylindrical _____

    _____

11. donning _____

    _____

12. dyspnea _____

    _____

13. handwashing _____

    _____

14. indicator _____

    _____

15. lap sponge _____

    _____

16. mask _____

    _____

17. neutral zone _____

    _____

18. NPO _____
_____

19. pathology _____
_____

20. PPE _____
_____

21. prep _____
_____

22. prone _____
_____

23. resident organisms _____
_____

24. scrub (sterile) attire _____
_____

25. sedation _____
_____

26. sterile team member _____
_____

27. supine _____
_____

28. surgeon's preference card _____
_____

29. surgical scrub _____
_____

30. transient organisms _____
_____

31. vital signs _____
_____

32. wraparound-style gown _____
_____

Surgical Preparation—Preoperative Phase

Sequence of Surgery:

1. Analyze the following events that occur in preparing the patient for surgery and place them in the correct sequence.

_____ A. General anesthesia initiated (induction, intubation, and maintenance).

_____ B. Surgical preparation of the site (skin prep) completed.

_____ C. Time-out/pause for the cause to verify patient, procedure, and site to prevent wrong-site surgery.

_____ D. Office visit—history and physical completed. Surgery and any preoperative preparation ordered.

_____ E. Positioning for surgical procedure completed.

_____ F. Preoperative medication given to reduce anxiety.

_____ G. Transported to the operating room (OR); transferred to OR table. Safety strap applied.

_____ H. Admission: preop checklist initiated: vital signs taken prior to preoperative medications; gown on; patient voids; IV started; any ordered preoperative lab work results on chart.

_____ I. Last moment patient can sign his/her own surgery consent form. Chart completed with all lab work, special consents, allergies, history, and physical. Patient is cleared to go for surgery. (Signing can occur any time from first office visit. After the next step, the patient can no longer sign the form.)

_____ J. Last routine moment for anesthesia preoperative assessment, preoperative medications ordered, risks/options for anesthesia discussed, and consent for anesthesia obtained. (Note: This can occur as a scheduled visit one to two days prior to surgery or immediately prior to the preoperative medication—which may occur for urgent surgery.)

_____ K. Surgery scheduled.

_____ L. Draping of the sterile site completed. Sterile field perimeters established.

2. Prioritize the surgical technologist in the scrub role (STSR) preoperative responsibilities in the order that they will be performed.

_____ A. Create and maintain the sterile field, known as opening the case.

_____ B. Prepare for and perform initial count once all items opened onto field.

_____ C. Wash hands and prepare the OR for the procedure (bed type, hemostasis unit, wipe down as needed, etc.).

_____ D. Don operating room attire and PPE.

_____ E. Gather instruments, equipment, and supplies—use preference card.

_____ F. Assist the operative team members to enter the sterile field (gown/glove surgeon).

_____ G. Scrub and don sterile attire.

_____ H. Organize the sterile field and instrumentation for use.

_____ I. Expose operative site with sterile drapes (draping).

_____ J. Report to main OR desk to obtain assignment.

_____ K. Participate in time-out to prevent wrong-site surgery.

_____ L. Pull up back table, Mayo stand, and ring stand. Establish the sterile perimeters of the field.

Role Responsibilities

Identify the role responsible for the following preoperative responsibilities. Note some responsibilities may have one or more persons who may share responsibility for the activity.

C = Circulator or S = Scrub or P = Physician

_____ 3. Obtaining the surgical procedure consent (explain risks and benefits).

_____ 4. Pulling the case utilizing the preference card.

_____ 5. Counting after all items have been opened onto the sterile field.

_____ 6. Completing surgical scrub—gown and glove closed technique.

_____ 7. Opening the sterile supplies for the case.

_____ 8. Organizing the sterile supplies for use.

_____ 9. Quiet during induction of general anesthesia—maintain environmental awareness to assist if laryngospasm occurs.

_____ 10. Assisting with intubation and Sellick's maneuver as needed.

_____ 11. Positioning the patient (especially with fractures).

_____ 12. Completing the surgical skin prep.

_____ 13. Verifying the surgical site and patient.

Hair Removal

_____ 14. True or False: The Centers for Disease Control and Prevention (CDC) recommends hair removal at all times due to the high number of microbes found on the hair shaft and follicle.

_____ 15. Choose the best method of hair removal.

   A. Wet shave with razor

   B. Clippers

   C. Depilatory

   D. Dry shave

_____ 16. Choose the best time to remove the hair.

   A. Immediately prior to the incision

   B. As close to the time of surgery as possible according to method used

   C. The night before prior to the bath to reduce contaminants

   D. Always just prior to the surgical prep

_____ 17. Choose the best answer regarding surgical shaves.

   A. Depilatory shave in preoperative holding is best.

   B. Clipper shave in OR is best.

   C. Wet shave performed in outpatient or inpatient room by the patient

   D. None of these—CDC recommends not removing the hair unless necessary.

_____ 18. OR Attire consists of _____ and _____.

Preoperative Preparation of the Patient

You may choose more than one answer.

_____ 19. Preoperative medications to prevent nausea and reduce anxiety are usually given:

   A. 15 minutes to 30 minutes prior to surgery.

   B. 1 to 2 hours prior to surgery.

   C. immediately prior to incision.

   D. immediately prior to induction.

_____ 20 Nail polish should be removed due to the use of

   A. noninvasive blood pressure monitor.

   B. invasive ABG.

   C. noninvasive pulse oximeter.

   D. nonivasive EKG monitor.

_____ 21. Identify which possessions the patient may take with him/her to the OR.

    A. Dentures

    B. Hearing aid

    C. Wigs

    D. Jewelry

    E. Both A and B.

_____ 22. What is ordered to prevent postoperative thromboembolism (resulting from the venous pooling in the lower legs)?

    A. Esmarch bandage

    B. Knee rest stirrups

    C. Sequential compression devices

    D. Pillow under knees for elevation

Identify the appropriate area of the surgical unit that requires or allows the attire described. (Note: More than one designation may be appropriate.)

N = Not recommended, U = Unrestricted, S = Semirestricted, and R = Restricted

_____ 23. Artificial nails during surgical procedures

_____ 24. OR attire, designated OR shoes, mask with eyewear

_____ 25. Dangling earrings or necklaces

_____ 26. Beard covered by mask and skull cap with eyewear

_____ 27. Street clothes can be worn

_____ 28. Shoes previously worn to work in the garden

_____ 29. OR attire, hat covering donned prior to scrubs ensure ALL hair is covered

_____ 30. Locker room designation of surgical unit and delivery areas

_____ 31. Scrubs worn in from home not covered by lab coat

_____ 32. Warm up jacket when circulating

_____ 33. Hallway when transporting patients into the OR for surgery

_____ 34. OR attire, shoe covers, mask, no eyewear during invasive surgery

_____ 35. Operating room designation during an invasive surgical procedure

_____ 36. Scrubs wet or soiled covered with impervious cover-ups prior to case

Fill in the Blank

Fill in the blank regarding staff and patients:

37. The major source of contamination in the OR is the _____ of patients and staff.

38. Surgeon skullcap–type hats are worn only if _____.

39. If personnel wear reusable head covers; they must be _____ daily and made of

_____.

40. Individuals with beards should wear _____.

41. Shoe covers are worn for _____ and must be changed when they become _____ or removed when _____.

Masks

42. Analyze the statement "the mask is worn either on or off." Discuss the rationale for the statement.

_____

_____

43. Describe a correct mask fit. _____

_____

44. Which mask is worn for a patient with tuberculosis? _____

_____

45. When are masks changed? _____

_____

Eyewear

46. Describe your options for protective eyewear. _____

_____

47. How can personal glasses be modified for wear during surgery? ____

_____

48. Why do you wear eyewear?_____

_____

49. Identify five ways to protect yourself from radiation. _____

_____

_____

_____

50. Double-gloving recommendation. Describe how to double glove. ____

_____

51. Why is it better to double glove than single glove?_____

_____

Preoperative OR Setup in the Room

1. When arranging furniture for the case, you must position your back table and Mayo(s) for the sterile field setup. Describe the basic concepts utilized when positioning the sterile field for setup.

_____

_____

_____

2. The doors to the OR should be kept open until you get ready to open sterile supplies, then they should be closed to prevent air currents and flies or flying insects from entering the room. Is this a true or false statement? Why?

_____

_____

_____

3. What equipment is routinely checked prior to the case to be sure it is functional?

_____

_____

_____

4. Diagram an example of the OR setup. Include any required furniture. Note the doorways entering the room and place your backtable appropriately.

Preference Card

Refer to the preference card in Chapter 12 of your textbook (Figure 12-7) to answer the following questions:

5. What items will be available in the room, but not necessarily opened or used during the initial setup of the case?

_____

6. What antibiotic will be used?

_____

7. When the circulator returns with the patient, you note that the patient is approximately 300 lbs. Which item will be opened due to this information?

_____

_____

8. The initial incision has been made; the surgeon asks for suction, which suction will you pass to the surgeon?

_____

9. Once the appendix has been grasped with a Babcock, you note material seeping from a hole in the side of the appendix. You can now anticipate what the surgeon will need to close the skin. What will you ask for?

_____

Opening Sterile Supplies

10. Prioritize the order in which the following items are opened. (Note: One or more items may be opened later by the circulator.)

_____ A. peel packed items

_____ B. back table pack

_____ C. scrub's gown and glove

_____ D. basin set and instruments

_____ E. peel packed long tubing with dangling ends

Matching—Scrub, Gown, and Glove Technique

Match the completion statement with the appropriate answer.

____ 11. STSR dons gown and gloves

____ 12. Clean under nails

____ 13. Specific time or count for scrub technique

____ 14. Assisted gowning/gloving technique

____ 15. Counted scrub technique

____ 16. To rescrub an area contaminated

____ 17. Circulator secures the gown

____ 18. When turning (to tie up front tie)

____ 19. Manufacturer's instructions

____ 20. Scrub technique progresses from

____ 21. Hand level when scrubbed

____ 22. Pinch in the middle to

____ 23. STSR dons gloves using

____ 24. When scrubbing or rinsing keep

A. Utilize 10 strokes to area

B. Closed glove technique

C. Pick up sterile towel, careful not to drip

D. Face the sterile field as you pass the tag or step away from the sterile field at least 12 or more inches

E. Hands above waist, below shoulders or in sight

F. With running water

G. Specified by facility policy

H. Fingertips up, hands above bent elbows

I. Uses 30 strokes for nails; 20 for other areas

J. Fingertips to 2 inches above elbow

K. Utilized for other teams members by STSR

L. At the neck edge and back tie

M. From a separate setup

N. Determines length of time/application technique for a specific antiseptic used

Preparation of the Sterile Field

25. Each item should have minimal handling, to facilitate the principle of moving an item once into place; the scrub must have a basic plan or a mental image of what the table and Mayo should look like when finished. Using your classroom image or the "setup" drawing provided to you by your instructor, diagram the basic Mayo, back table, and basin setup for a basic procedure.

Mayo Stand   Basin Setup

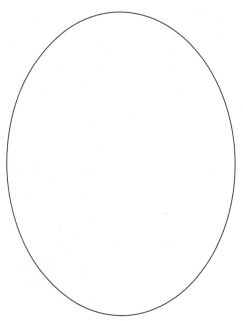

Back Table

Counts:

1. Prioritize the sequence of counts correctly.

    _____ A. Dressing sponges accounted for

    _____ B. Sponges (Kitners, Raytec, laps, etc.)

    _____ C. Instruments (tray 1, tray 2, etc., extra parts counted, then added items)

    _____ D. Sharps—suture, blades, hypodermics, ESU tip

2. Prioritize the order of counts to be completed. In what order are the counts required in the following scenario?

    _____ A. Closure of skin initiated

    _____ B. Closure of hollow organ (example: uterus)

    _____ C. The scrub nurse is relieved just after the initial incision.

    _____ D. When all items required on preference card are added to field.

    _____ E. Additional items added during delivery of the placenta (procedure) prior to any closing counts

    _____ F. Closure of cavity (example: abdominal)

3. Identify the flow of the closing counts from first to last.

   _____ A. Items on Mayo stand

   _____ B. Surgeon notified something missing

   _____ C. Items in use at sterile field

   _____ D. Kick bucket

   _____ E. Room search including trash

   _____ F. Back table

   _____ G. Recount starting at sterile field

   _____ H. X-ray taken

4. Identify how items are to be counted (method of counting).

   _____ A. Verify that circulator can see item

   _____ B. Circulator records the number on count sheet or board

   _____ C. Verbalize the numbers as you count them

   _____ D. State the name of the item to be counted

   _____ E. Circulator repeats the count

   _____ F. Separate items completely as they are counted for visualization

   _____ G. Repeat the total at the end of the count

   _____ H. Break the tag/band or remove stringer keeping the items together

5. Identify how items are placed on the Mayo stand:

   _____ A. Prepare a towel roll/instrument stand

   _____ B. Inspect instrument(s) as chosen—cleanliness, damage, and function

   _____ C. Mentally review the steps of the procedure and identify instruments likely to be used

   _____ D. Prepare a mental picture of final Mayo setup

   _____ E. Close items on first ratchet and place on towel roll in even numbers

   _____ F. Place sharps/load suture/load scalpel with care. Place sponges.

6. During what situation can counts be omitted? _____

Preoperative Holding: Transportation

7. When transporting a patient on a stretcher, the patient should be transported how?

   _____.

8. Describe how the patient is moved to the OR table. What is the minimum number of personnel for each situation? _____

   A. Awake mobile patient: _____

   B. Unconscious or immobile patient: _____

9. While the patient is in preoperative holding, the circulator will assess the patient; identify what relevant information is gathered to determine the patient's care during the procedure.

_____

_____

Patient Monitoring: Vital Signs

Temperature

1. Identify and define four mechanisms of heat loss:

   A. _____

   B. _____

   C. _____

   D. _____

2. Describe four benefits of maintaining a normal core temperature.

   A. _____

   B. _____

   C. _____

   D. _____

3. Analyze the effects of hypothermia. Describe at least five consequences of hypothermia.

   A. _____

   B. _____

   C. _____

   D. _____

   E. _____

4. Describe at least four methods of maintaining a normal core temperature.

   A. _____

   B. _____

   C. _____

   D. _____

5. Identify at least two conditions that can cause a rise in temperature.

   A. _____

   B. _____

6. Identify the temperature control area of the brain.

   _____

7. Analyze the normal temperatures:

   A. Identify the normal oral temperature for the two most common measurement scales.

   _____

   B. Identify the alternate methods or routes of taking the temperature.

   _____

   C. Compare the oral route temperature with the axillary and rectal routes. What is the difference?

   _____

Pulse:

8. Analyze the pulse descriptions in the following table.

Pulse Rate and Description	Age and Description	Identify the Pulse Rate Pattern; Normal or Abnormal	Possible Cause(s) or N/A
60 regular thready	2 years old, confused		
80 regular full	66 years old, sleeping		
110 regular bounding	45 years old, preop rate		
56 regular full	24-year-old triathlon contestant		
42 irregular thready	76-year-old complaining of chest pain		

9. Identify eight pulse points.

_____

_____

10. Define the following:

A. Dysrhythmia

_____

_____

B. PVC

_____

_____

Respirations

11. Identify the respiratory control area of the brain.

_____

12. The trigger for increasing respirations is the level of _____.

13. Analyze the respiratory descriptions in the following table:

Respiratory Rate and/or Description	Age and Description	Identify the Respiratory Pattern; Normal or Abnormal	Possible Cause(s) or N/A
No respirations	56-year-old man with chest pain		
32 respirations, regular and shallow	76-year-old man with COPD		
Unable to determine rate—fast, deep respirations; with periods of apnea	45-year-old, preop rate		
32 respirations no audible sounds and irregular and deep	2-month-old sleeping		

Respiratory Rate and/or Description	Age and Description	Identify the Respiratory Pattern; Normal or Abnormal	Possible Cause(s) or N/A
112 pulse; 28 deep regular respirations	7-year-old watching TV		
10 respirations slow and even	42-year-old man, home, sleeping		
8 respirations shallow and irregular	32-year-old female, on morphine sulfate		

14. Define the following.

   A. Eupnea _____

   _____

   B. Obstructive apnea _____

   _____

Blood Pressure

15. Define the following terms:

   A. Systolic _____

   _____

   B. Diastolic _____

   _____

16. Analyze the blood pressures described in the following table:

Blood Pressure (mm Hg)	Age and Description	Identify the Classification; Normal or Abnormal.
110/60	45-year-old, sleeping	
145/95	55-year-old, at 8:00 am in Wal-Mart for the fourth morning in a row.	
165/105	25-year-old with renal failure	
110/72	8-year-old, preop, vocalizes some fear	
50/25	2-month-old for inguinal hernia repair	

Urinary Catheterization

17. One of the most common HAI (hospital acquired infections, or nosocomial infections) results from urinary catheterization. Describe how to prevent contamination and retrograde flow of urine.

   _____

   _____

   _____

Analyze the procedural steps of urinary catheterization:

18. Why do you pretest the balloon?

_____

_____

19. Why is water used to inflate the balloon?

_____

_____

20. Why do you use 10 cc of water in a 5-cc capacity balloon?

_____

_____

21. Why is it important to secure the tubing and locate/control the drainage bag during transfer of the patient to the recovery stretcher?

_____

_____

_____

Positioning

1 Describe the goal of positioning.

_____

_____

_____

2. Identify the three basic positions.

_____

_____

_____

3. Identify the alternate name of the supine position.

_____

_____

4. Describe the anatomical position of supine position. Is the palm up or down if on arm boards? (Note: Use your description of supine position and definition in the back of the text to answer this question.)

_____

5. Analyze the Trendelenburg position. Describe the purpose(s) of this position.

_____

_____

6. Analyze the reverse Trendelenburg position. Describe the purpose(s) of this position.

_____

_____

7. Analyze the Fowler's position. Describe the purpose(s) of this position.

   _____

   _____

8. Analyze the lithotomy position and describe the purpose(s) of the position.

   _____

   _____

9. Describe what is needed to put the patient into the lithotomy position.

   _____

10. Describe how the table is set up for lithotomy prior to the patient entering the room.

    _____

11. Describe the position of the patient for lithotomy on the table. Where are the hips located?

    _____

12. How many people does it take to put the legs in stirrups? Describe how the legs are placed in stirrups.

    _____

    _____

13. Describe the uses of prone position.

    _____

    _____

    _____

14. Describe how the patient's arms are moved onto the arm boards.

    _____

    _____

    _____

15. Identify the alternate name for Kraske.

    _____

16. Describe how the prone position is modified for Kraske.

    _____

    _____

    _____

17. Describe the purpose(s) of the Kraske position.

    _____

    _____

    _____

18. Describe the uses of lateral position.

    _____

    _____

    _____

    _____

19. Identify the alternate name(s) for lateral position.

_____

_____

20. If the patient is having a right thoracotomy what position is he/she placed in?

_____

_____

21. What is the purpose of the axillary roll?

_____

_____

_____

22. Which leg is flexed to stabilize the patient on the OR table?

_____

23. Describe each variation of lateral, any positioning tools, and the use of each position.

_____

   A. Sims: _____

_____

   B. Kidney: _____

_____

24. When positioning the patient, considerations must be made to prevent complications. Describe what can be done to prevent shearing.

_____

_____

_____

25. Describe what can be done to prevent venous stasis with resultant possible thrombus formation and pulmonary embolus.

_____

_____

_____

26. When the patient is in the Fowler's position, there is a potential complication unique due to the sitting position. Identify the complication.

_____

_____

27. Pressure is a second consideration when positioning a patient. What areas have to be monitored for pressure?

_____

_____

_____

28. What can be done to prevent pressure injuries?

_____

_____

29. During supine positioning of the patient, care is made to check the patient after the patient is anesthetized. What areas must be assessed?

_____

_____

_____

30. During positioning of the patient prone or placement of the upper extremities in variations of supine, care is given to prevent pressure on the chest. Describe what possible problems can occur with pressure on this area.

_____

_____

_____

31. Who controls the timing when moving the patient?

_____

_____

_____

32. Why is it important for this person to direct the movement of the patient?

_____

_____

_____

33. Describe the potential hazard if the patient is not kept in anatomical alignment during movement (head and spine straight with control of all limbs).

_____

_____

_____

34. All movement of the patient is completed slowly including leveling of the operating room table and lifting of lower extremities. Describe what complications can occur with rapid movement.

_____

_____

_____

35. Describe what complications can occur due to contact with metallic parts of the table.

_____

_____

_____

36. Describe how to prevent a brachial plexus injury. In which position(s) is this likely to occur?

_____

_____

_____

37. Describe how to prevent an ulnar nerve injury. In which position(s) is this likely to occur?

_____

_____

_____

38. Describe how to prevent a peroneal nerve injury. In which position(s) is this likely to occur?

_____

_____

_____

39. Describe how to prevent a sciatic nerve injury. In which position(s) is this likely to occur?

_____

_____

_____

40. Describe how to prevent foot drop. In which position(s) is this likely to occur?

_____

_____

_____

41. Describe how to prevent back, knee, and hip pain from muscle strain or back injury that may occur with the lithotomy position.

_____

_____

_____

42. Describe how to prevent crushing injuries of the extremities when there is movement of the operating table such as dropping the foot section or flexing of the table for positions such as the lithotomy or the Kraske.

_____

_____

_____

43. Analyze what can be done to prevent patient falls during the surgical procedure. Describe what mechanisms can be used to prevent the patient from falling when recovering from anesthesia, sliding off the table during table rotations, or modifications such as Trendelenburg/reverse Trendelenburg.

_____

_____

_____

_____

_____

44. Describe the important checkpoints regarding the application of the safety strap.

_____

_____

Skin Prep:

45. Contaminated areas requiring surgical preparation are prepped last or as separate skin prep. Analyze the abdominal preparation for a routine exploratory laparotomy and identify which areas are prepped separately or last.

_____

46. Where does the preparation begin and how does it extend?

_____

47. Why is there great care in the prevention of pooling of the antiseptics under the patient?

_____

48. When applying an antiseptic, the most important principle to employ includes:

    A. following the manufacturer's recommendation for application

    B. using enough friction to remove all tape or skin oils

    C. removing all hair to prevent contamination

    D. always prepping any stoma first using a separate prep

Draping

1. When assisting the team member to gown and glove, present the first glove:

    A. Hooked onto surgeons other hand with fingers toward the surgeon—spread the hole.

    B. Cuffed over your spread fingers to protect your hand with a circular opening for the surgeon's hand to enter; be sure the thumb of the glove is toward the surgeon.

    C. For the left hand with thumb side toward surgeon; be sure there is a circular opening for surgeon

    D. Cuffed over your fingers—release once surgeon grasps the glove with his/her hand and pulls it on

2. Describe how to prepare the draping materials for a routine exploratory laparotomy.

    _____

    _____

    _____

3. Sometimes, the STSR will begin draping and must know how to place the "squaring off" towels. Describe how the towels are placed around the site.

    A. First towel _____

    B. Second towel _____

    C. Third towel _____

    D. Fourth towel _____

    Towels may be then be secured with towel clips, isolation/self adhering drapes, sutured in place, or stapled in place. Note if any item perforates the towel such as a suture/needle holder and/or towel clip is removed, it is passed off to the circulator as a contaminated item.

4. Circle the INCORRECT statement. When passing the main drape:

    A. Orient the drape, making sure head/foot segments are right

    B. Offer drape to surgeon with hands on top and fenestration over surgical site

    C. Open drape, keeping hands on top (in sight)

    D. Extend foot observing and stabilizing sheet to prevent shifting of sheet (do not pull against surgeon)

    E. Cuff drapes as you extend

    F. Drop end if anesthesia is too slow in taking your end so you can set up ESU and suction

Matching

Match the correct solution to the problem:

____ 5. Hole noted in sterile drape while opening drape

____ 6. Drape is upside down—feet and arm boards are exposed

____ 7. While anesthesia is taking drape—STSR's right glove is touched

____ 8. Small foreign body/hair noted on drape

____ 9. Allis clamp repositioned securing suction

____ 10. Nonperforating clamp used to secure suction

____ 11. Opening of legging misses foot and touches stirrup

____ 12. Draping of extremity is completed while double gloved

____ 13. Hole in glove from ESU pencil as you handle it

____ 14. Surgeon's sleeve touches IV pole

A. Replace drape, it is contaminated

B. Ask for half sheets to cover exposed areas

C. Cover hole with impermeable towel/drape

D. Ask for sterile sleeve cover or assist to regown/reglove

E. Pass off item, have circulator remove glove, reglove

F. Recommended removal of outer gloves and reglove

G. Not a problem—situation sterile

H. Pass off perforating clamp and cover with impermeable drape; nonperforating clamp is recommended

I. Remove with hemostat, pass hemostat to circulator, cover area

J. Remove contaminated outer right glove and reglove

15. Additional items that may be used to drape an extremity include:

_____

_____

_____

Pulling Up (Arranging the Sterile Field)

16. Describe the strategic considerations for positioning of the Mayo stand for the surgical procedure?

_____

_____

17. Describe how the STSR maneuvers the back table into place.

_____

_____

_____

18. Strategic placement of the back table allows the STSR to

_____

_____

19. In observing the area of the operative site to verify it is ready to begin the procedure, what items should be immediately available to the surgeon? (Note: Some items must be checked to be sure they are functional prior to the incision being made.)

_____

_____

_____

_____

_____

20. Once the STSR is pulled up into place and all team members have assumed their places at the field, the team will pause for a "time out" to prevent wrong-site surgery. Describe what is verified at this time.

_____

_____

_____

Surgical Procedure—Intraoperative Phase

1. Describe why it is important for the STSR to understand anatomy, normal variations, pathological or problematic variations, the normal steps of the procedure, and instrumentation for the procedure.

_____

_____

_____

_____

_____

Matching

Match the safe practice with the potential hazard.

_____ 2. Neutral zone

_____ 3. Double glove

_____ 4. Goggles/eyewear

_____ 5. Passing without touching surgeon

_____ 6. Lead apron; thyroid shield

_____ 7. Fiberoptic placement when on

_____ 8. Laser goggles

_____ 9. Labeling of medications and solutions

_____ 10. Counting

_____ 11. Gown glove separate setup

_____ 12. Separation of clean and dirty

_____ 13. ESU active electrode in holder

A. Foreign body retention

B. Accidental patient burn due to activation

C. Primary glove deterioration and possible contamination

D. Nonionizing radiation fire when activated on drapes

E. Retinal or corneal damage

F. Medication error prevention

G. Prevents distraction of surgeon from procedure

H. Radiation hazard exposure

I. Main instrument table contamination

J. Eye splash with blood or body fluids

K. Prevention of sharps injury

L. Prevention technique for bowel or cancer tissue

Passing Techniques:

14. Identify the hand signals in Figure 12-1.

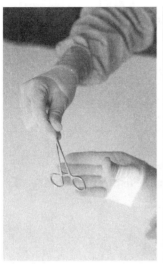 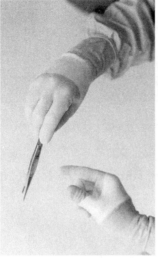 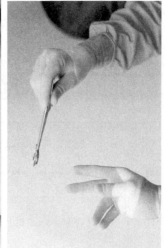 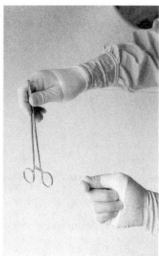

Figure 12-1

A. _____

B. _____

C. _____

D. _____

Matching

Analyze the passing techniques described in the textbook, and match the passing technique with the situation.

Item to be passed:	**Technique for passing**
_____ 15. RayTec/lap sponges	A. Moist laps or sponges used for packing inside patient
_____ 16. General rule for passing all items	B. Aligned with the curve of the surgeon's hand/fingers
_____ 17. Scalpel passed in neutral zone	C. Pencil style; be sure to remove hand ftom danger area up and way from blade
_____ 18. As passed to surgeon, counted	D. Draped behind hand to prevent surgeon grasping strand
_____ 19. Curved instruments	E. Do not obstruct surgeon's view of operative site
_____ 20. Laparoscopic/endoscopic instruments	F. Held by box lock; passed into palm to elicit grasp reflex
_____ 21. Suture passing, control of strand	G. Either surgeon or STSR hand is in the area; not both
_____ 22. Ringed instruments	H. Pass unfolded or lay open on field for surgeon use
_____ 23. Needle holder	I. Guide tip into port after passage of handle
_____ 24. Scalpel passed to surgeon's hand	J. Pass; needle tip up and same side as surgeon's thumb

Short Answer

Maintaining order, counts, and safety is essential; describe what the STSR responsibilities are for each of the following items.

25. ESU—active electrode: _____

26. Used sharps (include what is done for a full needle pad/box):

_____

27. Used sponges: _____

28. Medications/syringes: _____

29. Instruments: _____

Sequence of Surgery—Place the following segments of surgery in the correct order using numbers 1-10.

_____ 30. Closing sequence—Wound closure (suture and tissue forceps)

_____ 31. Opening sequence—Hemostasis (ESU handpiece or hemostats)

_____ 32. Closing sequence—Application of dressing

_____ 33. Opening sequence—Exposure (hand retractor to self-retaining retractor)

_____ 34. Closing sequence—Wound cleansing

_____ 35. Closing sequence—Counts (as each layer is closed)

_____ 36. Opening sequence—Pass skin knife

_____ 37. Closing sequence—Inspection of wound/hemostasis/irrigation

_____ 38. Procedure is performed—(What we came to do)

_____ 39. Opening Sequence—Dissection (scissors and tissue forceps)

Surgical Case Management—Postoperative Phase

After application of the sterile dressing:

1. Describe the rationale for preserving the sterile field after surgery, especially for such frequent bleeders such as a tonsillectomy and adenoidectomy (T&A) and carotid endarterectomy. In these cases, the scrub may not assist with drape removal in order to preserve the sterile field.

_____

_____

_____

_____

2. Describe how to remove the drape after the case.

_____

_____

_____

_____

3. Describe the sequence for removing your gown and gloves at the end of the procedure.

_____

_____

_____

_____

4. Breakdown of setup. Place the following events in the most likely sequence using numbers 1-13.

_____ A. Verify next case/arrange room and pull case into room

_____ B. Handwashing

_____ C. Instruments placed in water or water with enzyme

_____ D. Patient transported out

_____ E. Room setup with clean linen/suction for next case

_____ F. PPE Donned as needed

_____ G. Transport to decontamination

_____ H. Sharps disposed of/separated from other instruments

_____ I. All dirty items (suction, linen) broken down and furniture replaced

_____ J. Specimen cared for—passed off if not already completed.

_____ K. Turnover room cleaning—top to bottom; clean to dirty

_____ L. PPE removed

_____ M. Open sterile supplies for next case

Case Studies

CASE STUDY 1

Sean is a student STSR for a laparoscopic assisted vaginal hysterectomy (LAVH). As he reaches for a supply item being handed by the circulator, his left glove touches the outside of the packet.

1. Does Sean have a problem? What is it?

_____

_____

_____

_____

2. What steps need to be taken to correct the problem?

_____

_____

_____

_____

3. Describe the procedure(s) for changing a contaminated glove.

_____

_____

_____

_____

CASE STUDY 2

It is LuAnn's big day. She is scrubbing her first case as a student. She wants desperately to do everything right.

1. What type of surgical scrub should LuAnn perform? Why?

   _____

   _____

   _____

   _____

2. Describe the counted brush stroke method for a surgical scrub.

   _____

   _____

   _____

   _____

3. Identify the antiseptics available for use. When scrubbing, you should follow the manufacturer's directions for use; describe how to use the different antiseptics available at your local facilities. Which one will you choose to use and why?

   _____

   _____

   _____

   _____

4. Which method of self-gloving will LuAnn use after she has donned her sterile gown? Why?

   _____

   _____

   _____

   _____

Lab 12: Surgical Case Management

Introduction

The surgical technologist is responsible for many duties associated with the perioperative phases of surgery. This includes the nuts and bolts of what we do for our job to help the team along. This is the portion where students will get to do all the things we do to get ready for a case. Practice these pieces frequently; also make sure to introduce these pieces early. You can even start with the basics of handwashing the first week and work forward from there.

Game 1: What Is Sterile and What Is Not?

Time involved: One week for setup

Supplies: Paper and pencils

Instructors: Set up a sterile field. Have the students differentiate between the different areas of the operating room. Identify those that are considered sterile and nonsterile. Include the people that will be working within those areas, the equipment, the instruments, and the surrounding pieces of furniture. State the item. Instruct students to indicate on paper the name of the item and if it is sterile or nonsterile. Ask students to observe your movements and to let you know if there is a "break" in the sterile technique. You can show the students how easy it is to contaminate an area just by walking or by turning your back on the field. This can be a learning activity, pop quiz, or game.

Students: Make two lists. On one list you should place sterile areas and supplies and people. On the other list, place nonsterile pieces.

Game 2: Name that OR Attire

Time involved: One week for setup

Supplies: Paper and pencils, pieces of OR attire worn in and around surgery

Instructors: Set about the pieces of OR attire. Name for the students what is worn, when it is worn, how it is worn, and why it is worn. Then let the students name these pieces.

Students: Make a list of a surgical attire, then categorize it by who wears it, and when, how, and why it is worn.

Practical

A. Don OR attire

B. Open sterile supplies—back table pack

C. Open sterile supplies—small wrapped package onto sterile and nonsterile surfaces

D. Open sterile supplies—peel pack

E. Open sterile supplies—instrument set container system

F. Open sterile supplies—pour solution

G. Surgical scrub

H. Dry

I. Gown—self

J. Gown—other

K. Open glove—self

L. Closed glove—self

M. Glove—other

N. Disrobe to replace contaminated OR attire

O. Disrobe end of case

P. Cover Mayo stand

Q. Fill bulb syringe

R. Remove instrument set from container system

S. Back table setup

T. Mayo stand setup

U. Basic positioning

V.   Basic prepping

W.   Basic draping

X.   Instrument handling—load, pass, and unload a scalpel handle

Y.   Instrument handling—passing various instruments

Z.   Tear down

AA. Vital signs—temperature

BB. Vital signs—pulse

CC. Vital signs—respirations

DD. Vital signs—blood pressure

EE. Urinary catheterization—male

FF. Urinary catheterization—female

GG. Skin preps

Skill Assessment 12-1

Student Name	
SKILL	**OR Attire; Including Donning of Sterile Glove and Gown**
Instructions	Instructor will demonstrate skill. Practice skill set with your partner. When ready, notify instructor to schedule check-off. Skills assessment must be completed satisfactorily by _____ (due date).
Supplies	• External case or wrapping material—one double thickness wrap or two wrappers of appropriate material (if no tray top to secure items, three wrappers for inner wrap) • Internal chemical indicator • Outer chemical indicator (sterilization tape or label for case) • Internal protection such as towels, peel packs, or protective tips • Basic instrument count sheet • Tray • Instruments • Inspection supplies to test scissors, gauze • Cleaning supplies/water soluble lubricant prn

Note: Student must perform skill independently without prompting.

Practice with Partner Date: | **Skills Testing Date:**

PROCEDURAL STEPS			COMMENTS
1. Assembles equipment and supplies.	Correct	Needs Review	
2. Identifies traffic patterns in the OR including when the designations of Unrestricted; Semi-restricted and Restricted areas are used.	Correct	Needs Review	
3. Demonstrates appropriate attire for semi-restricted areas.	Correct	Needs Review	
4. Demonstrates appropriate attire for restricted areas including any appropriate PPE for the STSR or circulator roles.	Correct	Needs Review	
5. Organizes workspace for most effective ergonomics. Positions sterile setup correctly.	Correct	Needs Review	
6. Opens sterile gown/glove setup correctly.	Correct	Needs Review	
7. Demonstrates appropriate scrub technique. Utilizes antiseptic chosen appropriately.	Correct	Needs Review	
8. Demonstrates drying technique correctly.	Correct	Needs Review	
9. Demonstrates donning of sterile gown correctly.	Correct	Needs Review	
10. Demonstrate closed glove technique correctly.	Correct	Needs Review	
11. Demonstrates "turning" to tie up correctly.	Correct	Needs Review	
12. Maintains sterile technique; identifies and corrects any deviations correctly	Correct	Needs Review	
13. Identifies and maintains hands within sterile perimeters of gown correctly.	Correct	Needs Review	

Skill Assessment 12-1 (*continued*)

		Rating
Performance Evaluation Criteria	• Assembled all necessary supplies and equipment for skill testing. Arranges furniture for limited traffic.	
	• Discussed correctly traffic patterns (clean/dirty), designated areas of the OR including unrestricted (street clothes in locker rooms; delivery areas, etc), Semi-restricted (don hat first, covers all hair, scrubs, shoe covers or designated shoes) & restricted (adds mask, eyewear, jacket for circulator – to cover arms) areas. Discusses additional PPE use such as radiation monitoring devices, lead aprons, & shields/special footwear.	
	• Demonstrated correct opening of sterile gown/glove setup. Height appropriate for student. Positions gown packet so leading edge covered. Opens first fold away from self, sides, then last toward self. Controls ends. Flips gloves onto field without breaking technique. (unsterile hand does not cross over sterile field).	
	• Demonstrated correct surgical scrub technique. Prewash, Subungual areas using nail cleaner & running water, fingertips up, hands higher than elbows, elbows bent, body posture to prevent wet scrubs and contamination; identifies technique used correctly as counted (30 nails/20 all other), timed or application according to manufacturer's recommendation for antiseptic chosen.	
	• Demonstrated correct donning of sterile gown.	
	• Student prepared and performed procedure independently. Correctly maintained sterile technique. Identified any breaks in technique and corrected them appropriately. (If contaminated during scrubbing rescrubs area 10 strokes or as required by type of antiseptic/technique chosen.)	
	• Performed each step in appropriate sequence.	
	Overall Rating (Satisfactory; Must Redo; Fail):	
Instructor Comments		

Student Signature	*Date*
Instructor Signature	*Date*

Skill Assessment 12-1A

Student Name	
SKILL	**Scrubbing: Counted Method**
Instructions	Instructor will demonstrate skill. Practice skill set with your partner. When ready, notify instructor to schedule the check-off. Skills assessment must be completed satisfactorily by _____ (due date).
Supplies	• Scrub brush with nail pick and antiseptic • Scrubs, mask, eyewear

Note: Student must perform skill independently without prompting.

Practice with Partner Date:		**Skills Testing Date:**	
PROCEDURAL STEPS			**COMMENTS**
1. Assembles equipment and supplies. Prepares correctly.	Correct	Needs Review	
2. Demonstrates appropriate attire for restricted areas including any appropriate PPE for the STSR or circulator roles.	Correct	Needs Review	
3. Student is able to define surgical scrub.	Correct	Needs Review	
4. Student is able to state purpose for performing surgical scrub.	Correct	Needs Review	
5. Organizes workspace for most effective ergonomics. Positions sterile setup correctly.	Correct	Needs Review	
6. Inspects integrity of hands and arms.	Correct	Needs Review	
7. Opens brush package.	Correct	Needs Review	
8. Turns on water and adjusts temperature.	Correct	Needs Review	
9. Demonstrates routine hand washing. Wets hands and arms; applies soap; lathers.	Correct	Needs Review	
10. Cleans nails under running water using nail pick.	Correct	Needs Review	
11. Discards nail pick in garbage can and rinses.	Correct	Needs Review	
12. Secures and prepares brush (soap application and H20).	Correct	Needs Review	
13. Scrubs nails with 30 strokes.	Correct	Needs Review	
14. Scrubs all other areas and between webs of fingers using 20 strokes progressing from fingers to 2" above elbows. (If contaminates during the process of the scrub rescrubs area with 10 strokes.)	Correct	Needs Review	
15. Discards brush in garbage can and rinses without contamination.	Correct	Needs Review	
16. Proceeds to OR.	Correct	Needs Review	

Skill Assessment 12-1A (*continued*)

		RATING
Performance Evaluation Criteria	• Assembled all necessary supplies and equipment for skill testing. Arranges furniture for limited traffic.	
	• Defines the surgical scrub as the procedure taken to become a sterile team member within the established sterile field during an invasive surgical procedure. Discussed the purpose of the scrub correctly: To eliminate transient microbes and debris on the skin and reduce resident flora found on the hands and arms. This process does not render the hands sterile.	
	• Demonstrated correct opening of sterile gown/glove setup. Height appropriate for student. Positions gown packet so leading edge covered. Opens first fold away from self, sides, then last toward self. Controls ends. Flips gloves onto field without breaking technique (unsterile hand does not cross over sterile field).	
	• Demonstrated correct surgical scrub technique. Prewash, subungual areas using nail cleaner and running water, fingertips up, hands higher than elbows, elbows bent, body posture to prevent wet scrubs and contamination; identifies technique used correctly as counted (30 nails/20 all other), timed or application according to manufacturer's recommendation for antiseptic chosen.	
	• Demonstrated correct donning of sterile gown.	
	• Student prepared and performed procedure independently. Correctly maintained sterile technique. Identified any breaks in technique and corrected them appropriately. (If contaminates during scrubbing rescrubs area 10 strokes or as required by type of antiseptic/technique chosen.)	
	• Performed each step in appropriate sequence.	
	Overall Rating (Satisfactory; Must Redo; Fail):	
Instructor Comments		

Student Signature		***Date***
Instructor Signature		***Date***

Skill Assessment 12-1B

Student Name	
SKILL	**Donning Gown per Self (Self Gown)**
Instructions	Instructor will demonstrate skill. Practice skill set with your partner. When ready, notify instructor to schedule the check-off. Skills assessment must be completed satisfactorily by _____ (due date).
Supplies	• Gown pack (gown with towel wrapped envelop style) • Sterile gloves (appropriate size for student) • Scrub brush with nail pick and antiseptic or antiseptic and nail pick • Scrubs • Mask • Eyewear

Note: Student must perform skill independently without prompting.

Practice with Partner Date:		Skills Testing Date:	

PROCEDURAL STEPS			COMMENTS
1. Enter OR after surgical scrub with hands higher than elbows; away from the face and above the waist.	Correct	Needs Review	
2. Front of scrubs or sleeves are not wet (states if wet could cause strike-through).	Correct	Needs Review	
3. Secures towel: pinches in middle, does not drip onto sterile field.	Correct	Needs Review	
4. Opens towel and positions for drying.	Correct	Needs Review	
5. Bends at waist and dries first hand and arm without contaminating end of towel on front of scrubs.	Correct	Needs Review	
6. Transfer towel to opposite hand.	Correct	Needs Review	
7. Bends at waist and dries second hand and arm without contaminating end of towel on front of scrubs.	Correct	Needs Review	
8. Discards towel from appropriate height (keeps hands above the waist, drops into garbage can).	Correct	Needs Review	
9. Pinches gown in middle, away from neck edge. Picks up gown and steps back.	Correct	Needs Review	
10. Unfolds gown, being careful not to contaminate.	Correct	Needs Review	
11. Dons gown. Inserts arms in such a manner that hands remain in sight at all times, above the waist and away from the face. Hands do not protrude from end of cuffed edge. Circulator may assist by pulling gown up onto shoulders and securing neck edge and tying waist ties.	Correct	Needs Review	

Skill Assessment 12-1B (*continued*)

	12. Bends forward (observes front of gown to ensure it does not contaminate on leading edge of setup). Secures first glove and places upside down on gowned forearm/wrist (thumb to thumb).	Correct	Needs Review	
	13. Pulls on glove being careful to cover stocking cuff.	Correct	Needs Review	
	14. Secures and dons second glove. Adjusts gloves to cover stocking edge.	Correct	Needs Review	
	15. Grasps turnaround tie and passes "tabbed" string to circulator. Turns to left and grasps the tie only pulls tie free from tab and then proceeds to tie up.	Correct	Needs Review	
	16. Removes glove powder prn and proceeds with case setup.	Correct	Needs Review	
	17. Prepared gown/glove setup correctly. As first person to prepare field, did not don from the main instrument back table; used separate setup. Stated rationale correctly.	Correct	Needs Review	

		RATING
Performance Evaluation Criteria	• Assembled all necessary supplies and equipment for skill testing. Arranges furniture for limited traffic.	
	• Demonstrated correct opening of sterile gown/glove setup. Height appropriate for student. Positions gown packet so leading edge covered. Opens first fold away from self, sides, then last toward self. Controls ends. Flips gloves onto field without breaking technique (unsterile hand does not cross over sterile field).	
	• Demonstrated correct donning of sterile gown.	
	• Student prepared and performed procedure independently. Correctly maintained sterile technique. Identified any breaks in technique and corrected them appropriately.	
	• Stated rationale for gown/glove procedure for sterile personnel. First person dons gown/glove from separate setup other than main instrument table since an unsterile hand cannot reach over a sterile area. Subsequent persons are gowned and gloved by the assisted glove technique or don gown/glove from a separate setup.	
	• Performed each step in appropriate sequence.	
	Overall Rating (Satisfactory; Must Redo; Fail):	

Instructor Comments	
Student Signature	**Date**
Instructor Signature	**Date**

Skill Assessment 12-1C

Student Name	
SKILL	**Removal of Gown per Self (During Case)**
Instructions	Instructor will demonstrate skill. Practice skill set with your partner. When ready, notify instructor to schedule the check-off. Skills assessment must be completed satisfactorily by _____ (due date).
Supplies	• Gown pack (gown with towel wrapped envelop style) • Sterile gloves (appropriate size for student) • Scrub brush with nail pick and antiseptic or antiseptic and nail pick • Scrubs • Mask • Eyewear

Note: Student must perform skill independently without prompting.

Practice with Partner Date:		**Skills Testing Date:**		
PROCEDURAL STEPS				**COMMENTS**
1. Recognizes contamination of gloves/gown.		Correct	Needs Review	
2. State correct steps for replacement for situation. If outer gloves only: has circulator remove outer top glove(s) and replaces glove(s). If gloves pierced, both layers of gloves contaminated, or gloves and gown contaminated: replaces gloves and gowns.		Correct	Needs Review	
3. Disrobe during case:				
a. Steps away from field, requests glove/gown setup.		Correct	Needs Review	
b. Remains still while gown is unfastened in back by circulator.		Correct	Needs Review	
c. Faces circulator, and remains still while gown is removed.		Correct	Needs Review	
d. Turns palm up and presents one at a time to circulator (usually right hand first).		Correct	Needs Review	
e. Dons sterile gown and gloves using closed glove technique (rescrubs if necessary)		Correct	Needs Review	

Performance Evaluation Criteria	• Assembled all necessary supplies and equipment for skill testing. Arranges furniture for limited traffic. • Demonstrated correct removal of contaminated gloves and/or gown. Regowns and regloves correctly using closed glove technique. Able to state rationale for double gloving. • Student prepared and performed procedure independently. Correctly maintained sterile technique. Identified any breaks in technique and corrected them appropriately. • Stated rationale for regown and reglove procedure accurately for situation. Outer gloves only contaminated versus both gloves and/or gown. • Performed each step in appropriate sequence.	**RATING**
	Overall Rating (Satisfactory; Must Redo; Fail):	
Instructor Comments		

Student Signature	*Date*
Instructor Signature	*Date*

Skill Assessment 12-1D

Student Name	
SKILL	**Removal of Gown per Self (At end of Case)**
Instructions	Instructor will demonstrate skill. Practice skill set with your partner. When ready, notify instructor to schedule the check-off. Skills assessment must be completed satisfactorily by _____ (due date).
Supplies	• Gown pack (gown with towel wrapped envelop style) • Scrubs • Mask • Eyewear • Sterile gloves (appropriate size for student) • Scrub brush with nail pick and anti-septic or antiseptic and nail pick

Note: Student must perform skill independently without prompting.

Practice with Partner Date:	Skills Testing Date:		
PROCEDURAL STEPS			**COMMENTS**
1. Disrobes at end of case:			
a. All tasks requiring gown/glove are complete.	Correct	Needs Review	
b. Back of gown is unfastened (does not reach back per self; another team member unfastens or if disposable, fasteners may be torn).	Correct	Needs Review	
c. Grasps gown near shoulders and rolls away from self.	Correct	Needs Review	
d. Removes gown and places in proper receptacle.	Correct	Needs Review	
e. Removes first glove in glove to glove fashion. Inverts —*turns inside out*—glove slowly to prevent spattering. (Keeps glove balled in gloved hand.)	Correct	Needs Review	
f. Removes second glove skin to skin (fingers of bare hand inserted between bare forearm skin and glove). Inverts slowly to contain first glove inside second glove.	Correct	Needs Review	
g. Gloves placed in appropriate receptacle. Touches only inner surface of gloves with bare hands.	Correct	Needs Review	
2. Washes hands (standard precautions: 15 seconds with running water/all surfaces)	Correct	Needs Review	

Performance Evaluation Criteria	• Assembled all necessary supplies and equipment for skill testing. Arranged furniture for limited traffic. • Demonstrated correct removal of sterile gown and gloves at end of procedure correctly. • Student prepared and performed procedure independently. Correctly maintained sterile technique. Identified any breaks in technique and corrected them appropriately.	**RATING**

Skill Assessment 12-1D (*continued*)

	• Student prepared and performed procedure independently. Correctly maintained sterile technique. Identified any breaks in technique and corrected them appropriately. • Performed each step in appropriate sequence.	
	Overall Rating (Satisfactory; Must Redo; Fail):	
Instructor Comments		
	Student Signature	**Date**
	Instructor Signature	**Date**

Skill Assessment 12-1E

Student Name	
SKILL	**Scrubbing: Timed and Waterless Methods**
Instructions	Instructor will demonstrate skill. Practice skill set with your partner. When ready, notify instructor to schedule the check-off. Skills assessment must be completed satisfactorily by _____ (due date).
Supplies	• Nail pick, antiseptic of choice • Scrubs • Scrub brush for timed method (assembles • Mask, eyewear and opens with step 1)

Note: Student must perform skill independently without prompting.			
Practice with Partner Date:	**Skills Testing Date:**		
PROCEDURAL STEPS			**COMMENTS**
1. Assembles equipment and supplies. Prepares correctly.	Correct	Needs Review	
2. States purpose for performing surgical scrub. Able to state the common agents used; one advantage and one disadvantage of each. States important-to-follow manufacturer's recommended instructions for use.	Correct	Needs Review	
3. Inspects integrity of hands and arms. States that hands must be kept free from injury (water temperature too hot; never scrub too hard; remove all solution, etc.).	Correct	Needs Review	
4. Turns on water and adjusts temperature.	Correct	Needs Review	
5. Demonstrates routine hand washing. Wets hands and arms, applies soap, lathers.	Correct	Needs Review	
6. Cleans nails under running water using nail pick.	Correct	Needs Review	
7. Discards nail pick in garbage can and rinses.	Correct	Needs Review	
8. Timed Method (***States time is determined by hospital policy based on research and manufacturer's recommendations for application of the agent***):	Correct	Needs Review	
a. States minimum time according to APIC is 2 minutes with current research showing 2–3 minutes is sufficient but hospital policy and antiseptic manufacturer's recommendations for application are to be followed.	Correct	Needs Review	
b. Scrub begins with nails of hands then proceeds from 4 planes of fingers, hands, and forearm to 2" above elbows. (May alternate nails to nails/hand to hand; upper forearm to upper forearm and then lower forearm to elbows last.)	Correct	Needs Review	

Skill Assessment 12-1E (*continued*)

	c. Does not return to a previously scrubbed area. (If student contaminates during the process of the scrub, rescrubs area with 10 strokes.)	Correct	Needs Review	
	d. Keeps fingertips up, higher than elbows so scrubbing fluids will flow towards elbows.	Correct	Needs Review	
	e. Discards brush in trash can.	Correct	Needs Review	
	f. Keeping arms flexed, rinses from fingertips to elbows without contamination on sink or splashing of scrubs; rinses all scrub solution to prevent skin irritation; keeps fingertips up.	Correct	Needs Review	
	9. Waterless Scrub solutions (**States application time and method is determined by hospital policy based on research and manufacturer's recommendations for application of the agent**):	Correct	Needs Review	
	a. Completes 1–7 prior to beginning process; most solutions require that you dry your hands prior to application of the antiseptic solution.	Correct	Needs Review	
	b. Apply appropriate amount of the solution to all surfaces using friction to rub it into the subungual areas and creases.	Correct	Needs Review	
	c. Follows manufacturer's recommendations for solution regarding time and technique.	Correct	Needs Review	
	d. Allows solution to completely dry; does not fan arms and hands in the OR suite (creates air currents).	Correct	Needs Review	
	10. Continues to room for donning of gown/gloves, keeps arms above the waist, away from the face, fingertips up.	Correct	Needs Review	

RATING

| Performance Evaluation Criteria | • Assembled all necessary supplies and equipment for skill testing. Arranged furniture for limited traffic.
• Defined the surgical scrub as the procedure taken to become a sterile team member within the established sterile field during an invasive surgical procedure. Discussed the purpose of the scrub correctly: To eliminate transient microbes and debris on the skin and reduce resident flora found on the hands and arms. This process does not render the hands sterile.
• Stated rationale regarding care of hands to prevent cross-contamination. Inspection of hands/arms for any possible injury. Uses techniques to prevent skin irritation or injury. Water temperature not too hot; no excessive friction, all solution rinsed, completely dried prior to application of gloves, etc. | |

Skill Assessment 12-1E (*continued*)

	<ul><li>Demonstrated correct surgical scrub technique. Prewash, subungual areas using nail cleaner and running water, fingertips up, hands higher than elbows, elbows bent, body posture to prevent wet scrubs and contamination; identifies technique used correctly as timed or waterless solution application according to hospital policy and manufacturer's recommendation for antiseptic chosen.</li><li>Student prepared and performed procedure independently. Correctly maintained sterile technique. Identified any breaks in technique and corrected them appropriately. (If student contaminates during scrubbing, rescrubs area 10 strokes or as required by type of antiseptic/technique chosen.)</li><li>Performed each step in appropriate sequence.</li></ul>	
	Overall Rating (Satisfactory; Must Redo; Fail):	
Instructor Comments		
	Student Signature	*Date*
	Instructor Signature	*Date*

Skill Assessment 12-1F

Student Name	
SKILL	**Scrubbing: Other**
Instructions	Instructor will demonstrate skill. Practice skill set with your partner. When ready, notify instructor to schedule the check-off. Skills assessment must be completed satisfactorily by _____ (due date).
Supplies	• Scrub brush with nail pick and antiseptic • Scrubs • Mask • Eyewear

Note: Student must perform skill independently without prompting.				
Practice with Partner Date:		**Skills Testing Date:**		
PROCEDURAL STEPS				**COMMENTS**
1. Assembles equipment and supplies. Prepares correctly.	Correct	Needs Review		
2. Demonstrates appropriate attire for restricted areas including any appropriate PPE for the STSR or circulator roles.	Correct	Needs Review		
3. Student is able to define surgical scrub.	Correct	Needs Review		
4. Student is able to state purpose for performing surgical scrub.	Correct	Needs Review		
5. Organizes workspace for most effective ergonomics. Positions sterile setup correctly.	Correct	Needs Review		
6. Inspects integrity of hands and arms.	Correct	Needs Review		
7. Opens brush package.	Correct	Needs Review		
8. Turns on water and adjusts temperature.	Correct	Needs Review		
9. Demonstrates routine hand washing. Wets hands and arms, applies soap, lathers.	Correct	Needs Review		
10. Cleans nails under running water using nail pick.	Correct	Needs Review		
11. Discards nail pick in garbage can and rinses.	Correct	Needs Review		
12. Secures and prepares brush (soap application and water).	Correct	Needs Review		
13. Scrubs nails with 30 strokes.	Correct	Needs Review		
14. Scrubs all other areas and between webs of fingers using 20 strokes progressing from fingers to 2" above elbows. (If student contaminates during the process of the scrub, rescrubs area with 10 strokes.)	Correct	Needs Review		
15. Discards brush in garbage can and rinses without contamination.	Correct	Needs Review		
16. Proceeds to OR.				

Skill Assessment 12-1F (*continued*)

Performance Evaluation Criteria		RATING
	• Assembled all necessary supplies and equipment for skill testing. Arranged furniture for limited traffic.	
	• Defined the surgical scrub as the procedure taken to become a sterile team member within the established sterile field during an invasive surgical procedure. Discussed the purpose of the scrub correctly: To eliminate transient microbes and debris on the skin and reduce resident flora found on the hands and arms. This process does not render the hands sterile.	
	• Demonstrated correct opening of sterile gown/glove setup. Height appropriate for student. Positions gown packet so leading edge covered. Opens first fold away from self, sides, then last toward self. Controls ends. Flips gloves onto field without breaking technique (unsterile hand does not cross over sterile field).	
	• Demonstrated correct surgical scrub technique. Prewash, subungual areas using nail cleaner and running water, fingertips up, hands higher than elbows, elbows bent, body posture to prevent wet scrubs and contamination; identifies technique used correctly as counted (30 nails/20 all other), timed or application according to manufacturer's recommendation for antiseptic chosen.	
	• Demonstrated correct donning of sterile gown.	
	• Student prepared and performed procedure independently. Correctly maintained sterile technique. Identified any breaks in technique and corrected them appropriately. (If student contaminates during scrubbing, rescrubs area 10 strokes or as required by type of antiseptic/technique chosen.)	
	• Performed each step in appropriate sequence.	
	Overall Rating (Satisfactory; Must Redo; Fail):	
Instructor Comments		

Student Signature	*Date*
Instructor Signature	*Date*

Skill Assessment 12-1G

Student Name	
SKILL	**Removal of Gown per Self (During Case and at End of Case)**
Instructions	Instructor will demonstrate skill. Practice skill set with your partner. When ready, notify instructor to schedule the check-off. Skills assessment must be completed satisfactorily by _____ (due date).
Supplies	• Gown pack (gown with towel wrapped envelop style) • Sterile gloves (Appropriate size for student) • Scrub brush with nail pick and antiseptic or antiseptic and nail pick • Scrubs • Mask • Eyewear

Note: Student must perform skill independently without prompting.

Practice with Partner Date:		Skills Testing Date:	
PROCEDURAL STEPS			**COMMENTS**
1. Recognizes contamination of gloves/gown.	Correct	Needs Review	
2. State correct steps for replacement for situation. If outer gloves only, has circulator remove outer top glove(s) and replaces glove(s). If gloves pierced, both layers of gloves contaminated, or gloves and gown contaminated: replaces gloves and gowns.	Correct	Needs Review	
3. Disrobe during case:	Correct	Needs Review	
a. Steps away from field, requests glove/gown setup.	Correct	Needs Review	
b. Remains still while gown is unfastened in back by circulator.	Correct	Needs Review	
c. Faces circulator and remains still while gown is removed.	Correct	Needs Review	
d. Turns palm up and presents one at a time to circulator (usually right hand first).	Correct	Needs Review	
e. Dons sterile gown and gloves using closed glove technique (rescrubs if necessary).	Correct	Needs Review	
4. Disrobes at end of case:	Correct	Needs Review	
a. All tasks requiring gown/glove are complete.	Correct	Needs Review	
b. Back of gown is unfastened (does not reach back per self; another team member unfastens or if disposable, fasteners may be torn).	Correct	Needs Review	
c. Grasps gown near shoulders and rolls away from self.	Correct	Needs Review	
d. Removes gown and places in proper receptacle.	Correct	Needs Review	

Skill Assessment 12-1G (*continued*)

	e. Removes first glove in glove to glove fashion. Inverts—*turns inside out*—glove slowly to prevent spattering. (Keeps glove balled in gloved hand.)	Correct	Needs Review	
	f. Removes second glove skin to skin (fingers of bare hand inserted between bare forearm skin and glove). Inverts slowly to contain first glove inside second glove.	Correct	Needs Review	
	g. Gloves placed in appropriate receptacle. Touches only inner surface of gloves with bare hands.	Correct	Needs Review	
	5. Washes hands (standard precautions: 15 seconds with running water/all surfaces).	Correct	Needs Review	

		RATING
Performance Evaluation Criteria	• Assembled all necessary supplies and equipment for skill testing. Arranged furniture for limited traffic.	
	• Demonstrated correct removal of contaminated gloves and/or gown. Regowns and regloves correctly using closed glove technique. Able to state rationale for double gloving.	
	• Demonstrated correct removal of sterile gown at end of procedure correctly.	
	• Student prepared and performed procedure independently. Correctly maintained sterile technique. Identified any breaks in technique and corrected them appropriately.	
	• Stated rationale for regown and reglove procedure accurately for situation. Outer gloves only contaminated versus both gloves and/or gown.	
	• Performed each step in appropriate sequence.	
	Overall Rating (Satisfactory; Must Redo; Fail):	
Instructor Comments		

Student Signature	**Date**	
Instructor Signature	**Date**	

Skill Assessment 12-2

Student Name	
SKILL	**Opening Sterile Supplies**
Instructions	Instructor will demonstrate skill. Practice skill set with your partner. When ready, notify instructor to schedule the check-off. Skills assessment must be completed satisfactorily by _____ (due date).
Supplies	• 1/2 drape sheet or back table drape or drape pack • Basin wrapped or basin set • Instrument set • Wrapped items (irregular shaped or multiple items) • Peel-packed items • Scrubs, mask, eyewear • Furniture arranged correctly for "opening of supplies"

Note: Student must perform skill independently without prompting.

Practice with Partner Date:		Skills Testing Date:	
PROCEDURAL STEPS			**COMMENTS**
1. Demonstrates hand washing.	Correct	Needs Review	
2. Assembles equipment and supplies.	Correct	Needs Review	
3. Demonstrates appropriate attire for restricted areas including any appropriate PPE for the STSR.	Correct	Needs Review	
4. Organizes workspace for most effective ergonomics. Positions furniture correctly.	Correct	Needs Review	
5. Prepares furniture for opening. Places items on dry surface. Explains rationale for opening sequence.	Correct	Needs Review	
6. Demonstrates opening of back table drape correctly. Identifies sterile parameters correctly.	Correct	Needs Review	
7. Demonstrates opening of basin set correctly. Identifies sterile parameters correctly.	Correct	Needs Review	
8. Demonstrates opening of instrument set correctly. Identifies sterile parameters correctly.	Correct	Needs Review	
9. Demonstrates opening of wrapped items correctly. Identifies sterile parameters correctly.	Correct	Needs Review	
10. Demonstrates opening of peel packed items correctly. Identifies sterile parameters correctly.	Correct	Needs Review	
11. Guards sterile field assertively.	Correct	Needs Review	
12. Maintains sterile technique. Identifies correctly how to check the package integrity. Identifies and corrects any deviations correctly.	Correct	Needs Review	

Skill Assessment 12-2 (*continued*)

		Rating
Performance Evaluation Criteria	• Prepared correctly for skill. Washed hands and assembled all necessary supplies for skill testing.	
	• Demonstrated correctly restricted area attire.	
	• Prepared furniture for limited traffic (positions sterile field as far from door and major traffic area as possible).	
	• Demonstrated preparation for opening of sterile supplies. Removal of dust cover prn. Checks surfaces for moisture, inspects packaging for discoloration, integrity—no holes with seals intact, or expiration dates.	
	• Demonstrated correct opening of back table drape. Moves each end of table as necessary to open folds while preventing contamination (bend knees while opening large drape folds). Moves table back into place grasping table leg below drape and watching head position to keep 12" away from sterile field (bend knees). Opens in such a manner that unsterile hands never reach over sterile areas. Controls ends.	
	• Demonstrated correct opening of instrument set (varies according to method: wrapped or container system). _____	
	• Demonstrated correct opening of wrapped items. Opens first fold away from self, sides, then last fold toward self. Controls ends. Tosses item onto sterile back table or into basin without breaking technique. (Unsterile hand does not cross over sterile field.)	
	• Demonstrated protection of sterile field. Guards sterile field assertively. (Maintains field within sight and grouped loosely together. Instructs others to maintain distance. Keeps arms within sterile zone: above waist below shoulder and away from the face, keeps hands in sight at all times.)	
	• Student prepared and performed procedure independently. Correctly maintained sterile technique. Identified any breaks in technique and corrected them appropriately. (If student contaminates during scrubbing, rescrubs area 10 strokes or as required by type of antiseptic/technique chosen.)	
	• Performed each step in appropriate sequence.	
	Overall Rating (Satisfactory; Must Redo; Fail):	
Instructor Comments		

Student Signature	*Date*
Instructor Signature	*Date*

Skill Assessment 12-2A

Student Name	
SKILL	**Opening Sterile Supplies: Back Table**
Instructions	Instructor will demonstrate skill. Practice skill set with your partner. When ready notify instructor to schedule the check-off. Skills assessment must be completed satisfactorily by _____ (due date).
Supplies	• Half drape sheet or back table drape or drape pack • Scrubs, mask, eyewear • Furniture arranged correctly for "opening of supplies"

Note: Student must perform skill independently without prompting.

Practice with Partner Date:	Skills Testing Date:		
PROCEDURAL STEPS			**COMMENTS**
1. Demonstrates hand washing.	Correct	Needs Review	
2. Assembles equipment and supplies.	Correct	Needs Review	
3. Demonstrates appropriate attire for restricted areas including any appropriate PPE for the STSR.	Correct	Needs Review	
4. Organizes workspace for most effective ergonomics. Positions furniture correctly.	Correct	Needs Review	
5. Prepares furniture for opening. Places items on dry surface. Explains rationale for opening sequence.	Correct	Needs Review	
6. Demonstrates opening of back table drape correctly. Identifies sterile parameters correctly.	Correct	Needs Review	
7. Guards sterile field assertively.	Correct	Needs Review	
8. Maintains sterile technique. Identifies correctly how to check the package integrity. Identifies and corrects any deviations correctly.	Correct	Needs Review	

Performance Evaluation Criteria

RATING

- Prepared correctly for skill. Washed hands and assembled all necessary supplies for skill testing.
- Demonstrated correctly restricted area attire.
- Prepared furniture for limited traffic (positions sterile field as far from door and major traffic area as possible).
- Demonstrated preparation for opening of sterile supplies. Removal of dust cover prn. Checks surfaces for moisture, inspects packaging for discoloration, integrity—no holes with seals intact, or expiration dates.
- Demonstrated correct opening of back table drape. Moves each end of table as necessary to open folds while preventing contamination (bend knees while opening large drape folds). Moves table back into place grasping table leg below drape and watching head position to keep 12" away from sterile field (bend knees). Opens in such a manner that unsterile hands never reach over sterile areas. Controls ends.

Skill Assessment 12-2A (*continued*)

	• Demonstrated proper positioning of back table after opening the drape. Grasped legs below level of the drape to position the table 6-12" away from a stationary wall. Whiteboard for counts is not located on the wall above or close to the sterile field due to dust.	
	• Demonstrated proper control of the drape. Drape did not shift as it was opened; once drape drops over the edge only the top is sterile.	
	• Demonstrated protection of sterile field. Guards sterile field assertively. (Maintains field within sight and grouped loosely together. Instructs others to maintain distance. Keeps arms within sterile zone: above waist below shoulder and away from the face, keeps hands in sight at all times.)	
	• Student prepared and performed procedure independently. Correctly maintained sterile technique. Identified any breaks in technique and corrected them appropriately. (If student contaminates during scrubbing, rescrubs area 10 strokes or as required by type of antiseptic/technique chosen.)	
	• Performed each step in appropriate sequence.	
	Overall Rating (Satisfactory; Must Redo; Fail):	
Instructor Comments		
	Student Signature	**Date**
	Instructor Signature	**Date**

Skill Assessment 12-2B

Student Name	
SKILL	**Opening Sterile Supplies: Small**
Instructions	Instructor will demonstrate skill. Practice skill set with your partner. When ready, notify instructor to schedule the check-off. Skills assessment must be completed satisfactorily by _____ (due date).
Supplies	• Gown or other small wrapped items (irregular shaped or multiple items) • Scrubs, mask, eyewear • Furniture arranged correctly for "opening of supplies"

Note: Student must perform skill independently without prompting.	

Practice with Partner Date:	**Skills Testing Date:**		
PROCEDURAL STEPS			**COMMENTS**
1. Demonstrates hand washing.	Correct	Needs Review	
2. Assembles equipment and supplies.	Correct	Needs Review	
3. Demonstrates appropriate attire for restricted areas including any appropriate PPE for the STSR.	Correct	Needs Review	
4. Organizes workspace for most effective ergonomics. Positions furniture correctly.	Correct	Needs Review	
5. Prepares furniture for opening. Places items on dry surface. Explains rationale for opening sequence.	Correct	Needs Review	
6. Demonstrates opening of small wrapped items correctly. Identifies sterile parameters correctly.	Correct	Needs Review	
7. Demonstrates opening of a second small wrapped item correctly. Secures edges and tosses onto small wrapped sterile field in #6. Identifies sterile parameters correctly.	Correct	Needs Review	
8. Guards sterile field assertively.	Correct	Needs Review	
9. Maintains sterile technique. Identifies correctly how to check the package integrity. Identifies and corrects any deviations correctly.	Correct	Needs Review	

| **Performance Evaluation Criteria** | • Prepared correctly for skill. Washed hands and assembled all necessary supplies for skill testing. • Demonstrated correctly restricted area attire. • Prepared furniture for limited traffic (positions sterile field as far from door and major traffic area as possible). • Demonstrated preparation for opening of sterile supplies. Removal of dust cover prn. Checks surfaces for moisture, inspects packaging for discoloration, integrity—no holes with seals intact, or expiration dates. • Demonstrated correct opening of first wrapped item. Opens first fold away from self, sides, then last fold toward self. Opens in such a manner that unsterile hands never reach over sterile areas. Controls ends. | **RATING** |

Skill Assessment 12-2B (*continued*)

	• Identifies correctly sterile safety parameter as 1 inch or greater from contaminated edge or area where hand had touched during opening.	
	• Demonstrated correct opening of wrapped items. Opens first fold away from self, sides, then last fold toward self. Controls ends. Tosses item onto sterile back table or into basin without breaking technique. (Ensures that unsterile hand does not cross over sterile field.)	
	• Demonstrated protection of sterile field. Guards sterile field assertively. (Maintains field within sight and grouped loosely together. Instructs others to maintain distance. Keeps arms within sterile zone (above waist below shoulder and away from the face, keeps hands in sight at all times).	
	• Student prepared and performed procedure independently. Correctly maintained sterile technique. Identified any breaks in technique and corrected them appropriately. (If student contaminates during scrubbing, rescrubs area 10 strokes or as required by type of antiseptic/technique chosen.) • Performed each step in appropriate sequence.	
	Overall Rating (Satisfactory; Must Redo; Fail):	
Instructor Comments		
	Student Signature	**Date**
	Instructor Signature	**Date**

Skill Assessment 12-2C

Student Name	
SKILL	**Opening Sterile Supplies: Large Wrapped Items**
Instructions	Instructor will demonstrate skill. Practice skill set with your partner. When ready, notify instructor to schedule the check-off. Skills assessment must be completed satisfactorily by _____ (due date).
Supplies	• Large wrapped drape pack or large container to simulate bookwalter • Basin wrapped or basin set • Scrubs, mask, eyewear • Furniture arranged correctly for "opening of supplies"

Note: Student must perform skill independently without prompting.

Practice with Partner Date:	Skills Testing Date:		
PROCEDURAL STEPS			**COMMENTS**
1. Demonstrates hand washing.	Correct	Needs Review	
2. Assembles equipment and supplies.	Correct	Needs Review	
3. Demonstrates appropriate attire for restricted areas including any appropriate PPE for the STSR.	Correct	Needs Review	
4. Organizes workspace for most effective ergonomics. Positions furniture correctly.	Correct	Needs Review	
5. Prepares furniture for opening. Places items on dry surface. Explains rationale for opening sequence.	Correct	Needs Review	
6. Demonstrates opening of large draped item correctly. Identifies sterile parameters correctly.	Correct	Needs Review	
7. Demonstrates opening of basin set correctly. Identifies sterile parameters correctly.	Correct	Needs Review	
8. Guards sterile field assertively.	Correct	Needs Review	
9. Maintains sterile technique. Identifies correctly how to check the package integrity. Identifies and corrects any deviations correctly.	Correct	Needs Review	

Performance Evaluation Criteria	• Prepared correctly for skill. Washed hands and assembled all necessary supplies for skill testing. • Demonstrated correctly restricted area attire. • Prepared furniture for limited traffic. (positions sterile field as far from door and major traffic area as possible) • Demonstrated preparation for opening of sterile supplies. Removal of dust cover prn. Checks surfaces for moisture, inspects packaging for discoloration, integrity—no holes with seals intact, or expiration dates. • Demonstrated correct opening of large wrapped item. Moves to each end of table/cart as necessary to open folds while preventing contamination (bend knees while opening large drape folds). Opens in such a manner that unsterile hands never reach over sterile areas. Controls ends.	**RATING**

Skill Assessment 12-2C (*continued*)

	• Demonstrated correct opening of basin set. Opens first fold away from self, sides, then last fold toward self. Controls ends. (Unsterile hand does not cross over sterile field)	
	• Demonstrated protection of sterile field. Guards sterile field assertively. (Maintains field within sight and grouped loosely together. Instructs others to maintain distance. Keeps arms within sterile zone: above waist below shoulder and away from the face, keeps hands in sight at all times.)	
	• Student prepared and performed procedure independently. Correctly maintained sterile technique. Identified any breaks in technique and corrected them appropriately. (If student contaminates during scrubbing, rescrubs area 10 strokes or as required by type of antiseptic/technique chosen.) • Performed each step in appropriate sequence.	
	Overall Rating (Satisfactory; Must Redo; Fail):	
Instructor Comments		

	Student Signature	**Date**
	Instructor Signature	**Date**

Skill Assessment 12-2D

Student Name	
SKILL	**Opening Sterile Supplies: Peel-Packed Items**
Instructions	Instructor will demonstrate skill. Practice skill set with your partner. When ready, notify instructor to schedule the check-off. Skills assessment must be completed satisfactorily by _____ (due date).
Supplies	• 1/2 drape sheet or back table drape or basin wrapped or basin set • Peel-packed items • Scrubs, mask, eyewear • Furniture arranged correctly for "opening of supplies"

Note: Student must perform skill independently without prompting.

Practice with Partner Date:	Skills Testing Date:		
PROCEDURAL STEPS			**COMMENTS**
1. Demonstrates hand washing.	Correct	Needs Review	
2. Assembles equipment and supplies. Prepares peel packed items for skills assessment.	Correct	Needs Review	
3. Demonstrates appropriate attire for restricted areas including any appropriate PPE for the STSR.	Correct	Needs Review	
4. Organizes workspace for most effective ergonomics. Positions furniture correctly.	Correct	Needs Review	
5. Prepares furniture for opening. Places items on dry surface. Explains rationale for opening sequence.	Correct	Needs Review	
6. Demonstrates opening of drape/basin set or other area for peel packed items to be flipped correctly. Identifies sterile parameters correctly.	Correct	Needs Review	
7. Demonstrates assessment of the package correctly. Identifies sterile parameters of the peel pack correctly.	Correct	Needs Review	
8. Demonstrates opening of peel packed items correctly. Identifies sterile parameters correctly.	Correct	Needs Review	
9. Demonstrates flipping of item onto the sterile field correctly. Identifies sterile parameters correctly.	Correct	Needs Review	
10. Guards sterile field assertively.	Correct	Needs Review	
11. Maintains sterile technique. Identifies correctly how to check the package integrity. Identifies and corrects any deviations correctly.	Correct	Needs Review	

Skill Assessment 12-2D (*continued*)

		RATING
Performance Evaluation Criteria	• Prepared correctly for skill. Washed hands and assembled all necessary supplies for skill testing.	
	• Demonstrated correctly restricted area attire.	
	• Prepared furniture for limited traffic (positions sterile field as far from door and major traffic area as possible).	
	• Demonstrated preparation for opening of sterile supplies. Removal of dust cover prn. Checks surfaces for moisture, inspects packaging for discoloration, integrity—no holes with seals intact, or expiration dates.	
	• Demonstrated correct opening of back table drape. Moves each end of table as necessary to open folds while preventing contamination (bend knees while opening large drape folds). Moves table back into place grasping table leg below drape and watching head position to keep 12" away from sterile field (bend knees). Opens in such a manner that unsterile hands never reach over sterile areas. Controls ends.	
	• Demonstrated correct opening of peel packed items. Places hands to cover the width of the package to secure the item; hands are rolled so that thumbs are not over the seal. As seal is broken, package is steadied to prevent the item from sliding over the inner seal. Controls ends. Flips item onto sterile field or into basin without breaking technique. (Unsterile hand does not cross over sterile field.)	
	• Demonstrated protection of sterile field. Guards sterile field assertively. (Maintains field within sight and grouped loosely together. Instructs others to maintain distance. Keeps arms within sterile zone: above waist below shoulder and away from the face, keeps hands in sight at all times.)	
	• Student prepared and performed procedure independently. Correctly maintained sterile technique. Identified any breaks in technique and corrected them appropriately. (If student contaminates during scrubbing, rescrubs area 10 strokes or as required by type of antiseptic/technique chosen.)	
	• Performed each step in appropriate sequence.	
	Overall Rating (Satisfactory; Must Redo; Fail):	
Instructor Comments		
	Student Signature	*Date*
	Instructor Signature	*Date*

Skill Assessment 12-2E

Student Name	
SKILL	**Opening Sterile Supplies: Instrument Set**
Instructions	Instructor will demonstrate skill. Practice skill set with your partner. When ready, notify instructor to schedule the check-off. Skills assessment must be completed satisfactorily by _____ (due date).
Supplies	• Instrument set • Scrubs, mask, eyewear • Furniture arranged correctly for "opening of supplies"

Note: Student must perform skill independently without prompting.

Practice with Partner Date:		Skills Testing Date:	
PROCEDURAL STEPS			**COMMENTS**
1. Demonstrates hand washing.	Correct	Needs Review	
2. Assembles equipment and supplies.	Correct	Needs Review	
3. Demonstrates appropriate attire for restricted areas including any appropriate PPE for the STSR.	Correct	Needs Review	
4. Organizes workspace for most effective ergonomics. Positions furniture correctly.	Correct	Needs Review	
5. Prepares furniture for opening. Places items on dry surface. Explains rationale for opening sequence.	Correct	Needs Review	
6. Demonstrates opening of Instrument set correctly. Identifies sterile parameters correctly.	Correct	Needs Review	
7. Guards sterile field assertively.	Correct	Needs Review	
8. Maintains sterile technique. Identifies correctly how to check the package integrity. Identifies and corrects any deviations correctly.	Correct	Needs Review	

Performance Evaluation Criteria

- Prepared correctly for skill. Washed hands and assembled all necessary supplies for skill testing.
- Demonstrated correctly restricted area attire.
- Prepared furniture for limited traffic (positioned sterile field as far from door and major traffic area as possible).
- Demonstrated preparation for opening of sterile supplies. Removal of dust cover prn. Checks surfaces for moisture, inspects packaging for discoloration, integrity—no holes with seals intact, or expiration dates.
- Demonstrated correct opening of instrument set (varies according to method: wrapped or container system). If container system, break seals, lift lid and roll back keeping unsterile edge closest to self from crossing over the sterile instrument set; try to keep unsterile upper edge as flat as possible as it crosses as if a door swinging open.

RATING

Skill Assessment 12-2E (*continued*)

	• Demonstrated protection of sterile field. Guards sterile field assertively. (Maintains field within sight and grouped loosely together. Instructs others to maintain distance. Keeps arms within sterile zone (above waist below shoulder and away from the face, keeps hands in sight at all times).	
	• Student prepared and performed procedure independently. Correctly maintained sterile technique. Identified any breaks in technique and corrected them appropriately. (If student contaminates during scrubbing, rescrubs area 10 strokes or as required by type of antiseptic/technique chosen.)	
	• Performed each step in appropriate sequence.	
	Overall Rating (Satisfactory; Must Redo; Fail):	
Instructor Comments		
	Student Signature	*Date*
	Instructor Signature	*Date*

Skill Assessment 12-3

Student Name	
SKILL	**Donning of Sterile Gown and Gloves using Closed Glove Technique**
Instructions	Instructor will demonstrate skill. Practice skill set with your partner. When ready, notify instructor to schedule the check-off. Skills assessment must be completed satisfactorily by _____ (due date).
Supplies	• Gown pack (gown with towel wrapped envelope style) • Scrubs • Sterile gloves (appropriate size for student) • Mask • Eyewear

	Note: Student must perform skill independently without prompting.			
	Practice with Partner Date:	**Skills Testing Date:**		
	PROCEDURAL STEPS			**COMMENTS**
	1. Washes hands and assembles supplies.	Correct	Needs Review	
	2. Demonstrates appropriate attire for restricted areas including any appropriate PPE.	Correct	Needs Review	
	3. Organizes workspace for most effective ergonomics. Positions sterile setup correctly.	Correct	Needs Review	
	4. Opens sterile gown/glove setup correctly.	Correct	Needs Review	
	5. Demonstrates appropriate scrub technique. Utilizes antiseptic chosen appropriately.	Correct	Needs Review	
	6. Demonstrates drying technique correctly.	Correct	Needs Review	
	7. Demonstrates donning of sterile gown correctly.	Correct	Needs Review	
	8. Demonstrate closed glove technique correctly.	Correct	Needs Review	
	9. Demonstrates "turning" to tie up correctly.	Correct	Needs Review	
	10. Identifies and maintains hands within sterile perimeters of gown correctly.	Correct	Needs Review	
	11. Maintains sterile technique; identifies and corrects any deviations correctly.	Correct	Needs Review	
	12. Guards sterile field assertively.	Correct	Needs Review	

		Rating
Performance Evaluation Criteria	• Prepared correctly for skill. Washed hands and assembled all necessary supplies for skill testing. Arranges furniture for limited traffic.	
	• Discussed correctly restricted area (hat, scrubs, footwear, mask, and eyewear).	
	• Demonstrated correct opening of sterile gown/glove setup. Height appropriate for student. Positions gown packet so leading edge covered. Opens first fold away from self, sides, then last toward self. Controls ends. Flips gloves onto field without breaking technique. (Unsterile hand does not cross over sterile field.)	
	• Demonstrated correct surgical scrub. Inspects integrity of hands. Prewash, clean subungual areas using nail cleaner and running water; fingertips up, hands higher than elbows, elbows bent, body posture to prevent wet scrubs and contamination; scrubs to 2" above elbows; identifies technique used correctly as counted (30 nails/20 all other), timed or application according to manufacturer's recommendation for antiseptic chosen.	
	• Demonstrated correct drying technique (picks up by pinching in middle, no drips on surface, steps back, dries one hand/arm, changes hand, dries second hand/arm without contamination of end of towel on scrubs).	

Skill Assessment 12-3 (*continued*)

	• Demonstrated correct donning of sterile gown. (Pinches in middle, steps back, inserts arms keeping end of arms within sterile zone: above waist, within sight, below shoulder level, hands do not extend beyond end of stockinet cuff).	
	• Demonstrated closed glove technique correctly. (Places thumb to thumb; fingertips toward elbow. Covers opening with cuff; no contamination. Cuff completely covered.) Discusses double gloving for procedures.	
	• Demonstrated "turning" correctly. (Grasp ties correctly; passes to circulator; faces sterile field; ties securely)	
	• Demonstrated protection of sterile field. Guards sterile field assertively. (Maintains field within sight and grouped loosely together. Instructs others to maintain distance. Keeps arms within sterile zone: above waist, below shoulder and away from the face, keeps hands in sight at all times.)	
	• Student prepared and performed procedure independently. Correctly maintained sterile technique. Identified any breaks in technique and corrected them appropriately. (If contaminated during scrubbing, rescrubs area 10 strokes or as required by type of antiseptic/technique chosen.)	
	• Performed each step in appropriate sequence.	
	Overall Rating (Satisfactory; Must Redo; Fail):	
Instructor Comments		
	Student Signature	*Date*
	Instructor Signature	*Date*

Skill Assessment 12-4

Student Name	
SKILL	**Assisted Gowning Gloving of Team Member**
Instructions	Instructor will demonstrate skill. Practice skill set with your partner. When ready, notify instructor to schedule the check-off. Skills assessment must be completed satisfactorily by _____ (due date).
Supplies	• Gown pack (gown with towel wrapped envelope style) • Scrubs • Sterile gloves (appropriate size for student) • Mask • Gown pack and gloves for team member • Eyewear

Note: Student must perform skill independently without prompting.

Practice with Partner Date:		Skills Testing Date:	
PROCEDURAL STEPS			**COMMENTS**
1. Washes hands and assembles supplies.	Correct	Needs Review	
2. Demonstrates appropriate attire for restricted areas including any appropriate PPE.	Correct	Needs Review	
3. Organizes workspace for most effective ergonomics. Positions sterile setup correctly.	Correct	Needs Review	
4. Opens sterile gown/glove setups correctly.	Correct	Needs Review	
5. Demonstrates scrub, gown, and closed glove technique correctly. Gown/glove time: _____	Correct	Needs Review	
6. Demonstrates passing of towel to team member. Protects hands from contamination.	Correct	Needs Review	
7. Demonstrates presentation of gown to team member correctly. Protects hands.	Correct	Needs Review	
8. Demonstrates preparation of gown sleeves for gloving. (States some team members prefer gown left alone.)	Correct	Needs Review	
9. Demonstrates preparation, presentation, and application of right glove correctly.	Correct	Needs Review	
10. Demonstrates preparation, presentation, and application of left glove correctly.	Correct	Needs Review	
11. Demonstrates assisting with turning—wrap around back of gown correctly.	Correct	Needs Review	
12. Identifies and maintains hands within sterile perimeters of gown correctly.	Correct	Needs Review	
13. Maintains sterile technique; identifies and corrects any deviations correctly.	Correct	Needs Review	
14. Guards sterile field assertively.	Correct	Needs Review	

Performance Evaluation Criteria	• Prepared correctly. Washed hands and assembled all supplies for skill testing. Arranged for limited traffic. • Demonstrated correct opening of sterile gown/glove setup. Height appropriate for student. Positions gown packet so leading edge covered. Opens first fold away from self, sides, then last toward self. Controls ends. Flips gloves onto field without breaking technique. (Unsterile hand does not cross over sterile field.)	**Rating**

Skill Assessment 12-4 (*continued*)

• Demonstrated scrub, gown, and glove technique correctly. (Gowns and gloves in less than 2 minutes.)	
• Demonstrated towel passing correctly. (Opens and presents to team member; cuffs to prevent contamination.)	
• Demonstrated presentation of sterile gown correctly. (Opens with sterile side facing self and openings for arms visible to team member; cuffs over hands at shoulders; pushes gown onto team member's upper arms.)	
• Demonstrated glove application correctly. (Opens right glove, cuffs over fingertips, spreads fingers for visible hole, releases as team member's hand enters and cuff is covered. Opened left glove, hooked over team member's extended right fingertips, pulled to open hole, released when team member's hand entered and cuff was covered.)	
• Demonstrated "turning" correctly. (Grasps tag presented to STSR by team member; holds securely as team member turns; team member pulls the tag from tag holder.)	
• Demonstrated protection of sterile field. Guards sterile field assertively. (Maintains field within sight and grouped loosely together. Instructs others to maintain distance. Keeps arms within sterile zone: above waist below shoulder and away from the face, keeps hands in sight at all times.)	
• Student prepared and performed procedure independently. Correctly maintained sterile technique. Identified any breaks in technique and corrected them appropriately. (If tag drops; identified person must regown, reglove.) • Performed each step in appropriate sequence.	
Overall Rating (Satisfactory; Must Redo; Fail):	

Instructor Comments	
Student Signature	**Date**
Instructor Signature	**Date**

Skill Assessment 12-5

Student Name	
SKILL	**Removal of Gown and Gloves**
Instructions	Instructor will demonstrate skill. Practice skill set with your partner. When ready, notify instructor to schedule skills assessment check-off. Skills assessment must be completed satisfactorily by _____ (due date).
Supplies	• Opened gown pack (gown with towel wrapped envelope style) • Scrubs with gown and gloves on • Sterile gloves (appropriate size for student) • Mask, eyewear

Note: Student must perform skill independently without prompting.

Practice with Partner Date:	Skills Testing Date:		
PROCEDURAL STEPS			**COMMENTS**
1. Assembles equipment and supplies.	Correct	Needs Review	
2. States gown and/or gloves are contaminated during case. States would step away from sterile field and request new gown and gloves.	Correct	Needs Review	
3. Demonstrates removal of gown during case correctly. Remains still for circulator to remove.	Correct	Needs Review	
4. Demonstrates removal of contaminated gloves correctly. Presents hands palms up.	Correct	Needs Review	
5. Demonstrates gowning and gloving correctly from opened setup. States would double glove.	Correct	Needs Review	
6. Identifies and maintains hands within sterile perimeters of gown correctly.	Correct	Needs Review	
7. Maintains sterile technique; identifies and corrects any deviations correctly.	Correct	Needs Review	
8. Guards sterile field assertively.	Correct	Needs Review	
9. Demonstrates removal of gown at end of case correctly. Demonstrates how to break back ties.	Correct	Needs Review	
10. Demonstrates removal of gloves correctly.	Correct	Needs Review	
11. Demonstrates handwashing.	Correct	Needs Review	

| **Performance Evaluation Criteria** | • Assembled all necessary supplies and equipment for skill testing. Arranged furniture for limited traffic. • Demonstrated removal of contaminated gown and/or gloves during case correctly. Stated must step away from the sterile field. Remains still with back toward circulator while circulator unfastens back of gown. Faces circulator; remained still while gown is removed. Presents hands palms up for circulator to remove gloves usually right hand first then left. • Demonstrated regowning and regloving using closed glove technique correctly. • Demonstrated removal of gown and gloves at end of case correctly. Broke back tags or had circulator unfasten; grasped sleeves at shoulders and pulled forward, rolling gown into a ball containing contaminated areas; discarded into appropriate receptacle. Removed first glove by grasping palm of glove to be removed with opposite hand (glove to glove); pulled to remove first glove; balled glove into hand. Removed second glove by inserting finger inside cuff (skin to skin) and pushed down to remove glove; contained first glove inside second glove removed; discarded into appropriate receptacle. | **Rating** |

Skill Assessment 12-5 (*continued*)

	• Demonstrated handwashing correctly. Using soap, friction, and scrubbing webs of fingers.	
	• Demonstrated protection of sterile field. Guarded sterile field assertively. (Maintained field within sight and grouped loosely together. Instructed others to maintain distance. Kept arms within sterile zone: above waist below shoulder and away from the face, kept hands in sight at all times.)	
	• Student prepared and performed procedure independently. Correctly maintained sterile technique. Identified any breaks in technique and corrected them appropriately. (If tag dropped; identified person must regown, reglove.)	
	• Performed each step in appropriate sequence.	
	Overall Rating (Satisfactory; Must Redo; Fail):	
Instructor Comments		
	Student Signature	**Date**
	Instructor Signature	**Date**

Skill Assessment 12-6

Student Name	
SKILL	**Skill Practice: STSR Case Setup: Mayo Drape, Solution Preparation, Mayo Setup**
Instructions	Instructor will demonstrate skill. Practice skill set with your partner. When ready, notify instructor to schedule the check-off. Skills assessment must be completed satisfactorily by _____ (due date).
Supplies	• 1/2 sheet or back table drape; towels • Scrubs with gown and gloves on • Supplies: Mayo cover, bowl, saline, bulb syringe, labels, and marker • Mask, eyewear • Instrument set; other items as outlined on instructor diagram • Circulator team member

Note: Student must perform skill independently without prompting.

Practice with Partner Date:		Skills Testing Date:		
PROCEDURAL STEPS				**COMMENTS**
1. Assembles equipment and supplies.	Correct	Needs Review		
2. Prepares setup for practice correctly. Opens back table drape and other needed supplies.	Correct	Needs Review		
3. Demonstrates draping of Mayo stand correctly.	Correct	Needs Review		
4. Demonstrates towel preparation. Places towel on Mayo stand; secures edges. Prepares towel roll.	Correct	Needs Review		
5. Demonstrates minor instrumentation setup on Mayo as previously diagrammed by instructor.	Correct	Needs Review		
6. Maintains sterile technique; identifies and corrects any deviations correctly.	Correct	Needs Review		
7. Demonstrates pouring of solution into bowl correctly. Labels bowl prior to receiving solution.	Correct	Needs Review		
8. Demonstrates preparation of a bulb syringe correctly.	Correct	Needs Review		
9. Guards sterile field assertively.	Correct	Needs Review		
10. Demonstrates removal of gown at end of case correctly. Demonstrates how to break back ties.	Correct	Needs Review		
11. Demonstrates removal of gloves correctly.	Correct	Needs Review		
12. Demonstrates hand washing.	Correct	Needs Review		

Performance Evaluation Criteria	• Assembled all necessary supplies and equipment for skill testing. Arranged furniture for limited traffic.	**Rating**
	• Demonstrated pouring of solution. Identified solution, expiration date, and patient allergies. Labeled bowl. Solution (saline) poured into bowl without possible contamination of back table drape.	
	• Demonstrated application of Mayo stand cover correctly. Orient Mayo cover; insert hands and open Mayo cover opening while securing folded edges; approach Mayo stand and grasp Mayo stand in the opening; step on the footrest on side away from back table; slide Mayo cover onto Mayo stand; allow the Mayo cover to unfold as you slide it on. Secure the Mayo cover onto the Mayo stand to keep taut. Does not allow Mayo cover to drop below waist level.	

Skill Assessment 12-6 (*continued*)

	• Demonstrated placement of towels correctly. Prepares an instrument towel roll that is firm and relevant to the size needed. Places the towel roll on Mayo stand appropriately for setup as instructed.	
	• Demonstrated filling of bulb syringe correctly. Labels bulb syringe as instructed by instructor (open bulb, place label on green indentation and replace). Grasps bulb syringe similar to syringe with thumb on bulb and first two fingers on flanges. Compress bulb and stick open end into solution to draw into device. Hold upright and compress again to remove air, stick open end into solution repeatedly until completely filled. Replace in solution bowl until needed.	
	• Demonstrated instrument Mayo and back table setup as diagrammed by instructor. Removed instrument set from container or wrapper correctly, placed on back table after cleared by circulator. Inspected instruments for functionality and cleanliness as placed on setup. Practiced setup placement; moved items once into place.	
	• Student prepared and performed procedure independently. Correctly maintained sterile technique. Identified any breaks in technique and corrected them appropriately.	
	• Performed each step in appropriate sequence.	
	Overall Rating (Satisfactory; Must Redo; Fail):	
Instructor Comments		

Student Signature	**Date**	
Instructor Signature	**Date**	

Skill Assessment 12-6A

Student Name	
SKILL	**Skill Practice: STSR Case Setup: Draping the Mayo**
Instructions	Instructor will demonstrate skill. Practice skill set with your partner. When ready, notify instructor to schedule the check-off. Skills assessment must be completed satisfactorily by _____ (due date).
Supplies	• Towels • Supplies: Mayo cover • Scrubs with gown and gloves on • Mask, eyewear • Circulator team member

Note: Student must perform skill independently without prompting.

Practice with Partner Date:		Skills Testing Date:		
PROCEDURAL STEPS				**COMMENTS**
1. Assembles equipment and supplies.	Correct	Needs Review		
2. Prepares setup for practice correctly. Opens back gown/glove setup.	Correct	Needs Review		
3. Dons sterile gown and gloves. Accepts the Mayo cover from circulator.	Correct	Needs Review		
4. Demonstrates draping of Mayo stand correctly.	Correct	Needs Review		
5. Demonstrates towel preparation. Places towel on Mayo stand; secures edges. Prepares towel roll.	Correct	Needs Review		
6. Maintains sterile technique; identifies and corrects any deviations correctly.	Correct	Needs Review		
7. Guards sterile field assertively.	Correct	Needs Review		
8. Demonstrates removal of gown at end of case correctly. Demonstrates how to break back ties.	Correct	Needs Review		
9. Demonstrates removal of gloves correctly.	Correct	Needs Review		
10. Demonstrates hand washing.	Correct	Needs Review		

Performance Evaluation Criteria	**Rating**
• Assembled all necessary supplies and equipment for skill testing. Arranges furniture for limited traffic. • Demonstrated application of Mayo stand cover correctly. Orient Mayo cover; insert hands and open Mayo cover opening while securing folded edges; approach Mayo stand and grasp Mayo stand in the opening; step on the foot rest on side away from back table; slide Mayo cover onto Mayo stand; allow the Mayo cover to unfold as you slide it on. Secure the Mayo cover onto the Mayo stand to keep taut. Does not allow Mayo cover to drop below waist level. • Demonstrated placement of towels correctly. Prepares an instrument towel roll that is firm and relevant to the size needed. Places the towel roll on Mayo stand appropriately for setup as instructed. • Student prepared and performed procedure independently. Correctly maintained sterile technique. Identified any breaks in technique and corrected them appropriately. • Performed each step in appropriate sequence.	
Overall Rating (Satisfactory; Must Redo; Fail):	

Skill Assessment 12-6A (*continued*)

Instructor Comments	
Student Signature	**Date**
Instructor Signature	**Date**

Skill Assessment 12-6B

Student Name	
SKILL	**Skill Practice: STSR Case Setup: Pouring a Sterile Solution; Filling an Asepto**
Instructions	Instructor will demonstrate skill. Practice skill set with your partner. When ready, notify instructor to schedule the check-off. Skills assessment must be completed satisfactorily by _____ (due date).
Supplies	• Half sheet or back table drape • Supplies: bowl, saline, bulb syringe, labels, and marker • Scrubs with gown and gloves on • Mask, eyewear • Circulator team member

Note: Student must perform skill independently without prompting.

Practice with Partner Date:		**Skills Testing Date:**	
PROCEDURAL STEPS			**COMMENTS**
1. Assembles equipment and supplies.	Correct	Needs Review	
2. Prepares setup for practice correctly. Opens back table drape and other needed supplies.	Correct	Needs Review	
3. Demonstrates placement of bowel to accept solutions.	Correct	Needs Review	
4. Circulator demonstrates pouring of solution into bowl correctly. Labels bowl prior to receiving solution.	Correct	Needs Review	
5. Maintains sterile technique; identifies and corrects any deviations correctly.	Correct	Needs Review	
6. Demonstrates preparation of a bulb syringe correctly.	Correct	Needs Review	
7. Guards sterile field assertively.	Correct	Needs Review	
8. Demonstrates removal of gown at end of case correctly. Demonstrates how to break back ties.	Correct	Needs Review	
9. Demonstrates removal of gloves correctly.	Correct	Needs Review	
10. Demonstrates hand washing.	Correct	Needs Review	

| **Performance Evaluation Criteria** | • Assembled all necessary supplies and equipment for skill testing. Arranged furniture for limited traffic.
• Demonstrated correctly opening of setup including back table cover and wrapped bowls and supplies.
• Demonstrated pouring of solution. Identified solution, expiration date, and patient allergies. Labeled bowl. Solution (saline) poured into bowl without possible contamination of back table drape.
• Demonstrated filling of bulb syringe correctly. Labels bulb syringe as instructed by instructor (open bulb, place label on green indentation and replace). Grasps bulb syringe similar to syringe with thumb on bulb and first two fingers on flanges. Compress bulb and stick open end into solution to draw into device. Hold upright and compress again to remove air, stick open end into solution repeatedly until completely filled. Replace in solution bowl until needed.
• Student prepared and performed procedure independently. Correctly maintained sterile technique. Identified any breaks in technique and corrected them appropriately.
• Performed each step in appropriate sequence. | **Rating**

 |
| | **Overall Rating (Satisfactory; Must Redo; Fail):** | |

Skill Assessment 12-6B (*continued*)

Instructor Comments	
Student Signature	**Date**
Instructor Signature	**Date**

Skill Assessment 12-6C

Student Name	
SKILL	**Skill Practice: STSR Case Setup: Mayo Setup with Counts**
Instructions	Instructor will demonstrate skill. Practice skill set with your partner. When ready, notify instructor to schedule the check-off. Skills assessment must be completed satisfactorily by _____ (due date).
Supplies	• Half sheet or back table drape; towels • Supplies: Mayo cover, bowl, Ray-Tec (radiographic 4 × 4) • Instrument set; other items as outlined on instructor diagram • Scrubs with gown and gloves on • Mask, eyewear • Circulator team member

Note: Student must perform skill independently without prompting.

Practice with Partner Date:		Skills Testing Date:	
PROCEDURAL STEPS			**COMMENTS**
1. Assembles equipment and supplies.	Correct	Needs Review	
2. Prepares setup for practice correctly. Opens back table drape and other needed supplies.	Correct	Needs Review	
3. Demonstrates draping of Mayo stand correctly.	Correct	Needs Review	
4. Demonstrates towel preparation. Places towel on Mayo stand; secures edges. Prepares towel roll.	Correct	Needs Review	
5. Demonstrates minor instrumentation setup on Mayo as previously diagrammed by instructor.	Correct	Needs Review	
6. Demonstrates counting of Ray-Tec and instruments correctly.	Correct	Needs Review	
7. Maintains sterile technique; identifies and corrects any deviations correctly.	Correct	Needs Review	
8. Guards sterile field assertively.	Correct	Needs Review	
9. Demonstrates removal of gown at end of case correctly. Demonstrates how to break back ties.	Correct	Needs Review	
10. Demonstrates removal of gloves correctly.	Correct	Needs Review	
11. Demonstrates hand washing.	Correct	Needs Review	

| **Performance Evaluation Criteria** | • Assembled all necessary supplies and equipment for skill testing. Arranged furniture for limited traffic.
• Demonstrated removal of instrument set from sterilization packaging. Waited for circulator to indicate wrapper or container is dry, seal was intact, with no breaks in integrity.
• Demonstrated application of Mayo stand cover correctly. Orient Mayo cover; insert hands and open Mayo cover opening while securing folded edges; approach Mayo stand and grasp Mayo stand in the opening; step on the foot rest on side away from back table; slide Mayo cover onto Mayo stand; allow the Mayo cover to unfold as you slide it on. Secure the Mayo cover onto the Mayo stand to keep taut. Does not allow Mayo cover to drop below waist level. | **Rating**

 |

Skill Assessment 12-6C (*continued*)

• Demonstrated placement of towels correctly. Prepares an instrument towel roll that is firm and relevant to the size needed. Places the towel roll on mayo stand appropriately for setup as instructed.	
• Demonstrated counting of the Ray-Tec and instrument tray correctly.	
• Demonstrated instrument Mayo and back table setup as diagramed by instructor. Removed instrument set from container or wrapper correctly, places on back table after cleared by circulator. Inspected instruments for functionality and cleanliness as placed on setup. Practiced setup placement; moved items once into place.	
• Student prepared and performed procedure independently. Correctly maintained sterile technique. Identified any breaks in technique and corrected them appropriately.	
• Performed each step in appropriate sequence.	
Overall Rating (Satisfactory; Must Redo; Fail):	

Instructor Comments	

Student Signature	**Date**
Instructor Signature	**Date**

Skill Assessment 12-7

Student Name	
SKILL	**Preoperative Case Setup—Simulated Case**
Instructions	Instructor will demonstrate skill. Practice skill set with your partner. When ready, notify instructor to schedule check-off. Skills assessment must be completed satisfactorily by _____ (due date).
Supplies	• Gown and glove setup · • Drape pack and instrument set · • Other items peel packed or wrapped as identified on preference card · • Instrument set · • Breast biopsy or other simple simulation device · • Preference card

Note: Student must perform skill independently without prompting.

Practice with Partner Date:		Skills Testing Date:	
PROCEDURAL STEPS			**COMMENTS**
1. Researches case; describes instruments needed for case and major steps of procedure as outlined in textbook (incision, hemostasis, dissection, etc.).	Correct	Needs Review	
2. Washes hands; prepares room furniture for case.	Correct	Needs Review	
3. Assembles equipment and supplies using preference card. Prepares packs with all items needed.	Correct	Needs Review	
4. Demonstrates opening of sterile supplies. Opens back table drape and other needed supplies.	Correct	Needs Review	
5. Demonstrates surgical scrub, gown, and glove correctly.	Correct	Needs Review	
6. Demonstrates acceptance of sterile items from circulator correctly (instrument set, blade for scalpel, solutions).	Correct	Needs Review	
7. Demonstrates initial counts of sponges, suture, and instruments as per local policy once all items on field.	Correct	Needs Review	
8. Demonstrates draping of Mayo stand correctly.	Correct	Needs Review	
9. Demonstrate preparation of draping supplies and basin set correctly.	Correct	Needs Review	
10. Demonstrates minor instrumentation setup on Mayo as previously diagrammed by instructor.	Correct	Needs Review	
11. Demonstrates preparation of setup in a timely manner (less than 20 minutes).	Correct	Needs Review	
12. Maintains sterile technique; identifies and corrects any deviations correctly. Positions items to maintain sterile field close together and away from traffic.	Correct	Needs Review	
13. Guards sterile field assertively.	Correct	Needs Review	

Skill Assessment 12-7 (*continued*)

		Rating
Performance Evaluation Criteria	• Assembled all necessary supplies and equipment for skill testing. Arranged furniture for limited traffic.	
	• Demonstrated understanding of usual case sequence; able to identify a typical opening sequence, the procedure to be completed, and then the typical closing sequence and the instruments to pass for each task.	
	• Demonstrated ability to open sterile supplies utilizing the principles of sterile technique. Correctly maintained sterile technique. Identified any breaks in technique and corrected them appropriately.	
	• Demonstrated ability to perform the surgical scrub, gown and glove technique for the STSR correctly.	
	• Demonstrated ability to accept items from the circulator correctly including instrument set, blades, and solutions. Waited for verification instruments to dry; labeled all solutions; took blades using instrument.	
	• Demonstrated ability to count items correctly. Began with sponges (kitners, Ray-Tec 4 × 4, and lap sponges); sharps (suture, blades, hypodermic needles, etc.); instruments (as per local policy); other items small enough to fit into incision. Counted out loud with visual and verbal confirmation from circulator. Separated items completely so there is no chance of confusion or mistake.	
	• Demonstrated ability to drape the Mayo stand correctly. Faced sterile field; kept Mayo cover above waist level.	
	• Demonstrated instrument Mayo and back table setup as diagrammed by instructor. Inspected instruments for functionality and cleanliness as placed on setup. Practiced setup placement—moved items once into place when possible but not more than three times to the final place.	
	• Student prepared and performed procedure independently.	
	• Performed each step in appropriate sequence.	
	Overall Rating (Satisfactory; Must Redo; Fail):	

Case Prep: Student Diagram of Case Setup Planned

Mayo Stand

Back Table Setup

Basin Setup

Case Sequence	Opening Sequence	Steps	Instruments to pass for each step:
	Procedure	Steps	Instruments to pass for each step:
	Closing Sequence	Steps	Instruments to pass for each step:

Instructor Comments	

Student Signature	**Date**
Instructor Signature	**Date**

Skill Assessment 12-8

Student Name	
SKILL	**Skill Practice—Preoperative Case—Draping—Simulated Case—Segment 2**
Instructions	Instructor will demonstrate skill. Practice skill set with your partner. When ready, notify instructor to schedule the check-off. Skills assessment must be completed satisfactorily by _____ (due date).
Supplies	• Gown and glove setup for setup • Drape pack and instrument set • Other items peel packed or wrapped as identified on preference card • Instrument set • Breast biopsy or other simple simulation device • Preference card

Note: Student must perform skill independently without prompting.

Practice with Partner Date:		Skills Testing Date:		
PROCEDURAL STEPS				**COMMENTS**
1. Prepares draping supplies in correct order.	Correct	Needs Review		
2. Demonstrates correct assisted gowning, gloving for "surgeon."	Correct	Needs Review		
3. Demonstrates correct passing of towels for squaring off. Passes towel clips.	Correct	Needs Review		
4. Demonstrates correct presentation of drape to surgeon.	Correct	Needs Review		
5. Demonstrates application of drape correctly.	Correct	Needs Review		
6. Demonstrates correct placement of "doctor's tools" for surgeon to begin placement of light handles, ESU active electrode, and suction. Establishes neutral zone as per local policy.	Correct	Needs Review		
7. Demonstrates correct placement of Mayo stand, ring stand as needed, and back table.	Correct	Needs Review		
8. Demonstrates assistance with field preparation. Assists surgeon with tools not already placed, places two sponges in place to begin procedure. Ensures saline is on field and bulb syringe filled.	Correct	Needs Review		
9. Participates in "time-out" to verify surgical site and prevent wrong-site surgery.	Correct	Needs Review		
10. Maintains sterile technique; identifies and corrects any deviations correctly. Positions items to maintain sterile field as close together and away from traffic.	Correct	Needs Review		
11. Guards sterile field assertively.	Correct	Needs Review		

Skill Assessment 12-8 (*continued*)

		Rating
Performance Evaluation Criteria	• Demonstrated preparation of draping supplies correctly. (Prepared "doctor's tools"—towel with ESU active electrode, suction, light handles × 2, ESU scraper and holder. Placed drape, then four towels prepared correctly, opened surgeon's gloves, gown, drying towel. Ensured item used to secure squaring off towels such as towel clips, adhesive drape, etc., is ready.)	
	• Demonstrated assisted gowning and gloving technique correctly: Opened and presented towel to team member; cuffed to prevent contamination. Opened gown with sterile side facing self and openings for arms visible to team member; cuff over hands at shoulders; pushed gown onto team member's upper arms. Opened right glove, cuff over fingertips, spread fingers for visible hole, released as team member's hand entered and cuff is covered. Opened left glove, hooked over team member's extended right fingertips, pulled to open hole, released when team member's hand entered and cuff was covered. Grasped tag presented to STSR by team member; held securely as team member turned; team member pulled the tag from tag holder.	
	• Demonstrated passing of towels correctly. Towels prepared with 2" cuff, passed so first towel is placed with fold down on side of operative site immediately in front of surgeon; second and third towel placed with cuff down inferior and superior to wound, fourth towel is placed on opposite side of operative site. Passed device to secure towels such as towel clips or adhesive drape.	
	• Demonstrated placement of basic laparotomy drape correctly. Asked if surgeon wants adhesive strip covers off. Prepared drape correctly for style (head with arm board covers oriented correctly). Offered drape at the appropriate height compactly folded. As drape was placed with fenestration over operative site and unfolded, accepted drape and maintained hands on top, cuffed hands to prevent contamination, did not pull against surgeon or shift drape—maintained drape fenestration in original placement.	
	• Demonstrated placement of suction, ESU active electrode/holder, ESU scrapper, 2 sponges, and suction correctly. Secured items with nonperforating clamps/towel clips. Established neutral zone as per local policy.	
	• Demonstrated placement of sterile furniture correctly. Mayo foot pedal accessible to STSR, back table angled to eliminate turning back to surgical site, and basin with water accessible to keep instruments clean during surgical procedure. Ensured saline is labeled and received; bulb syringe labeled and loaded.	
	• Initiated "time-out" verification of surgical site, procedure, allergies, and patient.	
	• Demonstrated ability to maintain sterile technique. Identified any breaks in technique and corrected them appropriately.	
	• Student prepared and performed procedure independently.	
	• Performed each step in appropriate sequence.	
	Overall Rating (Satisfactory; Must Redo; Fail):	
Instructor Comments		
	Student Signature	**Date**
	Instructor Signature	**Date**

Skill Assessment 12-9

Student Name			
SKILL	**Skill Practice—Intraoperative Case Management—Simulated Case—Segment 4**		
Instructions	Instructor will demonstrate skill. Practice skill set with your partner. When ready, notify instructor to schedule skills assessment check-off. Skills assessment must be completed satisfactorily by _____ (due date).		
Supplies	• Gown and glove setup for setup • Drape pack and instrument set • Other items peel packed or wrapped as identified on preference card • Instrument set • Breast biopsy or other simple simulation device • Preference card		

Note: Student must perform skill independently without prompting.

Practice with Partner Date:	**Skills Testing Date:**		
PROCEDURAL STEPS			**COMMENTS**
1. Passes local medication correctly as needed.	Correct	Needs Review	
2. Passes scalpel correctly. According to surgeon technique may ask for skin marker first.	Correct	Needs Review	
3. Anticipates hemostasis needs by preparing to pass ESU active electrode or hemostats and ties as necessary.	Correct	Needs Review	
4. Anticipates dissection needs by preparing to pass Metzenbaum scissors and tissue forceps.	Correct	Needs Review	
5. Anticipates retraction needs by having appropriate-sized hand retractor to retract adipose layers and muscle layers as needed. Passes self-retaining retractor once all layers are exposed.	Correct	Needs Review	
6. Anticipates needs of procedure. Ensures Mayo is prepared with all anticipated instruments for procedure.	Correct	Needs Review	
7. Anticipates needs at end of procedure signifying closing segment. Ensures suction and irrigation are ready; passes hemostasis instrumentation (stick tie) or supplies as necessary.	Correct	Needs Review	
8. Anticipates needs as the layers of the wound are closed. Passes suture on needle holder and pickups correctly.	Correct	Needs Review	
9. Completes closing count(s) correctly.	Correct	Needs Review	
10. Applies dressing correctly.	Correct	Needs Review	
11. Identifies all instruments correctly.	Correct	Needs Review	
12. Passes instruments correctly for type of instrument. Elicits grasp reflex from surgeon.	Correct	Needs Review	
13. Anticipates associations correctly. Passes pickups with scissors and suture. If vessel seen passes hemostats × 2 scissors, and ties then suture scissors; or hemoclips × 2 and scissors.	Correct	Needs Review	

Skill Assessment 12-9 (*continued*)

	14. Maintains sterile technique; identifies and corrects any deviations correctly. Positions items to maintain sterile field as close together and away from traffic.	Correct	Needs Review	
	15. Guards sterile field assertively.	Correct	Needs Review	

		Rating
Performance Evaluation Criteria	• Demonstrated passing of medications correctly. Stated when passing, protected tip, monitored amount given, notified circulator at end of case amount given, recapped using scoop and pop technique or syringe/needle holding devices.	
	• Demonstrated passing of scalpel correctly according to local policy. Neutral zone no-hands technique or pencil-style passing.	
	• Demonstrated understanding of opening sequence. Described the opening sequence with usual instrumentation passed: incision, hemostasis, dissection, and retraction	
	• Demonstrated understanding of procedure sequence. All needed instrumentation for procedure placed on the Mayo stand during setup.	
	• Demonstrated understanding of closing sequence. Described the sequence of closing including establishing hemostasis, irrigation of wound (solution to pollution is dilution), closure of wound layers, counts, and dressing application.	
	• Demonstrated counting procedure for closing counts correctly. Began count at surgical site, Mayo stand, back table, and then Mayo. Described what to do for incorrect counts (notify surgeon, recount, search room, X-ray). Needle box and kick bucket used appropriately during procedure to maintain order for counted items.	
	• Demonstrated correct application of dressing as ordered on preference card. Cleaned site, applied dressing material, covered dressing with clean towel or lap sponge. Prepared for removal of drapes.	
	• Demonstrated knowledge of all instrumentation. Correctly identified all instruments. Responded appropriately to hand signals during surgical procedure.	
	• Demonstrated correct passing technique for each surgical instrument used during procedure. Forceps, ringed instruments, needle holders with suture, etc. No hand contact as instrument passed to distract surgeon. Ends of suture controlled appropriately.	
	• Demonstrated anticipation abilities for vessels seen (clamp, clamp, cut/Metz, tie, suture scissors), if suture passed, anticipates suture scissors needed next, passes pickups with scissors and suture.	
	• Demonstrated ability to maintain sterile technique. Identified any breaks in technique and corrected them appropriately.	
	• Student prepared and performed procedure independently.	
	• Performed each step in appropriate sequence.	
	Overall Rating (Satisfactory; Must Redo; Fail):	
Instructor Comments		

Student Signature	*Date*	
Instructor Signature	*Date*	

Skill Assessment 12-10

Student Name	
SKILL	**Skill Practice—Postoperative Procedure—Simulated Case—Segment 5**
Instructions	Instructor will demonstrate skill. Practice skill set with your partner. When ready, notify instructor to schedule the check-off. Skills assessment must be completed satisfactorily by _____ (due date).
Supplies	• Gown and glove setup for setup • Drape pack and instrument set • Other items peel packed or wrapped as identified on preference card • Instrument set • Breast biopsy or other simple simulation device • Preference card

Note: Student must perform skill independently without prompting.

Practice with Partner Date:		Skills Testing Date:		
PROCEDURAL STEPS				**COMMENTS**
1. Maintains sterile field until patient is removed from OR.	Correct	Needs Review		
2. Demonstrates assistance with drape removal as per local policy. Ensures dressing is protected during removal and all instruments accounted for.	Correct	Needs Review		
3. Demonstrates assistance with patient care as needed. Ensures specimen is accounted for and cared for. Assists with transfer of patient to stretcher as needed.	Correct	Needs Review		
4. Demonstrates safe breakdown of sterile field. Ensures all sharps are cared for properly.	Correct	Needs Review		
5. Demonstrates safe care of instruments as per local policy.	Correct	Needs Review		
6. Demonstrates disposal of biohazardous wastes correctly. Maintains standard precautions correctly.	Correct	Needs Review		
7. Demonstrates removal of gown and gloves correctly.	Correct	Needs Review		
8. Demonstrates handwashing correctly.	Correct	Needs Review		
9. Transports contaminated items correctly to appropriate decontamination area as per local policy.	Correct	Needs Review		
10. Returns as appropriate for room cleanup and turnover procedure. Resets room with suction, linen, and equipment.	Correct	Needs Review		

Performance Evaluation Criteria	• Demonstrated maintenance of sterile field until patient is removed from OR. Once dressing was covered, pushed Mayo stand and back table away from setup. Ensured at least scalpel and hemostats are available along with sterile Mayo cover if emergency tracheotomy or hemorrhage occurs. Described two case examples of importance such as T&A and carotid endarterectomy. • Demonstrated assistance with drape removal as per local policy. Removed contaminated outer gloves. Ensured dressing is covered to protect dressing as drape is removed. Ensured all instruments accounted for. Cleaned around site, removed sterile protection from dressing. Assisted circulator with securing dressing.	**Rating**

Skill Assessment 12-10 (*continued*)

	• Demonstrated assistance with patient care as needed. Ensured specimen is accounted and cared for. Assisted with transfer of patient to stretcher as needed.	
	• Demonstrated safe breakdown of sterile field. Ensured all sharps separated from rest of instruments. Ensured all needles accounted for and disposed of properly.	
	• Demonstrated safe care of instruments as per local policy. Soaked in water or enzyme solution in covered container or transport cart system.	
	• Demonstrated disposal of biohazardous wastes correctly. Maintained standard precautions correctly. Saline, suction, contaminated disposables, and linen.	
	• Demonstrated removal of gown and gloves correctly.	
	• Demonstrated safe infection control techniques for room turnover and setup. Demonstrated handwashing technique correctly.	
	• Student prepared and performed procedure independently.	
	• Performed each step in appropriate sequence.	
	Overall Rating (Satisfactory; Must Redo; Fail):	
Instructor Comments		

Student Signature	Date
Instructor Signature	Date

Skill Assessment 12-11

Student Name	
SKILL	**Skill Practice—Vital Signs**
Instructions	Instructor will demonstrate skill. Practice skill set with your partner. When ready, notify instructor to schedule check-off. Skills assessment must be completed satisfactorily by _____ (due date).
Supplies	• Watch with second hand • Stethoscope • Paper and pen to record vital signs • Thermometer with protective • Blood pressure cuff device

Note: Student must perform skill independently without prompting.

Practice with Partner Date:		Skills Testing Date:	
PROCEDURAL STEPS			**COMMENTS**
1. Washes hands.	Correct	Needs Review	
2. Assembles supplies and equipment.	Correct	Needs Review	
3. Identifies patient, self, and explains procedure.	Correct	Needs Review	
4. Positions patient as necessary.	Correct	Needs Review	
5. Demonstrates temperature monitoring correctly.	Correct	Needs Review	
6. Identifies temperature monitoring techniques.	Correct	Needs Review	
7. Describes normal values for temperature and explain implications for variations. Hyperthermia and hypothermia.	Correct	Needs Review	
8. Demonstrates pulse monitoring correctly.	Correct	Needs Review	
9. Identifies pulse and pressure points.	Correct	Needs Review	
10. Describes normal values for pulse measurement including rate, rhythm, and volume. Defines tachycardia, bradycardia, dysrhythmia, ventricular tachycardia, ventricular fibrillation, and asystole.	Correct	Needs Review	
11. Demonstrates respiratory monitoring correctly.	Correct	Needs Review	
12. Describes respiratory rate, rhythm, and breath sounds. Defines apnea, dyspnea, orthopnea, eupnea, and Cheyne Stokes respirations.	Correct	Needs Review	
13. Demonstrates blood pressure monitoring correctly.	Correct	Needs Review	
14. Identifies methods of measuring blood pressure.	Correct	Needs Review	
15. Describes normal parameters for blood pressure and the implications of an abnormality.	Correct	Needs Review	
16. Demonstrates recording of vital signs correctly.	Correct	Needs Review	
17. Maintains infection control measures to prevent contamination of equipment. Washes hands after completion of activity.	Correct	Needs Review	

Skill Assessment 12-11 (*continued*)

		Rating
Performance Evaluation Criteria	• Demonstrated infection control measures correctly. Washed hands prior to procedure, decontaminated equipment prior to use, protected thermometer prior to use, cleaned equipment after use.	
	• Assembled all supplies and equipment needed including paper and pencil to record vital signs.	
	• Demonstrated effective patient communication. Identified self to patient, identified patient correctly, and explained procedure correctly. Patient cooperated and followed directions during procedure.	
	• Demonstrated vital signs monitoring correctly. Obtained temperature, pulse, respirations, and blood pressure correctly as validated by instructor.	
	• Demonstrated knowledge of normal parameters of vital signs. Stated correct temperature for oral 98.6°F, axillary 97.6°F, and rectal 99.6°F. Identified correct range for adult pulse: 60–80 bpm. Stated correct range for respiration 12–20 per minute. Stated normal range for blood pressure systolic <120 mm Hg and diastolic <80 mm Hg.	
	• Demonstrated knowledge of abnormal pathology. Described hyperthermia and hypothermia (temperature greater than 99.6°F or less than 97.6°F). Described tachycardia, bradycardia, dysrhythmia, ventricular tachycardia, ventricular fibrillation, and asystole. Described apnea, dyspnea, orthopnea, eupnea, and Cheyne Stokes respirations. Described hypertension and hypotension.	
	• Described methods of obtaining temperature (noninvasive touch, skin sticker, axillary, ear, and invasive oral, rectal, core (bladder or esophageal); methods of pulse measurement and arterial pressure points (radial, brachial, carotid, apical, femoral, and dorsalis pedis known as pedal pulse or posterior tibial with pressure points of temporal artery and popliteal artery), and methods of measuring blood pressure (radial or femoral invasive arterial monitoring or noninvasive monitoring listening for Korotkoff's sounds).	
	• Student prepared and performed procedure independently.	
	• Performed each step in appropriate sequence.	
	Overall Rating (Satisfactory; Must Redo; Fail):	
Instructor Comments		
	Student Signature	*Date*
	Instructor Signature	*Date*

Skill Assessment 12-12

Student Name				
SKILL	**Open Glove Technique**			
Instructions	Instructor will demonstrate skill. Practice skill set with your partner. When ready, notify instructor to schedule the check-off. Skills assessment must be completed satisfactorily by _____ (due date).			
Supplies	• Sterile gloves (appropriate size for student)			

	Note: Student must perform skill independently without prompting.			
	Practice with Partner Date:	**Skills Testing Date:**		
	PROCEDURAL STEPS			**COMMENTS**
	1. Washes hands.	Correct	Needs Review	
	2. Assembles equipment and supplies.	Correct	Needs Review	
	3. Organizes workspace for most effective ergonomics. Positions sterile setup correctly.	Correct	Needs Review	
	4. Describes situations in which open glove technique will be necessary.	Correct	Needs Review	
	5. Opens sterile glove correctly. States parameters of sterile field and examples of contamination.	Correct	Needs Review	
	6. Demonstrates glove removal of first glove correctly. States reason for picking glove straight up.	Correct	Needs Review	
	7. Demonstrates glove application of first glove correctly.	Correct	Needs Review	
	8. Demonstrates glove removal of second glove from wrapper correctly.	Correct	Needs Review	
	9. Demonstrates glove application of second glove.	Correct	Needs Review	
	10. Maintains sterile technique; identifies and corrects any deviations correctly.	Correct	Needs Review	
Performance Evaluation Criteria	• Prepared correctly for skill. Washed hands and assembled all necessary supplies for skill testing. • Discussed correctly situations in which open glove technique will be necessary. (Surgical skin prep, catheterization, removal of items from high-level disinfection, dressing changes, etc.) • Demonstrated correct opening of sterile glove setup. Height appropriate for student. Positioned glove packet on dry surface. Removes outer wrapper. Opened inner wrapper and secured open to ensure folds of wrapper do not close. Controlled wrapper ends. Stated that wrapper has a 1" or more safety margin from edge or where touched by unsterile hand. Stated that if wrapper closes back on gloves; it is contaminated (possible contamination from contact with unsterile hand and table surface). • Demonstrated correct glove removal of first glove. Selects glove; pinched in cuffed area; removes straight up and steps back to pull on. (Stated reason for picking glove straight up is to prevent dragging of gloved fingers over the 1" safety margin.)			**Rating**

Skill Assessment 12-12 (*continued*)

	• Demonstrated correct glove application of first glove. Oriented glove to pull on. Grasped edge of cuff over thumb area and pulled glove on. Touched only folded cuff of glove and kept hands above waist level.	
	• Demonstrated correct glove removal of second glove. Scooped second glove with gloved four fingers inside cuff; removed straight up and stepped back. Gloved thumb is kept well away from exposed skin.	
	• Demonstrated glove application of second glove. Oriented gloved to open hand to pull on. Pulled glove on keeping thumb well away from exposed skin. Made minor adjustments keeping sterile gloved fingers to sterile areas only.	
	• Demonstrated correct sterile technique. Correctly maintained sterile technique. Identified any breaks in technique and corrected them appropriately. (If contaminated during gloving, discarded gloves and repeated process.) Guarded sterile field assertively. (Maintained field within sight. Kept hands within sterile zone: above waist, below shoulder, and away from the face, kept hands in sight at all times.)	
	• Student prepared and performed procedure independently. • Performed each step in appropriate sequence.	
	Overall Rating (Satisfactory; Must Redo; Fail):	
Instructor Comments		
	Student Signature	*Date*
	Instructor Signature	*Date*

Skill Assessment 12-13

Student Name	
SKILL	**Urinary Catheterization (Male or Female)**
Instructions	Instructor will demonstrate skill. Practice skill set with your partner. When ready, notify instructor to schedule check-off. Skills assessment must be completed satisfactorily by _____ (due date).
Supplies	• Sterile gloves (appropriate size for student) • Catheterization mannequin • Catheterization kit (sterile drape, gloves, lubricant, antiseptic, Foley catheter usually 14 or 16 French, 10 cc water, drainage bag) • Tape • Trash receptacle for discarded sponges

Note: Student must perform skill independently without prompting.

Practice with Partner Date: **Skills Testing Date:**

PROCEDURAL STEPS			COMMENTS
1. Washes hands.	Correct	Needs Review	
2. Assembles equipment and supplies.	Correct	Needs Review	
3. Organizes workspace for most effective ergonomics. Positions sterile setup correctly.	Correct	Needs Review	
4. Describes knowledge of urinary catheterization. Defines urinary catheterization. States purpose or indications for urinary catheterization. Discusses appropriate size. Describes the difference between straight catheterization and retention catheterization. States reason for water in balloon.	Correct	Needs Review	
5. Demonstrates correct patient care. Identifies self, patient, allergies, and explains procedure. Positions patient correctly for male or female. Positions light for adequate visualization. Protects privacy.	Correct	Needs Review	
6. Opens sterile catheterization kit correctly.	Correct	Needs Review	
7. Demonstrates open glove technique correctly.	Correct	Needs Review	
8. Demonstrates draping of the patient correctly.	Correct	Needs Review	
9. Demonstrates preparation of supplies correctly. Organizes supplies, pretests balloon, prepares lubrication and prep solutions.	Correct	Needs Review	
10. Demonstrates cleansing of urethral meatus correctly. Describes difference for male and female correctly.	Correct	Needs Review	
11. Demonstrates catheter insertion correctly. Describes difference for male or female correctly. States what to do if resistance is encountered. Inflates balloon correctly.	Correct	Needs Review	
12. Demonstrates postprocedure patient care correctly. Secures catheter correctly. Secures drainage bag appropriately for situation. Repositions patient.	Correct	Needs Review	
13. Disposes of setup correctly. Washes hands.	Correct	Needs Review	

Skill Assessment 12-13 (*continued*)

	14. Documents procedure correctly.	Correct	Needs Review	
	15. Maintains sterile technique; identifies and corrects any deviations correctly.	Correct	Needs Review	

		Rating
Performance Evaluation Criteria	• Prepared correctly for skill. Washed hands and assembled all necessary supplies for skill testing.	
	• Demonstrated knowledge of urinary catheterization and genitourinary anatomy. Discussed correctly indications for urinary catheterization will be needed (decompression, drainage, irrigation, control of bleeding). Discussed appropriate size. Described difference in straight catheterization (using Robinson catheter) and retention catheterization (inflation of balloon for continuous drainage). Described reason for water for inflation to prevent compromise of balloon integrity.	
	• Demonstrated patient care correctly. Identified and explained correctly. Checked for allergies to antiseptics or latex. Positioned patient supine for male or frog-legged for female.	
	• Demonstrated correct opening of sterile setup. Height appropriate for student. Opened away from self first, toward self last.	
	• Demonstrated correct draping of patient. Discussed differences for male or female.	
	• Female—placed bottom drape under buttocks—touched only area to come in contact with patient's buttocks. Maintained center sterile. Placed fenestrated drape over perineum visualizing labia.	
	• Male—placed fenestration over penis. Bottom drape can be placed over thighs to extend sterile area as needed.	
	• Demonstrated correct preparation of supplies. Prepared antiseptic, K-Y jelly/lubricant, tested balloon. Attached drainage bag. Left syringe attached to Foley balloon port.	
	• Demonstrated correct cleansing of urethral meatus.	
	• Female—retracted labia with nondominant hand, exposing urethral meatus. Hand remained in place for all of procedure. Used at least three sponges from clitoris toward anus on each side of urethral meatus and once down middle to prep entire labia minora. Discarded each one in trash.	
	• Male—grasped shaft of penis with nondominant hand (hand remained in place). Retracted foreskin during cleansing and replaced when completed. Used sponges and started at urethral meatus and cleansed in circular motion entire glans penis. Discarded used sponge in trash.	
	• Demonstrated correct insertion of catheter. Grasped about 2 inches from tip, controlled catheter to prevent accidental contamination. Lubricated tip with K-Y Jelly.	
	• Female—inserted tip slowly until urine was flowing, then advanced another 2 inches. Inflated 5-cc balloon with 10 cc water. If any balloon resistance felt, stopped, withdrew fluid, and advanced catheter further (may be in bladder neck). Once balloon was inflated, pulled back slightly until resistance felt to move catheter balloon to neck of the bladder. If no urine was seen, removed and inspected perineum (possible vagina insertion). Replaced catheter and catheterized correct meatus. If still unable to catheterize, notified surgeon.	
	• Male—inserted catheter approximately 7–9 inches until urine was flowing, then advanced another 2 inches and inflated 5-cc balloon with 10 cc water. Once balloon was inflated, pulled back slightly until resistance felt to move catheter balloon to neck of the bladder. If resistance felt during insertion (prostate usually), withdrew slightly and advanced again slowly. If resistance still felt, withdraws and notifies surgeon. (Obtains Coude Foley prn.)	

Skill Assessment 12-13 (*continued*)

	• Demonstrated correct securing of catheter. Ensured Foley catheter was attached securely to drainage bag. Drainage bag was kept below level of bladder to prevent reflux (contamination). If raised above level of bladder, tubing was kinked to prevent reflux into bladder. During surgery, tubing usually placed under leg with padding (small towel over tubing to prevent pressure) and bag placed so anesthesia can view. Catheter may be taped to patient's thigh if transported postop with catheter.	
	• Demonstrated correct sterile technique. Correctly maintained sterile technique. Identified any breaks in technique and corrected them appropriately. Guarded sterile field assertively. Maintains sterility of catheter during preparation and insertion. Used sponges not placed back on sterile field.	
	• Student prepared and performed procedure independently.	
	• Performed each step in appropriate sequence.	
	Overall Rating (Satisfactory; Must Redo; Fail):	
Instructor Comments		
	Student Signature	**Date**
	Instructor Signature	**Date**

Skill Assessment 12-14

Student Name	
SKILL	**Surgical Skin Prep**
Instructions	Instructor will demonstrate skill. Practice skill set with your partner. When ready, notify instructor to schedule check-off. Skills assessment must be completed satisfactorily by _____ (due date).
Supplies	• Sterile gloves (appropriate size for student) • Skin prep kit (basin × 2, cotton tip applications, sponges, sterile towels × 2, gloves, antiseptic, forceps if 4 × 4 used) • Mannequin protected for solution • Trash receptacle for discarded sponges • Unsterile towels

Note: Student must perform skill independently without prompting.

Practice with Partner Date:		Skills Testing Date:	
PROCEDURAL STEPS			**COMMENTS**
1. Washes hands.	Correct	Needs Review	
2. Assembles equipment and supplies.	Correct	Needs Review	
3. Organizes workspace for most effective ergonomics. Positions sterile setup correctly.	Correct	Needs Review	
4. Describes knowledge of skin prep. States purposes for skin prep. Discusses antiseptics and precautions for each. Discusses possible complications and prevention techniques.	Correct	Needs Review	
5. Demonstrates correct patient care. Identifies self, patient, allergies, and explains procedure (for awake patients). Positions patient correctly. Protects privacy. Limits exposure to prevent excessive heat loss. Positions light for adequate visualization. Applies unsterile towels to limit pooling. Ensures ESU or EKG pads are protected.	Correct	Needs Review	
6. Inspects skin. Notifies surgeon of any "infections." Removes any gross soil, adhesives, or oils correctly. Discusses hair removal considerations. Discusses skin marking.	Correct	Needs Review	
7. Opens sterile supplies/skin prep kit correctly.	Correct	Needs Review	
8. Demonstrates open glove technique correctly.	Correct	Needs Review	
9. Demonstrates draping of the patient correctly.	Correct	Needs Review	
10. Demonstrates preparation of supplies correctly. Organizes supplies and prepares prep solutions.	Correct	Needs Review	
11. Demonstrates cleansing of surgical site and surrounding areas correctly. Describes difference for contaminated areas correctly.	Correct	Needs Review	
12. Demonstrates blotting correctly. Removes scrub solution for Betadine correctly.	Correct	Needs Review	
13. Demonstrates postprocedure patient care correctly. Removes towels correctly.	Correct	Needs Review	
14. Disposes of setup correctly. Washes hands.	Correct	Needs Review	
15. Documents procedure correctly.	Correct	Needs Review	
16. Maintains sterile technique; identifies and corrects any deviations correctly.	Correct	Needs Review	

Skill Assessment 12-14 (*continued*)

		Rating
Performance Evaluation Criteria	• Prepared correctly for skill. Washed hands and assembled all necessary supplies for skill testing.	
	• Demonstrated knowledge of surgical skin prep. Discussed correctly purpose(s): remove transient organisms, reduce resident organisms. Discussed appropriate antiseptics and precautions for each: Iodophors/Betadine—check for allergies to iodine/shellfish and deactivated by blood; Chlorhexidine gluconate—ototoxic, no eyes or mucous membrane contact with residual effects and not deactivated by blood; alcohol—flammable; combination Betadine/alcohol or chlorhexidine/alcohol solutions have precautions of both components. Discussed possible complication includes chemical irritation or EXU or laser burns. Prevention is to limit pooling of chemicals and allow any flammable solutions to completely dry prior to drape application.	
	• Demonstrated patient care correctly. Identified and explained correctly. Checked for allergies to antiseptics or latex. Positioned patient correctly for surgical procedure and prep indicated. Limited exposure; utilized blankets to conserve heat. Applied unsterile towels correctly to limit pooling. Ensured ESU dispersive pad and EKG pads are protected from surgical solutions.	
	• Demonstrated correct inspection of surgical site. Discussed hair removal—preferred method of clippers if absolutely necessary (no hair removal is best). Discussed skin inspection for infections, open lesions, adhesives, or gross soil. Discussed mechanisms to remove with degreaser, adhesive remover, soap and water, etc., as necessary. Discussed situations when surgeon will premark the skin in preoperative holding and prep should not remove skin markings.	
	• Demonstrated correct opening of sterile setup. Height appropriate for student. Opened away from self first, toward self last.	
	• Demonstrated correct preparation of supplies. Organized setup and antiseptics correctly.	
	• Demonstrated correct draping of patient. Sterile towels placed to demarcate area of prep and absorb solutions.	
	• Demonstrated correct cleansing of surgical site and surrounding areas.	
	• Described difference for contaminated areas correctly. (Umbilicus, groin, axilla, skin folds, stomas, etc., have a higher microbial count and are cleansed first with a separate setup or last.) Umbilicus is prepped using cotton tip applicators, which are discarded as used (first as separate prep); groin or axilla is cleansed last. (Contaminated areas can be isolated during prep withsponges soaked in antiseptic solution.)	
	• Began cleansing at superior end of the incision site and extended down the incision line then outward to the periphery in a circular motion. Discarded used sponge in trash. Hand did not come in contact with the skin during prep. If area missed, prepped with the next sponge. Did not go back from periphery toward incision.	
	• Scrubbed with scrub solutions used friction and circular motion. Paint with antiseptics—keep sponge in contact with skin from incision site outward using same circular motion. Use as many "paint sticks/applicators" as necessary to paint the contaminated areas (example: Betadine/alcohol prep solution for knee surgery may require at least two prep sticks—one begins at incision to toes and other upward to groin).	
	• Demonstrated blotting correctly. Removed scrub solution for Betadine correctly. Stated that scrub solutions contain detergents, which can interfere with wound healing and must be removed.	
	• Demonstrated postprocedure patient care correctly. Removed towels correctly without contamination.	

Skill Assessment 12-14 (*continued*)

	• Demonstrated correct sterile technique. Correctly maintained sterile technique. Identified any breaks in technique and corrected them appropriately. Guards sterile field assertively. Used sponges are not placed back on sterile field.	
	• Student prepared and performed procedure independently.	
	• Performed each step in appropriate sequence.	
	Overall Rating (Satisfactory; Must Redo; Fail):	
Instructor Comments		
	Student Signature	*Date*
	Instructor Signature	*Date*

Surgical Procedures

Diagnostic Procedures

After studying this chapter, the reader should be able to:

A 1. Apply knowledge of anatomy and physiology to determine which diagnostic examinations will be useful.

P 2. Indicate the sources of patient data.

O 3. Compare and contrast techniques used to establish the diagnosis.

4. Determine which diagnostic procedures will require surgical intervention.

5. Recognize the major indications for surgical intervention.

S 6. Demonstrate knowledge of the surgical technologist's role in caring for each specific type of specimen.

Select Key Terms

Define the following, using your textbook glossary or a medical dictionary if needed:

1. angina _____

_____

2. auscultation _____

_____

3. biopsy _____

_____

4. capnography _____

_____

5. C-arm _____

_____

6. cholangiography _____

_____

7. contrast media _____

_____

8. CSF _____

_____

9. cystoscopy _____

_____

10. ECG _____

_____

11. EEG _____

_____

12. frozen section _____

_____

13. -gram _____

_____

14. Gram stain _____

_____

15. -graph _____

_____

16. indwelling _____

_____

17. isotope scanning _____

_____

18. obstruction _____

_____

19. palpation _____

_____

20. prosthesis _____

_____

21. roentgenography _____

_____

22. sign _____

_____

23. symptom _____

_____

24. urinalysis (UA) _____

_____

25. ultrasonography _____

_____

History and Physical

1. What is considered the first step in determining the etiology of a patient's condition? Why?

   _____

   _____

2. Three types of visualization may be used by the examiner during a physical examination. Name the three types, explain how they differ, list any special equipment that may be needed for each, and give at least one example of each type.

   A. _____

   B. _____

   C. _____

3. Will pressure readings from a Swan-Ganz catheter placed in the pulmonary artery be useful in diagnosing pulmonary embolism?

   _____

4. What are the arteries that can be used to insert a Swan-Ganz pulmonary artery catheter?

   _____

   _____

Diagnostic Imaging

1. What type of examination is necessary to identify an atelectasis (collapsed lung)?

   _____

2. Identify six purposes of radiographic exams in the operating room.

   A. _____

   B. _____

   C. _____

   D. _____

   E. _____

   F. _____

3. During a portable x-ray of the surgical site, what is the duty of the surgical technician in the scrub role?

   _____

4. What piece of radiographic equipment is shown in Figure 13-1?

   _____

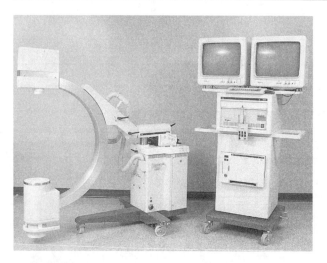

Figure 13-1

5. What is the advantage of fluoroscopy?_____

_____

_____

6. List four intraoperative applications for fluoroscopy.

A. _____

B. _____

C. _____

D. _____

7. List the steps, in order, for percutaneous placement of a femoral artery catheter using the Seldinger technique.

A. _____   E. _____

B. _____   F. _____

C. _____   G. _____

D. _____   H. _____

8. Identify the structures seen in Figure 13-2.

A. _____   D. _____

B. _____   E. _____

C. _____

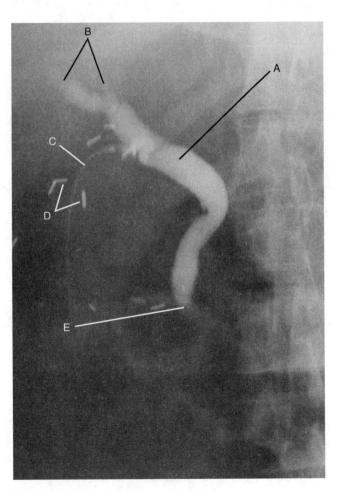

Figure 13-2

9. What type of radiography can be used to visualize the structures of the biliary tract?

_____

10. Why is contrast media used? _____

_____

11. Describe the process of shooting an intraoperative cholangiogram (IOC).

_____

_____

12. What pathologic condition(s) is/are detected with the use of cholangiography?

_____

_____

13. A bone scan is an example of what type of scan? The term "hot spot" refers to what aspect of the scan, and what condition might be indicated by its presence?

_____

_____

14. A six-month-old is scheduled to undergo a CT scan with general anesthesia. What is the most likely reason that general anesthesia will be administered?

_____

_____

15. The patient is suspected to have a spinal cord tumor. Will an MRI or a CT scan be more useful in visualizing the soft tissue tumor?

_____

_____

16. Why is ultrasonography ideal for examination of a fetus?

_____

_____

17. What is the one condition that a metaiodobenzylguanidine (MIBG) scan is useful in diagnosing?

_____

_____

18. Name the two methods of administering radiation therapy. What is the purpose of administering radiation therapy?

_____

_____

Matching

Match the type of diagnostic imaging to the usage.

_____ 19. Real-time manipulation of fractures

_____ 20. AP view with cassette in OR

_____ 21. Highlights chemical brain activity

_____ 22. Needle localization breast biopsy

_____ 23. Multidirectional soft tissue imaging

_____ 24. Useful to diagnose adrenal gland tumors

_____ 25. Detects cerebral bleeding faster

_____ 26. Useful during cardiac valve surgery

_____ 27. Clearly outlines vertebral bone structure

_____ 28. Used for planning prior to endarterectomy

A. Portable X-ray

B. Mammography

C. Fluoroscopy

D. Angiography

E. CT Scan

F. MRI

G. Myelography

H. PET Scan

I. Echocardiography

J. MBIG Scan

Laboratory Reports

1. Identify the normal lab value range for the test.

   A. Hematocrit _____

   B. WBC _____

   C. Hemoglobin (female) _____

   D. RBC (female) _____

   E. Oxygen saturation (ABG—arterial blood gas) _____

   _____

   F. pH of blood (ABG—arterial blood gas) _____

Matching: Tissue Specimens

Match the following.

_____ 2. Bullet—preserve markings

_____ 3. Fluid aspirated for examination

_____ 4. Smear slide requiring fixative

_____ 5. Most common preservative for permanent

_____ 6. Prevents desiccation (drying out)

_____ 7. Study of tissue

_____ 8. Orientation to check margins

_____ 9. No preservative—sent dry

_____ 10. Excised tissue for frozen section or permanent

_____ 11. Study of cells

A. Histology (define)

B. Cytology (define)

C. Suture marker

D. Formalin

E. Saline

F. Aspiration biopsy

G. Brush biopsy

H. Incisional biopsy

I. Calculi

J. Gloved handling only

True or False

_____ 12. The frozen section that results is considered a final diagnosis.

_____ 13. Frozen sections should be sent moistened with saline.

_____ 14. Amputated limbs are always sent to the morgue for disposal via incinerator.

_____ 15. Counted sponges are never passed off with the specimen.

_____ 16. Cerebral spinal fluid obtained from a spinal tap should not have red blood cells. Cloudy or bloody fluid can indicate a preliminary diagnosis.

_____ 17. The scrub person has a responsibility to correctly identify and ensure specimens are labeled correctly.

_____ 18. Right and left specimens are routinely placed in the same container.

_____ 19. Permanent sections are routinely placed in the preservative saline to send to the pathologist.

_____ 20. Frozen sections are sent dry for immediate review by the pathologist to determine the need for further surgery or postoperative surgery.

_____ 21. Calculi are placed in formalin to preserve their integrity.

Short Answer

22. What is the purpose of performing a Gram stain?

_____

_____

23. A "culture and sensitivity" has been ordered. The organism has been "cultured" and identified. What is determined by the "sensitivity" portion of the examination?

_____

_____

24. Which bacteria are more sensitive to the culture process and may die if too much time is taken to place the swab in the culture tube? Aerobic or anaerobic?

_____

_____

Other Studies

1. The electrical activity of the heart represents the cardiac cycle. Identify what part of the cardiac cycle A, B, and C represent. Refer to Figure 13-3.

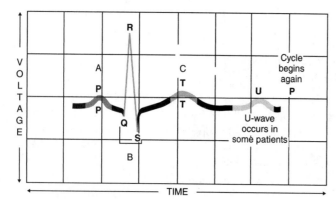

Figure 13-3

A. Represents _____

B. Represents _____

C. Represents _____

Matching

Match the test with the usage.

____	2. Useful to detect diabetic vessel abnormalities	A. Pulse oximetry
____	3. End tidal levels of carbon dioxide	B. EEG
____	4. 24-Hour monitoring of ECG	C. EMG
____	5. Noninvasive measurement of oxygen	D. Holter monitor
____	6. Display brain activity	E. Spirometry
____	7. Useful in OR to detect blood flow	F. Capnography
____	8. Useful to detect lung capacity	G. Endoscopy
____	9. Display skeletal muscle activity	H. Phleborheography
____	10. Useful to diagnose DVT (deep venous thrombosis)	I. Plethysmography DVT
____	11. View internal structures	J. Doppler sonography

Short Answer

12. Terms for further discussion: Discuss these terms with your instructor and write in the definition.

   A. Scout film:

   _____

   _____

   B. Diagnostic procedure versus a therapeutic procedure versus a palliative procedure:

   _____

   _____

   C. Invasive procedure versus noninvasive procedure:

   _____

   _____

Critical Thinking

Use your critical thinking skills to identify the appropriate answer.

13. You are cleaning up after the last routine case of the day and the phone rings in the OR suite. The surgeon is calling and states, "I have an emergency patient with a gunshot wound to the chest." It is after hours and there is only one team for the 3:00–11:00 PM shift. There is a call team available for emergencies. Which case will go next in your room? The urgent case posted to follow that was posted this morning or the new emergency case? What about the other case, what will happen to it?

   _____

Case Studies

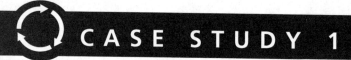

CASE STUDY 1

Pauline, a 56-year-old female, has been scheduled for a breast biopsy with needle localization and frozen section, possible modified radical mastectomy. She had a mammogram, which showed a nonpalpable mass in the upper right quadrant of her breast near the nipple.

1. What type of biopsy will Pauline most likely have?

   _____

   _____

2. During the procedure, the surgeon asks for a culture swab. What tests will be done and why?

   _____

   _____

3. The lab technician calls back to the room to report the results of the gram stain. He reports seeing milky fluid on the swab but no microorganisms seen. The surgeon continues with obtaining the specimen and sends it down for the frozen section. (1) Who will perform the frozen section? (2) What is the purpose of the frozen section? (3) How is the specimen sent to the lab? (4) How will the frozen section be processed?

   1. _____

   2. _____

   3. _____

   4. _____

4. The frozen section is returned as positive for cancer cells. The surgeon instructs the staff to prep and redrape for a mastectomy. He comments that the patient will have radiation therapy after the procedure. How does radiation kill cells?

   _____

   _____

CASE STUDY 2

Lynn has just sustained a fall off a stepladder. She fell backward, striking her head against the wall. She temporarily lost consciousness but is now awake, alert, and oriented. Lynn was transferred to the emergency department at the local hospital by ambulance with a cervical collar in place. She responds appropriately to verbal commands and is able to move all four extremities. She has a history of craniofacial fractures with stainless steel implants.

(continues)

CASE STUDY 2 *(continued)*

1. Lynn is complaining of a headache. The surgeon is concerned that her intracranial pressure may be increasing, so speed is an issue. Which diagnostic imaging test will be ordered to see if she has any intracranial bleeding? Why is an MRI not likely to be ordered for Lynn?

   _____

   _____

   _____

   _____

2. What diagnostic examination is most likely to be performed to view a vertebral bone injury prior to removal of the cervical collar? How is the amount of x-ray exposure measured?

   _____

   _____

   _____

   _____

3. What type of physician specialist will be needed to interpret the results of the diagnostic examination?

   _____

   _____

   _____

   _____

Lab 13 Diagnostic procedures

Introduction

The Diagnostic Procedures portion of this lab will give the student a better understanding of what diagnostic procedures can be performed along with the different tests and their corresponding values. Understanding what is being done and what is to be gained from learning about the diagnostics will further enhance the student understanding of the patient and what further procedures may need to be performed. This is one of those labs that should be taught right along with some of the specialties but also be brought in early. The student will have to use a lot of memorization skills to just get the basic procedures and values down. Introducing a little bit at a time over a longer period will give the students better chances for success. Add pieces each and every week until their memory catalog grows to fully encompass your expectations.

Game 1: What Are the Values?

Time involved: One week for setup

Supplies: Paper and pencil, note cards

Instructors: Playing "What Are the Values?" can be accomplished in several different ways. The largest part of learning these tests and their values is to break them down into easy pieces. Assign one test at a time (CBC, EKG, UA, etc.) and have the students learn those values. When it then comes time for the game, you will know that they have had time to digest the information. The basics of the game are for you to say a known value. The student should then be able to say if it is high, normal, or low. You can mix and match as needed or ask the students to name a value that is high, normal, or low for each of the tests and procedures. You can also ask about different tissues and which diagnostic procedures would be used for that area such as bone versus muscle or other soft tissues, and heartbeats versus brainwave activity. Setup can be a little quicker because you can use different test values that are already printed in different material. Make sure you do give the students time to study the material beforehand. Knowing that the students are learning the information here in the lab will make the classroom portion go a little quicker.

Students: On one side of a note card make a list of all the tests performed, and on the other side make a list of the values. Study these to help you better understand the values and also to see what problems occur or may occur when a value is out of sync. Study the categories of how, what, where, and when tests can be grouped or used. Making note cards can be a big help but also thinking about the how, where, when, and why a test is used will give you better options and skills on anticipating the surgeon's needs. If you know a patient has low clotting factors, you can anticipate more bleeding and possibly the need for more hemostatic agents.

Practical

a. Handling specimens—from physician

b. Handling specimens—permanent

c. Handling specimens—frozen

d. Handling specimens—fluid

Skill Assessment 13-1

Student Name	
SKILL	**Seldinger Technique**
Instructions	Instructor will demonstrate assembly. Practice procedure with your partner. When ready, notify instructor to schedule the check-off. Skills assessment must be completed satisfactorily by _____ (due date).
Supplies	• Ray-Tec • #11 blade • Needle/cannula with stylet and syringe (may simulate insertion of needle with syringe containing vascular irrigation fluid or dry or simple insertion of needle) • Guidewire • Catheter (simulation tubing smaller than vessel simulation tubing) • Syringe with needle ×2 and local anesthetic (Xylocaine ___%) • Syringe and contrast media (simulation—bottle labeled with contrast media used locally—Hypaque, Renografin, Omnipaque, ___). • Vascular irrigation solution (heparin mixed as per local facility ___ units of heparin in ___ cc of normal saline or other irrigant ___) • Labels (skin marker and blank labels/Steri-strips or preprinted labels) • Normal saline for dilution as necessary • X-ray gown (simulation = gown with word LEAD APRON) • Vessel simulation (tubing with red fluid secured to prevent rolling under a disposable towel) • Basic instrument tray (various hemostats, scissors, tissue forceps, ringed instruments appropriate to local facility)

Note: Student must perform skill independently without prompting.

Practice with Partner Date:		Skills Testing Date:		
PROCEDURAL STEPS				**COMMENTS**
1. Assembles and prepares supplies and lab for practice.		Correct	Needs Review	
2. Identifies appropriate X-ray precautions.		Correct	Needs Review	
3. Identifies correctly classification and precautions for medications: local anesthetic, heparin, and contrast media. Labels correctly. States drug, strength, and any additives when passing.		Correct	Needs Review	
4. Demonstrates adequate case preparation. Setup is organized with supplies and instrumentation in order of use.		Correct	Needs Review	
5. Demonstrates safe preparation, handling, and passing of sharps.		Correct	Needs Review	
6. Demonstrates anticipation of procedure sequence. Passes local anesthetic, knife, hemostat, needle/cannula setup, guidewire, catheter, then contrast media (if angiography simulation).		Correct	Needs Review	
7. Maintains work area neat and organized. Immediately retrieves free ends of suture and disposes in "trash bag."		Correct	Needs Review	
8. Breaks down setup and stores appropriately.		Correct	Needs Review	

Skill Assessment 13-1 (*continued*)

		Rating
Performance Evaluation Criteria	• Assembled necessary supplies and equipment. • Identified and safely passed each instrument/Asepto, which elicited grasp reflex for "surgeon." • Demonstrated safe preparation and passing of pharmacy preparations (local, contrast media, and vascular irrigation solution). • Demonstrated safe passing of sharps. • Demonstrated knowledge of Seldinger technique and medications. Anticipated correctly each step of procedure. • Demonstrated attention to detail—work area setup is completed, as instructed, and maintained in an organized, clean, and safe manner. If not, needs improvement with: _____ • Student prepared and performed procedure independently. • Performed each step in appropriate sequence.	
	Overall Rating (Satisfactory; Must Redo; Fail):	
Instructor Comments		

Student Signature	Date
Instructor Signature	Date

Skill Assessment 13-2

Student Name	
SKILL	**Intraoperative Cholangiogram Technique**
Instructions	Instructor will demonstrate assembly. Practice procedure with your partner. When ready, notify instructor to schedule the check-off. Skills assessment must be completed satisfactorily by _____ (due date).
Supplies	• Ray-Tec • Hook scissors or #11/#12 knife blade if open procedure • Cholangiogram catheter and syringe of normal saline • Syringe and contrast media (simulation—bottle labeled with contrast media used locally—Hypaque, Renografin, Omnipaque, ___). Solution prepared full strength or half and half as directed by instructor. • Labels (skin marker and blank labels/Steri-strips or preprinted labels) • Normal saline • X-ray gown (simulation = gown with word LEAD APRON); identifies safeguarding of sterile field: half sheet for portable X-ray to cover field or C-arm drape if fluoroscopy used • Hemoclip appliers or if simulated open procedure cystic duct clamp (T catheter clamp) • Cystic duct/common bile duct simulation (tubing secured to prevent rolling) • Basic instrument tray (various hemostats, scissors, tissue forceps, ringed instruments appropriate to local facility)

Note: Student must perform skill independently without prompting.

Practice with Partner Date:	Skills Testing Date:		
PROCEDURAL STEPS			**COMMENTS**
1. Assembles and prepares supplies and lab for practice.	Correct	Needs Review	
2. Identifies appropriate X-ray precautions.	Correct	Needs Review	
3. Identifies correctly classification and precautions for contrast media. Labels correctly. Prepares syringe with contrast media (no air bubbles—may look like a stone on X-ray). States drug and strength when passing.	Correct	Needs Review	
4. Demonstrates adequate case preparation. Setup is organized with supplies and instrumentation in order of use.	Correct	Needs Review	
5. Demonstrates safe preparation, handling, and passing of sharps.	Correct	Needs Review	
6. Demonstrates anticipation of procedure sequence. Passes scissors/knife, hemoclip, catheter with saline setup to check placement and possible leakage, and if secure contrast media (no air bubbles). Identifies preparation of field to safeguard sterility during X-ray as used locally.	Correct	Needs Review	

Skill Assessment 13-2 (*continued*)

	7. Identifies next step if "obstruction" visualized on field: Prepare for CBDE (common bile duct exploration) or patient will be scheduled for ERCP (endoscopic retrograde cholangiogram). CBDE needs choledochoscope, irrigation fluid, Fogarty catheter or stone basket, and T-tube with bile drainage bag postop.	Correct	Needs Review	
	8. Maintains neat and organized work area.	Correct	Needs Review	
	9. Breaks down setup and stores appropriately.	Correct	Needs Review	

		Rating
Performance Evaluation Criteria	• Assembled necessary supplies and equipment	
	• Identified and safely passed each instrument/Asepto, which elicited grasp reflex for "surgeon."	
	• Demonstrated safe preparation and passing of pharmacy preparations (local, contrast media, and vascular irrigation solution)	
	• Demonstrated safe passing of sharps.	
	• Demonstrated knowledge of Seldinger technique and medications. Anticipated correctly each step of procedure.	
	• Demonstrated attention to detail—work area is set up as instructed and maintained in an organized, clean, and safe manner. If not, needs improvement with: _____.	
	• Student prepared and performed procedure independently.	
	• Performed each step in appropriate sequence.	
	Overall Rating (Satisfactory; Must Redo; Fail):	
Instructor Comments		

Student Signature	*Date*	
Instructor Signature	*Date*	

CHAPTER 14

General Surgery

OBJECTIVES

After studying this chapter, the reader should be able to:

A 1. Recognize the relevant anatomy and physiology of the abdominal wall, digestive system, hepatic and biliary system, pancreas, spleen, thyroid, and breast.

P 2. Indicate the pathology and related terminology of each system or organ that prompts surgical intervention.

3. Evaluate preoperative diagnostic procedures and tests.

4. Indicate special preoperative preparation procedures related to general surgery procedures.

O 5. Recall the names and uses of general surgery instruments, supplies, and drugs.

6. Recall the names and uses of special equipment related to general surgery.

7. Propose the intraoperative preparations of the patient specific to the general surgery procedure.

8. Summarize the surgical steps of illustrative general surgery procedures in this chapter.

9. Identify the purpose and expected outcomes of the illustrative procedures.

10. Determine the immediate postoperative care of the patient and possible complications of the illustrative procedures.

S 11. Determine any specific variations related to the preoperative, intraoperative, and postoperative care of the general surgery patient.

Select Key Terms

Define the following, using the textbook glossary or a medical dictionary:

1. absorption _____

_____

2. anastomosis _____

_____

3. ascites _____

_____

4. bile _____

_____

5. chole- _____

_____

6. chyle _____

_____

7. chyme _____

_____

8. -cysto _____

_____

9. -docho- _____

_____

10. -ectomy _____

_____

11. excision _____

_____

12. incision _____

_____

13. lysis _____

_____

14. necrosis _____

_____

15. -oma _____

_____

16. -ostomy _____

_____

17. -otomy _____

_____

18. parietal _____

_____

19. peristalsis _____
_____

20. peritoneum _____
_____

21. portal venous system _____
_____

22. -stasis _____
_____

23. stenosis _____
_____

24. ulcer _____
_____

25. viscera _____
_____

Anatomy

Identify the nine regions and four quadrants of the abdomen as shown in Figure 14-1.

Nine Regions (Figure 14-1A):

1. _____
2. _____
3. _____
4. _____
5. _____
5. _____
7. _____
8. _____
9. _____
10. Which section contains the majority of the small intestines?
_____

Four Quadrants (Figure 14-1B):

11. _____
12. _____
13. _____
14. _____

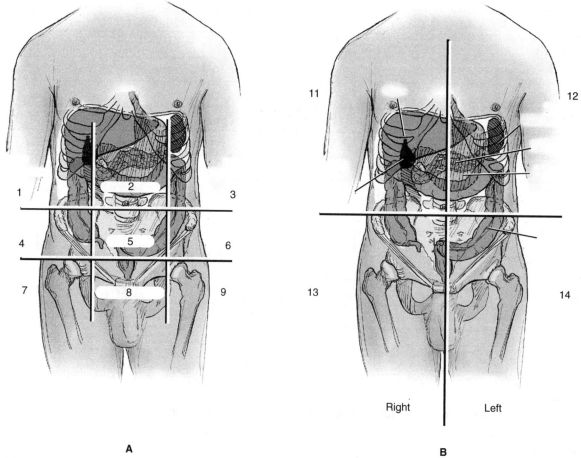

A   **B**

Figure 14-1

Matching

Using Figure 14-1, match the quadrant of the abdomen with the organ that it is located in.

_____ 15. Splenic flexure   A. RUQ

_____ 16. Appendix   B. LUQ

_____ 17. Most of stomach   C. RLQ

_____ 18. Liver   D. LLQ

_____ 19. Head of pancreas

_____ 20. Sigmoid colon

_____ 21. Tail of pancreas

_____ 22. Spleen

_____ 23. Duodenum

_____ 24. Cecum

25. Gallbladder _____

26. Left ovary _____

Short Answer

27. Linea alba literally means _____ _____ and will be found in the _____ abdominal wall.

28. Identify where the bilateral abdominocrural creases are located.

_____

29. Identify the two layers of the peritoneum.

_____

30. What is the primary function of the peritoneum?

_____

31. Identify the three regions of the retroperitoneal space and the organs that are located in each.

A. _____

_____

B. _____

_____

C. _____

_____

32. Trace the alimentary pathway by placing the following structures and segments in the correct numerical order.

A. Upper gastrointestinal tract. Use numbers 1–15.

a. ____ Uvula

b. ____ Body of stomach

c. ____ Cardia of stomach

d. ____ Cardiac sphincter

e. ____ Mouth

f. ____ Pharynx

g. ____ Duodenum (biliary tree connects here)

h. ____ Epiglottis

i. ____ Esophagus

j. ____ Fundus of stomach

k. ____ Ileum

l. ____ Pyloric sphincter

m. ____ Pylorus of stomach

n. ____ Jejunum

o. ____ Ileocecal valve

B. Lower gastrointestinal tract. Begin at the small intestine and use numbers 1–10:

a. _____ Hepatic flexure

b. _____ Anus

c. _____ Ascending colon

d. _____ Rectum

e. _____ Sigmoid colon

f. _____ Splenic flexure

g. _____ Transverse colon

h. _____ Cecum

i. _____ Descending colon

j. _____ Ileocecal valve

C. Biliary tree. Trace the flow of bile from the organ of creation to the organ of storage to area of use. Use numbers 1–10.

a. _____ Common bile duct

b. _____ Liver

c. _____ Duodenum

d. _____ Sphincter of Oddi

e. _____ Right and left hepatic ducts

f. _____ Cystic duct

g. _____ Ampulla of Vater

h. _____ Gallbladder

i. _____ Cystic duct

j. _____ Common hepatic duct

33. Identify the structures and segments of the stomach using Figure 14–2.

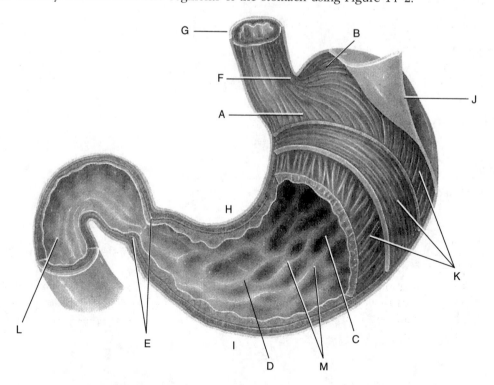

Figure 14-2

A. _____

B. _____

C. _____

D. _____

E. _____

F. _____

G. _____

H. _____

I. _____

J. _____

K. _____

L. _____

M. _____

34. Anatomy of the stomach

   A. Identify the five major segments of the stomach and the purpose of each section.

   _____

   _____

   _____

   _____

   B. The sphincter of the stomach that is labeled F is called the _____ _____ and prevents gastric reflux. The sphincter labeled E is called the _____ _____ and controls the exit of food from the stomach. The bolus of food is mixed in the stomach into a liquid substance called _____ as it exits the stomach.

   C. The shape of the stomach labeled H is the called the _____ _____ and the shape labeled I is called the _____ _____. These are important areas of innervation and blood flow.

   _____

   _____

   D. The folds of the stomach labeled M are called _____.

   E. Identify the location and purpose of the greater and lesser omentum.

   _____

   _____

35. Parasympathetic innervation to the stomach is provided by the _____ nerve. This nerve and the main left and right gastric arteries run primarily along the _____ _____ of the stomach. The left gastroepiploic artery is located primarily along the _____ _____ of the stomach.

36. The four layers of the wall of the digestive tract are the _____, _____, _____, and _____.

37. Relate each organ to the function of digestion. For information not in Chapter 14 of textbook, use your medical dictionary to fill in the blanks.

   A. The enzyme amylase secreted in the oral cavity begins digestion of the food substance _____.

   B. The enzyme pepsinogen (pepsin) secreted in the stomach begins digestion of the food substance

   _____

   C. Bile secreted in the duodenum works to emulsify the food substance _____.

   Define emulsification: _____

   _____

   D. The enzyme lipase begins digestion of the food substance

   _____

   E. The small intestine is responsible for the digestion and absorption of _____.

   F. The large intestine is responsible for absorption of _____.

   G. The movement of food through the intestines by the muscles of the alimentary canal is called _____.

38. What is the purpose of the mesentery? _____

   _____

39. Describe the typical location of the appendix. What is the purpose of the mesoappendix?

   _____

   _____

40. Identify the structures labeled in Figure 14-3.

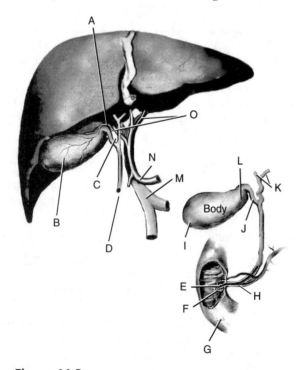

Figure 14-3

A. _____

B. _____

C. _____

D. _____

E. _____

F. _____

G. _____

H. _____

I. _____

J. _____

K. _____

L. _____

M. _____

N. _____

O. _____

41. The three segments of the gallbladder manipulated during removal include:

_____

_____

_____

42. The biliary tree outlined during an intraoperative cholangiogram may include:

_____

_____

43. What is the function of the Sphincter of Oddi?

_____

_____

44. Identify the duct(s) that transport enzymes from the pancreas to duodenum.

_____

_____

45. The pancreas is classified as both a(n) _____ and _____ gland.

46. Where are the islets of Langerhans located, and what is their function?

_____

_____

47. What is the largest parenchymal organ in the normal abdominal cavity? Identify the blood supply of this organ.

_____

_____

48. List the functions that are performed by the cells of the liver.

A. _____

B. _____

C. _____

D. _____

E. _____

F. _____

49. List the significant tissues and landmarks of the groin area.

_____

_____

_____

_____

Short Answer

50. An indirect hernia occurs at the _____ ring and may extend to the _____ ring.

51. List the structures pictured in Figure 14-4A.

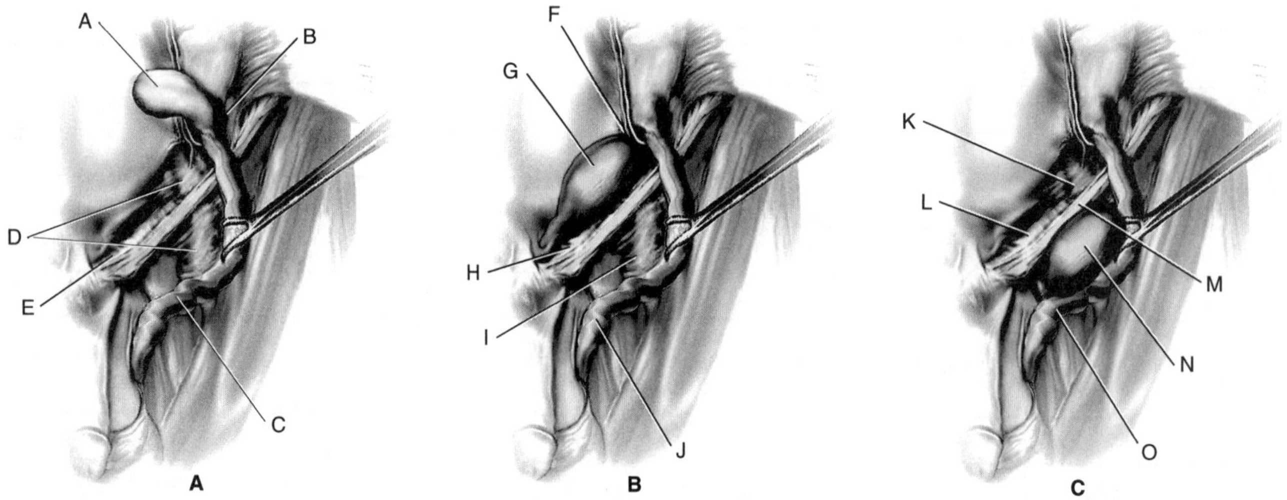

Figure 14-4

A. _____

B. _____

C. _____

D. _____

E. _____

52. A direct hernia occurs within _____

_____

53. List the structures pictured in Figure 14-4B.

F. _____

G. _____

H. _____

I. _____

J. _____

54. A femoral hernia occurs as a defect in the _____ _____.

55. List the structures pictured in Figure 14-4C.

K. _____

L. _____

M. _____

N. _____

O. _____

56. Inguinal hernias occur _____ the abdominocrural crease; femoral hernias occur

_____ the abdominocrural crease.

57. Define varicose veins:

_____

_____

58. Identify where varicose veins can occur:

_____

_____

59. Why is lymphatic drainage important in the mammary gland?

_____

_____

60. Identify the major function of the thyroid gland.

_____

_____

61. What nerve requires careful dissection during thyroid surgery?

_____

_____

62. Describe the parathyroid glands.

_____

_____

63. What happens if all parathyroid glands are removed?

_____

_____

Pathology

Match the condition with the description.

_____ 1. Sac or pouch/enlargement of intestinal wall

_____ 2. Mucosal growth considered a precursor to dysplasia

_____ 3. Telescoping of intestine within itself

_____ 4. Twisting of bowel

_____ 5. Occurs in the sacrococcygeal area with sinus formation

_____ 6. Difficulty swallowing due to motility disorder

_____ 7. Hiatal hernia causing mucosal trauma

_____ 8. Perianal abscess

_____ 9. Congenital outpouching located in the ileum

_____ 10. Chronic condition with weight loss, abscess, or bleeding

A. Dysphagia

B. Reflux disease

C. Diverticulum

D. Meckel's diverticulum

E. Crohn's disease

F. Volvulus

G. Intussception

H. Polyp

I. Pilonidal disease

J. Fistula-in-ano

Match the procedure with the condition.

_____ 11. Surgical intervention for prolonged intubation

_____ 12. Splenomegaly

_____ 13. Severely increased basal metabolic rate (BMR)

_____ 14. Elevated WBC count, rebound tenderness

_____ 15. Multicentric ductal carcinoma, male or female

_____ 16. Severe Crohn's disease

_____ 17. Cancer in the head of the pancreas removed

_____ 18. Stage I or stage II cancer without axillary node involvement

_____ 19. Laceration of the spleen

_____ 20. Defect in abdominal wall affecting structures of spermatic cord, Scarpa's fascia, cremaster muscle

A. Whipple

B. McVay repair

C. Radical mastectomy

D. Tracheostomy

E. Splenorrhaphy

F. Appendectomy

G. Right hemicolectomy

H. Splenectomy

I. Thyroidectomy

J. Mastectomy

Short Answer

21. What are the two types of choleliths, and what is the composition of each?

    A. _____

    B. _____

22. Peptic ulcers are most frequently found in which location?

    _____

    _____

23. Define hernia.

    _____

    _____

Matching

Match the type of hernia with the definition.

_____ 24. Includes both direct and indirect hernias   A. Femoral

_____ 25. Occurs usually at esophageal hiatus   B. Direct

_____ 26. A direct or indirect hernia usually in men   C. Indirect

_____ 27. Acquired defect that occurs in Hesselbach's triangle   D. Incarcerated

_____ 28. Occurs congenital or acquired due to obesity or pregnancy   E. Ventral

_____ 29. Entrapment of organs, which cannot be returned to abdomen   F. Pantaloon

_____ 30. Most common in females/may entrap lymph nodes   G. Strangulated

_____ 31. Occurs on anterior abdominal wall   H. Umbilical

_____ 32. Usually congenital along spermatic cord   I. Diaphragmatic

_____ 33. Entrapment that compromises vascularity   J. Inguinal

34. Thrombocytopenia is a deficiency of _____ in the blood.

35. Which diagnostic tools will be useful in determining liver pathology?

    _____

    _____

36. List four of the causes of varicose veins of the lower extremity.

    _____

    _____

    _____

    _____

37. Define gynecomastia, and describe the surgical treatment that may be recommended to treat the condition.

_____

_____

38. Overactivity of the thyroid gland is referred to as _____ or _____

_____

39. What is meant by the term "staging" in reference to malignant tumors?

_____

_____

Operation

Matching
Match the instrument with the usage.

_____ 1. Biopsy needle or Tru-Cut for liver biopsy

_____ 2. Maintains or enlarges size of esophagus

_____ 3. Manipulates vagus trunk during vagotomy

_____ 4. Grasps bowel such as appendix

_____ 5. Liver resection or liver laceration—
Yankauer tip

_____ 6. Direct visualization placement of umbilical port

_____ 7. Enlarges size of cystic duct and CBD

_____ 8. Decompress an engorged gallbladder

_____ 9. Used for insertion of vascular access device

_____ 10. Extends incision in vessel or duct

_____ 11. Removal of stones from duct

_____ 12. Fistula incision guide

_____ 13. Premoistened to manipulate spermatic cord/esophagus

_____ 14. Clamps for occlusion of intestines

_____ 15. Grasping hemorrhoids

A. Bakes dilator

B. Randall forceps

C. Babcock tissue forceps

D. Allen clamp

E. Probe/grooved director

F. Maloney dilators/bougie

G. Ochsner GB trocar

H. Buie Pile forceps

I. Penrose drain

J. Nerve hook

K. Franklin Silverman

L. Hasson Trocar

M. Cell saver required

N. Potts Smith scissors

O. J-shaped guidewire

Match the most likely position with the procedure.

_____ 16. Cholecystectomy

_____ 17. Esophagectomy

_____ 18. Pilonidal cystectomy

_____ 19. Herniorrhaphy or mastectomy

_____ 20. Endoscopic hernia repair

A. Supine

B. Trendelenburg

C. Reverse Trendelenburg

D. Kraske

E. Lateral

Short Answer

21. Identify the incisions in Figure 14-5.

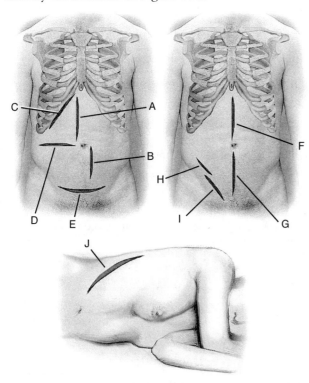

Figure 14-5

A. _____

B. _____

C. _____

D. _____

E. _____

F. _____

G. _____

H. _____

I. _____

J. _____

Matching

Match the closure device to its usage.

____ 22. Closure mucosal layer of intestinal anastomosis

____ 23. Circular GI anastomosis—check the donuts

____ 24. Used to reinforce defect (stapled or sutured in place)

____ 25. Vessel or duct closure using applier to place clip(s)

____ 26. Securely closes tissue around a catheter/inverts stump

____ 27. Closure serosal layer of intestinal anastomosis

____ 28. Single application for resection of diseased bowel

____ 29. Clamp, clamp, cut, _____ to control bleeding

____ 30. Used to reestablish negative pressure after procedure

____ 31. Liver laceration or biopsy to control bleeding

A. Mesh

B. Chest tube secured with silk

C. Pursestring stitch

D. GIA or linear stapler

E. EEA or intraluminal stapler

F. Large chromic blunt needle

G. Hemoclip or ligating clip

H. 3-0 absorbable continuous suture

I. Tie (2-0 or 3-0 ilk)

J. 3-0 Silk interrupted suture

Match the procedure with the description

____ 32. Diagnosis neuromuscular diseases

____ 33. Gastroduodenostomy (antrectomy)

____ 34. Reconstruction of gastric sphincter to release chyme

____ 35. Repair of the diaphragm and fundus wrapping

____ 36. Removal of breast, pectoralis major, and axillary nodes

____ 37. Lobectomy—careful of recurrent laryngeal nerve

____ 38. Omental wrap, stapling/suture repair

____ 39. Gastrojejunostomy (antrectomy/duodenectomy)

____ 40. Preferred method—also known as parietal cell

____ 41. Use of self-retaining Foley, Pezzer for feeding

____ 42. Obliteration of varicose veins

____ 43. Mobilization of jejunum—anastomosis/side branch

____ 44. Creation of permanent stoma for breathing

____ 45. Removal of breast tissue and axillary nodes

____ 46. Pancreaticojejunostomy with gastrojejunostomy and choledochojejunostomy

A. Whipple

B. Sclerotherapy

C. Billroth I

D. Gastrostomy

E. Splenorrhaphy

F. Tracheostomy

G. Radical mastectomy

H. Muscle biopsy

I. Billroth II

J. Thyroidectomy

K. Nissen fundoplication

L. Highly selective vagotomy

M. Roux-en-Y

N. Pyloroplasty

O. Modified radical mastectomy

Short Answer

47. Is the Maloney dilator inserted under sterile conditions? Why?

_____

_____

48. List two reasons for performing a gastrostomy.

A. _____

B. _____

49. Explain what is meant by the phrase "mobilize the bowel."

_____

_____

50. List the three basic configurations for intestinal anastomosis.

A. _____

B. _____

C. _____

51. What ligament is used as an anatomical landmark to identify the end of the duodenum and the beginning of the jejunum?

_____

52. Describe the technique used to care for instrumentation and supplies that have been exposed to the inside of the intestinal tract.

_____

_____

53. Identify the types of colon resections in Figure 14-6.

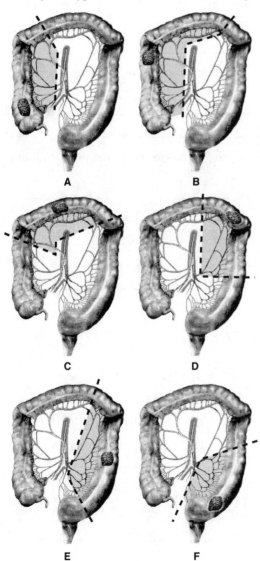

A

B

C

D

E

F

Figure 14-6

A. _____

B. _____

C. _____

D. _____

E. _____

F. _____

54. What is a stoma?

_____

_____

55. Describe the difference between an end colostomy and a loop colostomy.

_____

_____

56. What is the purpose of a T-tube? Describe stab wound placement of the drain.

_____

_____

57. Why is it important to expel all air from the cholangiogram system prior to an intraoperative cholangiogram?

_____

_____

58. What is the reason for providing a second setup to perform a breast reconstruction following a modified radical mastectomy due to a malignancy?

_____

_____

59. Why is it important for the STSR to maintain the sterile field until the patient is extubated and breathing freely following a thyroidectomy?

_____

_____

60. What instruments and supplies will be needed to enter the common bile duct for CBDE?

_____

_____

Matching

Match the incision with the procedure.

____ 61. Paramedial incision; heals stronger

____ 62. Right subcostal/Kocher

____ 63. Thoracoabdominal

____ 64. Inguinal oblique incision

____ 65. Median incision, more likely to herniated

____ 66. McBurney incision

A. Appendectomy

B. Trauma—quicker

C. Cholecystectomy

D. Esophagoduodenostomy

E. Herniorrhaphy

F. Sigmoid surgery

67. Bassini-Shouldice repair is performed to correct which condition?

_____

_____

Match the scrub precaution to the surgical procedure.

____ 68. Separation of clean and dirty; clean closure necessary

____ 69. Have extra laps ready and cell saver for immediate use

____ 70. Pass scissors with T-tube for possible alteration

____ 71. Trach tray available for possible swelling postop

____ 72. As soon as received from surgeon prepare for reuse

____ 73. No air bubbles in contrast media

____ 74. Check balloon; send obturator with patient postop

____ 75. Lubrication required for instrumentation entering orifice

____ 76. Have culture tubes ready; anaerobic to medium quickly

____ 77. Care with instruments/tissue to prevent seeding; keep sharp blade

A. Liver laceration

B. Tracheostomy

C. Bowel resection

D. Use of linear stapler

E. CBDE

F. Hemorrhoidectomy

G. Mastectomy

H. Cholecystectomy with IOC

I. Thyroidectomy

J. Appendectomy

Short Answer

78. Identify the retractors in Figure 14-7.

A. _____

B. _____

C. _____

D. _____

E. _____

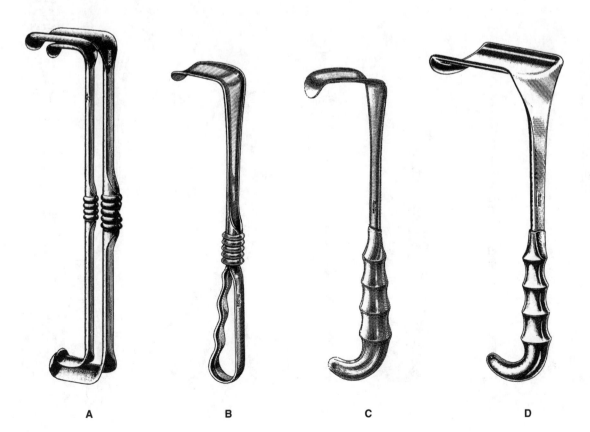

A   B   C   D

Figure 14-7

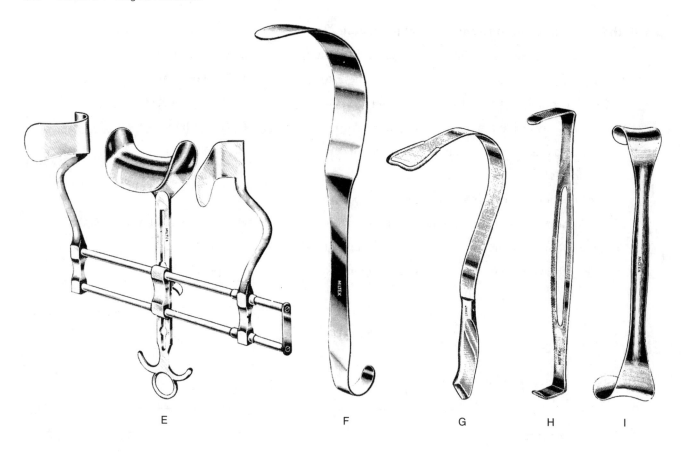

E   F   G   H   I

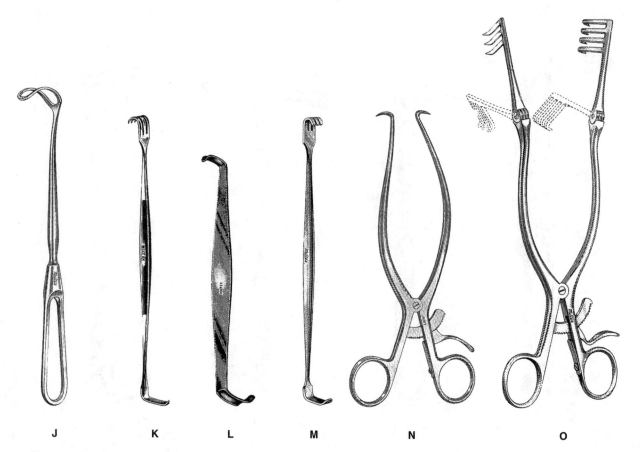

J   K   L   M   N   O

Figure 14-7 (continued)

F. _____

G. _____

H. _____

I. _____

J. _____

K. _____

L. _____

M. _____

N. _____

O. _____

79. Identify the instruments in Figure 14-8:

A. _____

B. _____

C. _____

D. _____

E. _____

F. _____

G. _____

H. _____

I. _____

J. _____

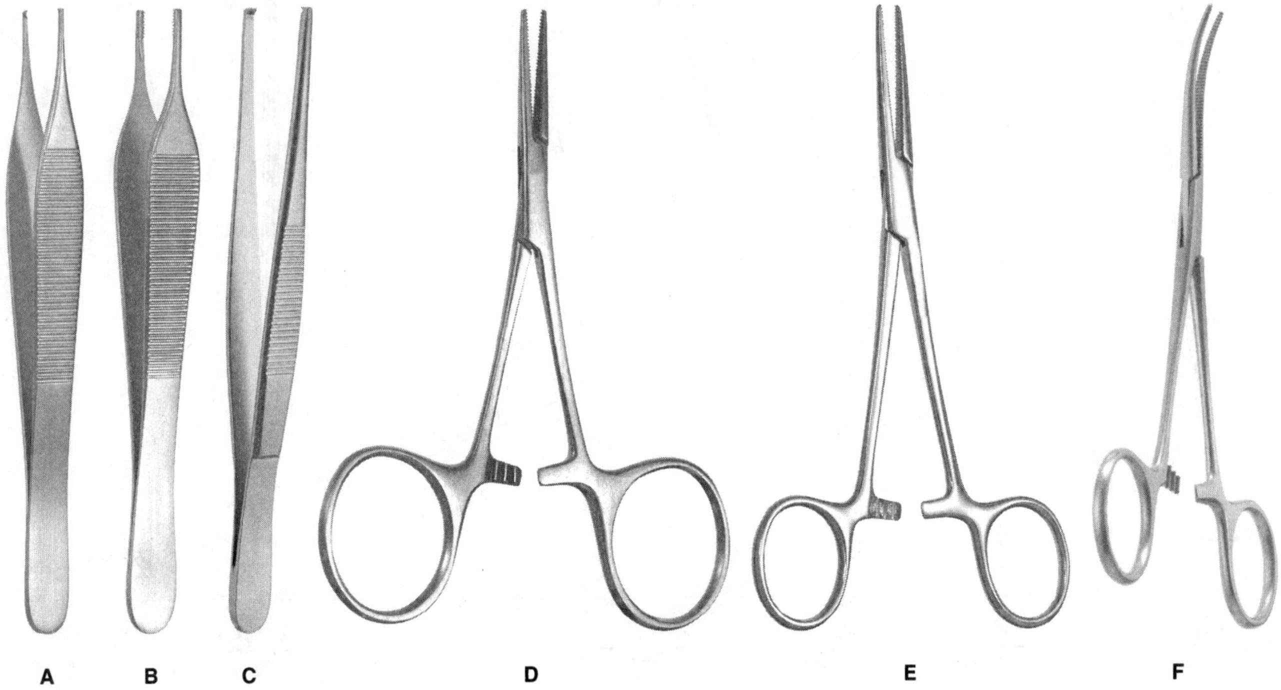

Figure 14-8

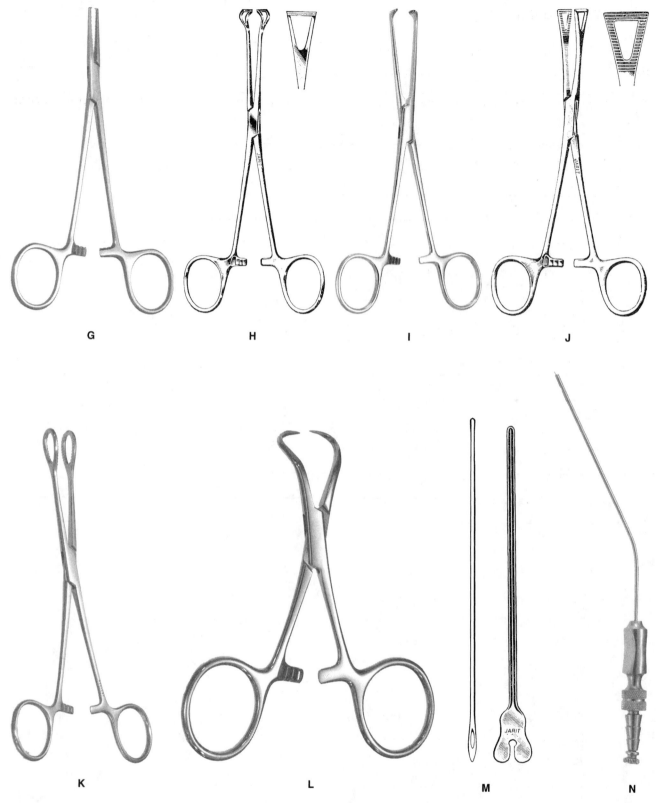

Figure 14-8 (*continued*)

K. _____

L. _____

M. _____

N. _____

Specific Variations

Student Name: _____   Date: _____

Instructor: _____

The student will be provided with basic patient information (real or simulated) and is expected to complete the following case study.

1. Procedure name: _____

   _____

   _____

2. Definition of procedure: _____

   _____

   _____

   _____

   _____

3. What is the purpose of the procedure?

   _____

   _____

   _____

   _____

4. What is the expected outcome of the procedure?

   _____

   _____

   _____

   _____

5. Patient age: _____

6. Gender: _____

7. Additional pertinent patient information: _____

   _____

   _____

   _____

8. Probable preoperative diagnosis: _____

   _____

   _____

   _____

   _____

9. How was the diagnosis determined?

   _____

   _____

_____

_____

_____

10. Discuss the relevant anatomy.

_____

_____

_____

_____

_____

_____

11. List the general and procedure-specific equipment that will be needed for the procedure.

_____

_____

_____

_____

_____

_____

12. List the general and procedure-specific instruments that will be needed for the procedure.

_____

_____

_____

_____

_____

_____

13. List the basic and procedure-specific supplies that will be needed for the procedure.

Pack _____

Basin _____

Gloves _____

Blades _____

Drapes _____

Drains _____

Dressings _____

Suture: Type of Suture, Needle (if applicable), and Anticipated Tissue Usage

_____

_____

_____

_____

_____

_____

Pharmaceuticals

_____

_____

_____

_____

Miscellaneous

_____

_____

_____

_____

_____

14. Operative preparation: _____

_____

_____

_____

_____

_____

15. What type of anesthesia will likely be used? Why?

_____

_____

_____

_____

16. List any special anesthesia equipment that may be needed.

_____

_____

_____

_____

_____

17. Patient position during the procedure: _____

_____

_____

_____

_____

18. What supplies will be necessary for positioning?

_____

_____

_____

_____

_____

19. What type of shave/skin preparation will be necessary (if any)?

_____

_____

_____

_____

20. Define the anatomic perimeters of the prep.

_____

_____

_____

_____

_____

_____

21. List the order in which the drapes will be applied, and describe any specific variations.

_____

_____

_____

_____

_____

_____

_____

22. List any practical considerations.

_____

_____

_____

_____

_____

_____

_____

23. List the procedural steps, and describe the preparatory and supportive actions of the STSR during each step (use additional space if necessary).

_____

_____

_____

_____

_____

_____

24. What is the postoperative diagnosis?

_____

_____

_____

_____

_____

_____

25. Describe the immediate postoperative care.

_____

_____

_____

_____

_____

_____

26. What is the patient's long-term prognosis?

_____

_____

_____

_____

_____

_____

27. What are the possible complications?

_____

_____

_____

_____

_____

_____

28. Comments or questions: _____

_____

_____

_____

_____

_____

29. What is the most valuable information you obtained from preparing this surgical procedure case study?

_____

_____

_____

_____

Case Studies

CASE STUDY 1

Lin Su is a 21-year-old female college student. She was admitted to the college's health center for right lower quadrant pain, nausea, and low grade fever. She was diagnosed with acute appendicitis, and surgery was scheduled.

1. Describe the causes of appendicitis. Is the appendix ever removed when appendicitis is not involved?

_____

_____

_____

2. Describe the signs and symptoms of appendicitis. Describe the significance of perforation.

_____

_____

_____

_____

3. Describe how a McBurney's incision is made for an open procedure. A laparoscopic appendectomy will require an infraumbilical incision for the Hasson trocar; where is this incision made?

_____

_____

_____

CASE STUDY 1 *(continued)*

4. Describe how the appendix/mesoappendix is ligated and how the appendiceal stump is inverted.

_____

_____

_____

_____

5. Describe what precautions you take with the instruments, lap sponges, and supplies that come in contact with the appendix.

_____

_____

_____

_____

6. The appendix was perforated; the surgeon states he is going to have this wound heal by third intention healing. He then asks for a Penrose drain. From information in previous chapters regarding wound healing, describe what this means to the patient.

_____

_____

_____

_____

CASE STUDY 2

Jon and Linda are both 41-year-old computer programmers. They are in the preoperative holding area. Each is scheduled for a hernia repair in the groin area.

1. Evaluate the chances that Jon's hernia is a femoral hernia and compare that to Linda's chance.

_____

_____

_____

_____

2. Jon's hernia is said to be incarcerated. What does this mean? Why will his case go first?

_____

_____

_____

_____

(continues)

↻ CASE STUDY 2 *(continued)*

3. If Linda has a femoral hernia, the hernia exists below what anatomical marker? The basic principle includes a repair of the defect.

_____

_____

_____

_____

4. Describe the anatomy of Hesselbach's triangle. Analyze the types of hernia. Which inguinal hernia occurs in Hesselbach's triangle? Describe the chances that Jon's hernia is this type of hernia.

_____

_____

_____

_____

5. Jon's hernia was described in the postoperative report as an indirect hernia. Is it probable that the hernia was congenital in nature? Describe how the hernia sac is removed.

_____

_____

_____

_____

6. The surgery is over and you are placing the dressing, the patient begins to wake up and does not like the endotracheal tube. You notice that his stomach is contracting and he is coughing hard. The surgeon instructs you to place some pressure on the suture line (reinforce the suture line). What do you think will happen if a stitch breaks?

_____

_____

_____

_____

CASE STUDY 3

Libby Brown is a 55-year-old female scheduled for an abdominal peritoneal resection of the colon due to a mass identified and biopsied during a routine colonoscopy. During her interview she described chronic changes in bowel elimination patterns. Her initial examination indicated a positive occult blood test.

1. Describe the position that the patient will be placed in. What type of stirrups will be utilized—C-shaped high lithotomy stirrups or Allen stirrups?

   _____

   _____

   _____

   _____

2. The surgeon is worried about the length of the surgery and asks for sequential compression devices to be placed on her legs. Describe why.

   _____

   _____

   _____

   _____

3. Describe the setup for this procedure. Why are two setups necessary? How do you set up Ray-Tec for use during this procedure?

   _____

   _____

   _____

   _____

4. During the procedure the surgeon is afraid that he has accidently injured the ureter. What diagnostic dye can be given intravenously to check for leakage intraoperatively? (Use information provided in previous chapters regarding pharmacology.)

   _____

   _____

   _____

   _____

Lab 14: General Surgery

Introduction

General surgery is one of the larger surgery specialties that you will learn. This is not to say that these are the biggest cases you will learn to do, but that these cases tend to be part of a large surgical specialty that is practiced just about everywhere from large hospitals to small surgical centers. Learning the surgery step by step in lecture will help you in the lab portion. This is where you will learn the "hands-on" of the specialty and the instruments that will be used for each piece of the surgery.

Game: General Surgery on Felt Mayo Stands

Time involved: 1–2 weeks setup.

Instructors: Make a list of instruments you expect students to know as part of the general surgery lab. Have the students trace the real instruments onto the felt if possible; if not, have them find pictures they can cut out and trace onto the felt or other material. I like felt because it tends to be durable, but paper or cardboard can be substituted. There should be no need for multiple cutouts of the same instruments if students are given the chance to show how many of those instruments they would have on the Mayo by way of a numbered marker (a piece of paper with a number designation on it). The students are given a list of surgeries that they are expected to know. **Note:** This can also be made easier if you have photos of these Mayo stand setups that the students can study.

Students: You will need several pieces of felt, paper, or cardboard. The largest piece should be cut to the size of a regular Mayo stand. The student will proceed to cut out the pieces as close to life-sized instruments as possible using felt or some other material. Label the backsides of the cutouts for easy reference.

Supplies: Felt (or paper or cardboard), real instruments, or pictures that have been printed and cut out from the computer, felt-tip marker, scissors, measuring tool

How the game is played

The students are given a list of surgeries that they are expected to know. The instructor will then assign one of those surgeries to the student in the lab. The student will then be expected to complete a Mayo stand setup utilizing the instruments they have cut out in a specified time frame. Score the students according to placement of instruments, time needed for setup, correct instrumentation, and correct number of instruments.

Practical: Set up general surgery cases

Utilizing a full lab/OR setup, assign the students to different surgical cases. Having been given a number of cases to learn, the students will then be expected to set up some of these cases under the supervision of the instructor. They should utilize as much of the OR equipment as needed including backtable, Mayo stand, ring stands, and instrument trays and pans. The student should be scored on correct placement of supplies, utilizing economy of time and motion (pick it up and place it one time), correct order of instruments, correct number of instruments, aseptic technique, time to set up, and order of use for instruments and supplies; a mock surgery should be performed so that the student can work on anticipating the needs of the surgeon.

Skill Assessment 14-1

Student Name	
SKILL	**General Surgery—Application of Clean Concept**
Instructions	Instructor will demonstrate assembly. Practice procedure with your partner. When ready, notify instructor to schedule the check-off. Skills assessment must be completed satisfactorily by _____ (due date).
Supplies	• Bowel isolation technique: ○ Items to isolate contamination: towels or lap sponges to place around the contaminated area ○ Basin or additional tray to place contaminated instruments and staplers in or on ○ Once items are used on the contaminated area, they are not returned to mayo unless you have a completely new/2nd Mayo stand to use for "clean closure" • Clean closure technique ○ Change of gown/gloves for all team members who came in contact with contaminated areas ○ Change of gown/gloves for all team members who came in contact with contaminated areas ○ Clean setup—minimal items include replacement lap sponges, suction tubing with tip, Bovie pencil, and replacement closure instruments used during the contaminated segment of procedure • Policy/guidelines handout used by local facilities or physicians regarding clean setup preferences. • Basic instrument tray (various hemostats, scissors, tissue forceps, and ringed instruments appropriate to local facility)

Note: Student must perform skill independently without prompting.

Practice with Partner Date:		Skills Testing Date:	
PROCEDURAL STEPS			**COMMENTS**
1. Assembles and prepares supplies and lab for practice.	Correct	Needs Review	
2. Identifies surgical procedures that require a separation of clean and dirty technique to prevent contamination by microbes or possible seeding of cancerous tissue.	Correct	Needs Review	
3. Identifies alternative methods of isolating "contaminated" instruments. Identifies other examples such as using sponges or instruments to contact skin (unable to sterilize) and use of skin knife for incision or extension of incision only.	Correct	Needs Review	
4. Demonstrates adequate case preparation. Setup is organized with supplies and instrumentation in order of use according to local policy/guidelines.	Correct	Needs Review	
5. Demonstrates safe preparation, handling, and passing of contaminated items.	Correct	Needs Review	

Skill Assessment 14-1 (*continued*)

	6. Demonstrates anticipation of procedure sequence to setup up closure clean setup.	Correct	Needs Review	
	7. Maintains work area neat and organized.	Correct	Needs Review	
	8. Breaks down setup and stores appropriately.	Correct	Needs Review	

		Rating
Performance Evaluation Criteria	• Assembled necessary supplies and equipment.	
	• Identified types of cases requiring isolation technique including any surgical instrumentation or supplies that come in contact with the gastrointestinal tract; vaginal tract; cancerous tissue; skin knife versus deep knife; material with microbe such as feces or purulent tissue.	
	• Demonstrated isolation of contaminated instruments and supplies as identified by local guidelines.	
	• Demonstrated safe preparation of "clean setup" for closure of surgical wound (towels for field, changing out Bovie and suction).	
	• Anticipated correctly each step of procedure.	
	• Demonstrated attention to detail—work area was set up as instructed and maintained in an organized, clean, and safe manner. If not, needs improvement with: _____	
	• Student prepared and performed procedure independently.	
	• Performed each step in appropriate sequence.	
	Overall Rating (Satisfactory; Must Redo; Fail):	
Instructor Comments		
	Student Signature	***Date***
	Instructor Signature	***Date***

CHAPTER 15

Obstetric and Gynecologic Surgery

OBJECTIVES

After studying this chapter, the reader should be able to:

A 1. Recognize the relevant anatomy and physiology of the female reproductive system.

P 2. Summarize the pathology of the female reproductive system that prompts surgical intervention, and the related terminology.

3. Determine any special preoperative obstetric/gynecologic diagnostic procedures/tests.

O 4. Determine any special preoperative preparation procedures related to obstetric/gynecologic procedures.

5. Indicate the names and uses of obstetric and gynecologic instruments, supplies, and drugs.

6. Indicate the names and uses of special equipment related to obstetric/gynecologic surgery.

7. Determine the intraoperative preparation of the patient undergoing an obstetric or gynecologic procedure.

8. Summarize the surgical steps of obstetric/gynecologic procedures.

9. Interpret the purpose and expected outcomes of the obstetric/gynecologic procedure.

10. Recognize the immediate postoperative care and possible complications of the obstetric/gynecologic procedure.

S 11. Assess any specific variations related to the preoperative, intraoperative, and postoperative care of the obstetric/gynecologic patient.

Select Key Terms

Define the following, using your textbook glossary or a medical dictionary if needed:

1. adnexa _____

2. bony pelvis _____

3. breech _____

4. cesarean section _____

5. corpus luteum _____

6. CPD _____

7. curettage _____

8. DUB _____

9. dystocia _____

10. episiotomy _____

11. exenteration _____

12. fimbria _____

13. fistula _____

14. gravida _____

15. LEEP _____

16. ligament _____

17. marsupialization _____

18. myoma _____

19. occiput anterior _____

_____

20. parity _____

_____

21. perineum _____

_____

22. Pfannenstiel _____

_____

23. vestibule _____

_____

Anatomy

1. Identify the structures of the female reproductive organs shown in Figure 15-1.

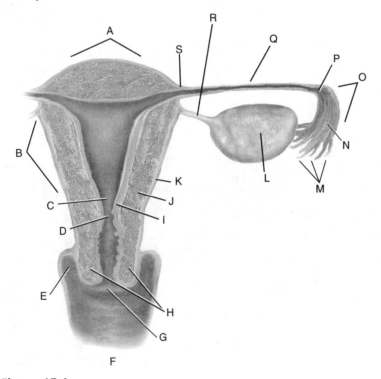

Figure 15-1

A. _____

B. _____

C. _____

D. _____

E. _____

F. _____

G. _____

H. _____

I. _____

J. _____

K. _____

L. _____

M. _____

N. _____

O. _____

P. _____

Q. _____

R. _____

S. _____

2. Identify the structures of the bony pelvis shown in Figure 15-2.

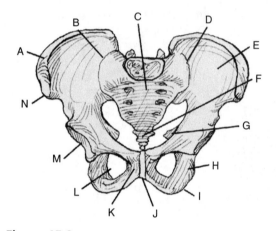

Figure 15-2

A. _____

B. _____

C. _____

D. _____

E. _____

F. _____

G. _____

H. _____

I. _____

J. _____

K. _____

L. _____

M. _____

N. _____

3. Identify the supporting structures of the female anatomy shown in Figure 15-3.

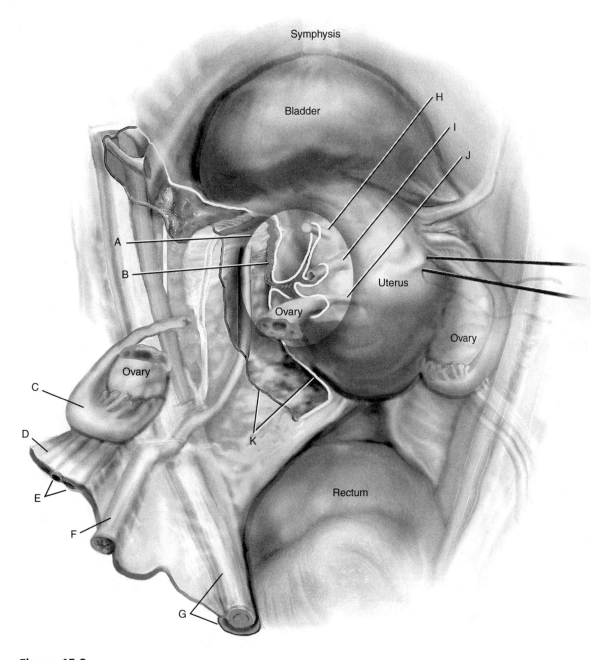

Figure 15-3

A. _____

B. _____

C. _____

D. _____

E. _____

F. _____

G. _____

H. _____

I. _____

J _____

K. _____

4. Identify the supporting structures and spaces of the female anatomy shown in Figure 15-4.

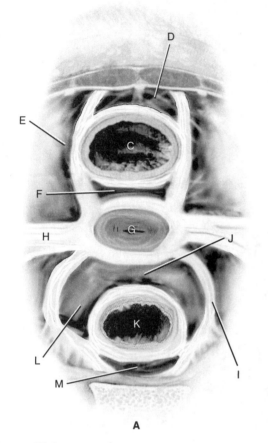

A

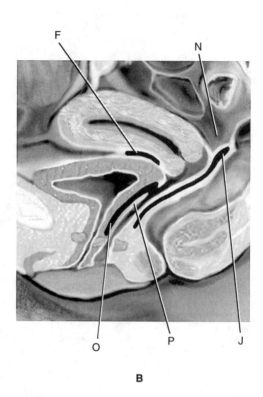

B

Figure 15-4

A. _____

B. _____

C. _____

D. _____

E. _____

F. _____

G. _____

H. _____

I. _____

J. _____

K. _____

L. _____

M. _____

N. _____

O. _____

P. _____

5. What is the fornix?

_____

_____

6. Describe the locations of the internal and external cervical os.

_____

_____

7. List the three layers of the uterine wall.

A. _____

B. _____

C. _____

8. Where are the Bartholin's glands located? What is their function?

_____

_____

9. List the structures contained within the broad ligament.

A. _____

B. _____

C. _____

D. _____

E. _____

F. _____

10. What are the other two names for the fallopian tubes?

_____

_____

11. Describe the location of the ovaries.

_____

_____

12. Name the two hormones from the anterior pituitary that stimulate the ovarian cycle.

_____

_____

13. Name the two hormones that are produced by the ovary.

_____

_____

14. What is the main muscle of the pelvic floor? Name its three components.

   A. _____

   B. _____

   C. _____

15. Branches of which nerve and artery provide sensation and blood flow to the perineum and external genitalia?

   _____

   _____

Matching

Match the external structure with the description.

_____ 16. Rounded prominent longitudinal flaps

_____ 17. Area between the vaginal opening and anus

_____ 18. The external female genitalia

_____ 19. Cavity between the labia minora containing the urethral meatus

_____ 20. Secretes lubrication

_____ 21. Rounded prominence over symphysis pubis

_____ 22. Erectile structure of the female anatomy

_____ 23. Two flat cutaneous flaps containing sebaceous glands

_____ 24. Rectal orifice

_____ 25. Thin fold of membrane just inside the vaginal orifice

A. Vestibule

B. Clitoris

C. Mons pubis

D. Bartholin's glands

E. Perineum

F. Hymen

G. Anus

H. Labia minora

I. Labia majora

J. Vulva

True or False

_____ 26. The uterus is pear-shaped with a fundus, body, and cervix.

_____ 27. The ligaments connecting to the pelvic wall include the cardinal, ovarian, and broad.

_____ 28. The posterior vaginal wall is longer than the anterior vaginal wall.

_____ 29. The normal cervix lies anterior to the fundus of the uterus.

_____ 30. The junction between the cervix and vagina is called the cul de sac of Douglas.

_____ 31. The Graafian follicle releases the oocyte.

_____ 32. The corpus luteum is responsible for releasing estrogen to maintain the endometrial lining.

_____ 33. The pituitary gland releases LH and FSH to stimulate the development of an oocyte or ovum.

_____ 34. Blood flow is supplied to the uterus via branches of the internal iliac artery.

_____ 35. The isthmus of the fallopian tube is important in the prevention of endometriosis.

Pathology

1. Are Braxton-Hicks contractions an indication that delivery of the fetus is imminent?

   _____

   _____

Matching

Match the term with the definition.

_____	2. Used for prevention of perineal lacerations	A. Effacement
_____	3. Fetus head too large for maternal birth canal	B. Gravida
_____	4. Mother and infant relationship	C. Dilation
_____	5. Largest diameter of head encircled by vulvular ring	D. Presentation
_____	6. Number of times giving birth	E. Para
_____	7. Descent of presenting part of fetus in relation to ischial spines	F. Crowning
_____	8. Opening of the cervix	G. Station
_____	9. Fetal part overlying pelvic inlet	H. Episiotomy
_____	10. Cervix softens and thins	I. Bonding
_____	11. Number of pregnancies	J. CPD

Vaginal Delivery

12. Identify the stages of a vaginal delivery:

Stage one: _____

_____

Stage two: _____

_____

Stage three: _____

_____

Stage four: _____

_____

13. What surgical intervention is commonly done during a normal vaginal delivery?

_____

14. Cord blood is collected routinely with every delivery. Why?

_____

_____

15. What does "fetal distress" mean?

_____

_____

16. What is the most common reason for performing a cesarean section?

_____

_____

17. Define cystocele, and give two reasons why a cystocele may occur.

_____

_____

18. What procedure is commonly performed with a colposcopy? What condition can be diagnosed?

_____

_____

19. List the possible sites for ectopic pregnancy.

_____

_____

20. What is meant by the term incompetent cervix? What procedure is performed to treat the condition during pregnancy?

_____

_____

21. Define leiomyoma.

_____

_____

22. What are the symptoms of endometriosis?

_____

_____

23. Is ultrasound useful in diagnosing a malignancy?

_____

_____

24. What is the most common symptom of uterine cancer?

_____

_____

25. Define two placental conditions that may necessitate a cesarean section. Find the two conditions in your textbook and look up their definitions in your medical dictionary.

_____

_____

26. Amenorrhea is the condition of

_____

_____

27. What is a pedunculated lesion?

_____

_____

Operation

1. In what position will the patient be placed to accomplish a D&C? In addition to the basic position, which position may be used to enhance the surgeon's view of the anatomy?

_____

_____

2. Explain the usefulness of the Trendelenburg position during pelvic surgery.

_____

_____

3. Describe the complications that the patient may experience from an undiagnosed or improperly closed perineal laceration.

_____

_____

4. Name two types of suction devices that may be used to clear a neonate's airway.

_____

_____

5. What are the advantages to a "classic" approach for a cesarean section?

_____

_____

6. Name the three approaches that are available for tubal sterilization.

A. _____

B. _____

C. _____

Matching

Match the medication or gas appropriately.

____ 7. White stain for abnormal tissue   A. Lugol's solution

____ 8. Prevention of adhesions   B. Acetic acid (vinegar)

____ 9. Schiller test—abnormal no stain   C. Nitrous oxide or CO_2

____ 10. Causes uterine contraction   D. Monsel's solution

____ 11. Hemostasis agent   E. 10% Dextran 70

____ 12. Cryotherapy to remove lesion   F. Methergine/Pitocin

Short Answer

13. What is used to manipulate the vaginal mucosa during the anterior colporrhaphy?

_____

_____

14. What are the advantages of the LAVH approach?

_____

_____

15. What is the importance of draining the bladder prior to D&C or other pelvic procedures?

_____

_____

16. Why is a Foley catheter placed prior to a cesarean section?

_____

_____

17. List the structures that will be removed during a total pelvic exenteration.

_____

_____

18. What safety measures must be implemented when a laser is in use?

_____

_____

19. List the drape components that are necessary to drape a patient in the lithotomy position. Describe the draping sequence.

_____

_____

20. What structure(s) is/are removed during a TAH?

_____

_____

21. List three transverse incisions used for gynecological surgery.

_____

_____

Matching

Match the pathological condition with the treatment.

_____ 22. Microsurgical reanastomosis with dextran

_____ 23. Excision of fibroids to preserve uterus for conception

_____ 24. Rectocele

_____ 25. Bartholin's cyst

_____ 26. Incomplete spontaneous abortion or menorrhagia

_____ 27. Desires sterilization

_____ 28. Endometrial visualization

_____ 29. External genitalia with in situ neoplasia

_____ 30. Incompetent cervical os

_____ 31. Endocervical suspicious lesions or dysplasia

_____ 32. Cystocele

_____ 33. Ruptured ectopic pregnancy

A. Colpotomy tubal ligation

B. Shirodkar cerclage

C. Tuboplasty

D. Emergency salpingotomy

E. Anterior colporrhaphy

F. Posterior colporrhaphy

G. Cold conization

H. Hysteroscopy

I. Vulvectomy

J. Marsupialization

K. Dilation and curettage

L. Myomectomy

Short Answer

34. Identify the vaginal retractors shown in Figure 15-5

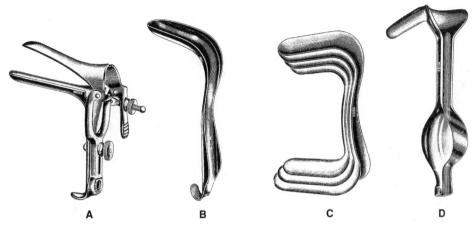

Figure 15-5

A. _____

B. _____

C. _____

D. _____

35. Identify the cervical and uterine instruments shown in Figure 15-6.

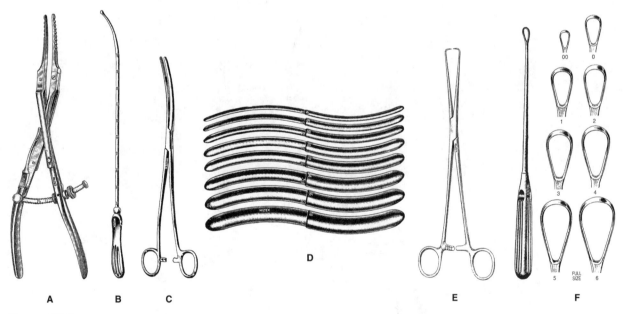

Figure 15-6

A. _____

B. _____

C. _____

D. _____

E. _____

F. _____

36. Identify the retracting instruments shown in Figure 15-7.

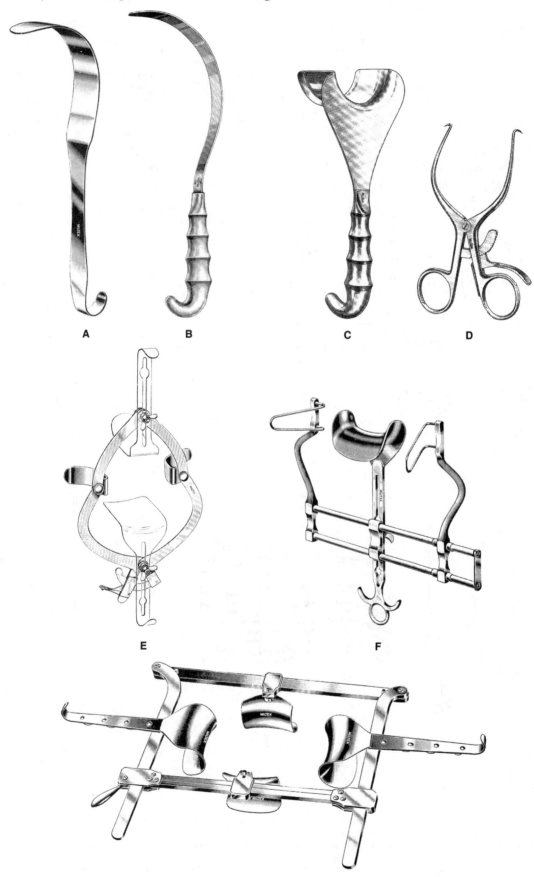

Figure 15-7

A. _____

B. _____

C. _____

D. _____

E. _____

F. _____

G. _____

37. Identify the retracting instruments shown in Figure 15-8.

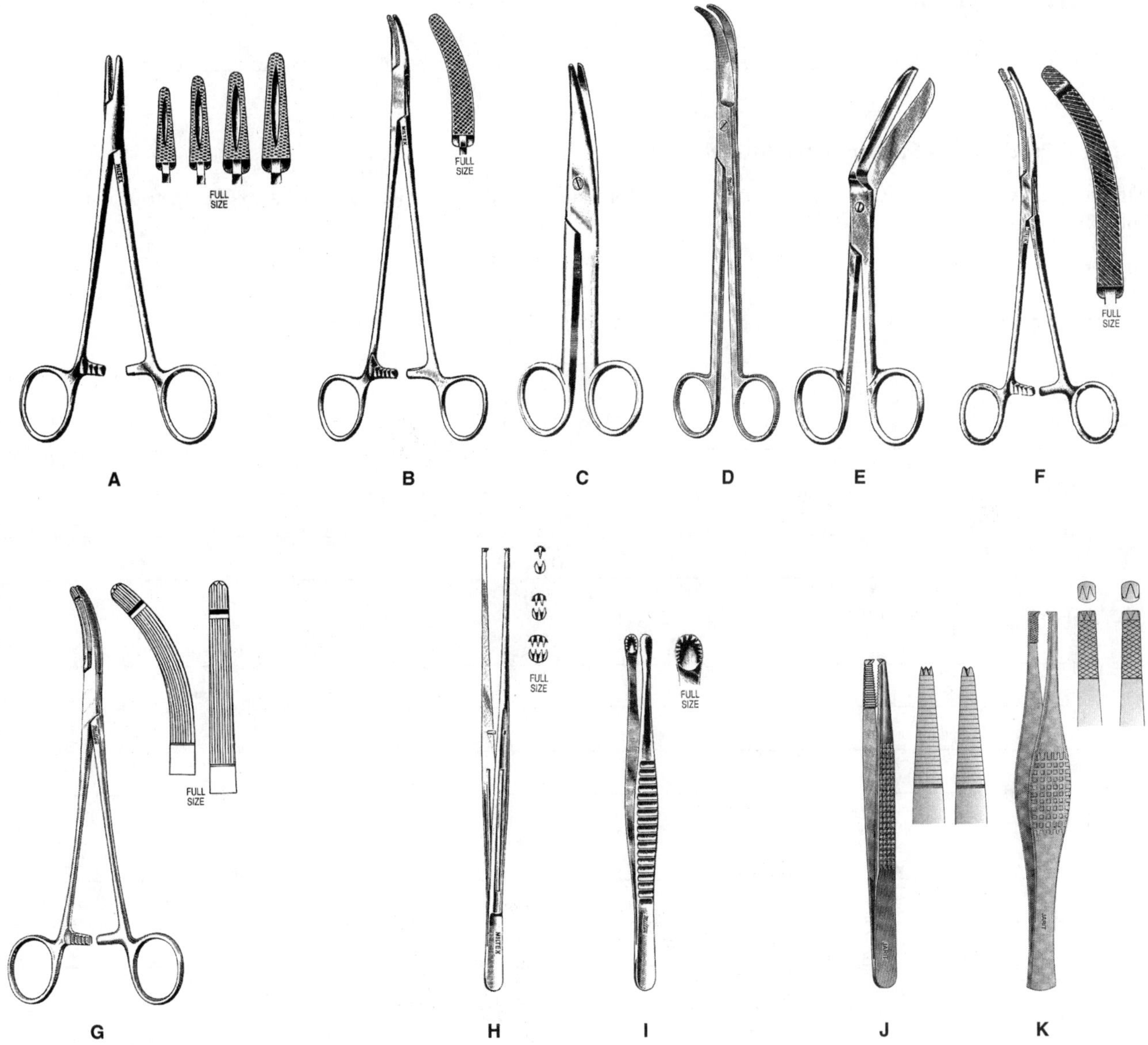

Figure 15-8

A. _____

B. _____

C. _____

D. _____

E. _____

F. _____

G. _____

H. _____

I. _____

J. _____

K. _____

Specific Variations

Student Name _____ Date _____

Instructor _____

Surgical Procedure—Student Case Study Report

The student will be provided with basic patient information (real or simulated) and is expected to complete the following case study.

1. Procedure name:

    _____

    _____

2. Definition of procedure:

    _____

    _____

    _____

    _____

3. Purpose of the procedure:

    _____

    _____

    _____

    _____

4. Expected outcome of the procedure:

    _____

    _____

    _____

    _____

5. Patient age: _____

6. Gender: _____

7. Additional pertinent patient information:

    _____

    _____

    _____

8. Probable preoperative diagnosis:

_____

_____

_____

_____

_____

9. How was the diagnosis determined?

_____

_____

_____

_____

_____

10. Discuss the relevant anatomy.

_____

_____

_____

_____

_____

_____

11. List the general and procedure-specific equipment that will be needed for the procedure.

_____

_____

_____

_____

_____

_____

12. List the general and procedure-specific instruments that will be needed for the procedure.

_____

_____

_____

_____

_____

_____

13. List the basic and procedure-specific supplies that will be needed for the procedure.

Pack _____

Basin _____

Gloves _____

Blades _____

Drapes _____

Drains _____

Dressings _____

Suture—Type of Suture, Needle (if applicable), and Anticipated Tissue Usage

_____

_____

_____

_____

_____

_____

Pharmaceuticals

_____

_____

_____

_____

Miscellaneous

_____

_____

_____

_____

_____

14. Operative preparation:

_____

_____

_____

_____

_____

15. What type of anesthesia will likely be used? Why?

_____

_____

_____

_____

_____

16. List any special anesthesia equipment that may be needed.

17. Patient position during the procedure:

18. What supplies will be necessary for positioning?

19. What type of shave/skin preparation will be necessary (if any)?

20. Define the anatomic perimeters of the prep.

21. List the order in which the drapes will be applied, and describe any specific variations.

22. List any practical considerations.

_____

_____

_____

_____

_____

_____

23. List the procedural steps, and describe the preparatory and supportive actions of the STSR during each step (use additional space if necessary).

_____

_____

_____

_____

24. What is the postoperative diagnosis?

_____

_____

_____

_____

25. Describe the immediate postoperative care.

_____

_____

_____

_____

_____

26. What is the patient's long-term prognosis?

_____

_____

_____

_____

_____

27. What are the possible complications?

_____

_____

_____

_____

_____

28. Comments or questions:

_____

_____

_____

_____

_____

29. What is the most valuable information you obtained from preparing this surgical procedure case study?

_____

_____

_____

_____

Case Studies

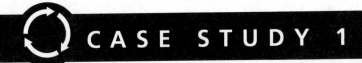
CASE STUDY 1

Shannon is a 23-year-old primipara who has just been admitted to the labor and delivery unit room 3 for Dr. Templeton. She has had a normal pregnancy, and sonograms confirm only one fetus with a cephalic presentation. Her cervix is dilated to 4 cm and is 40% effaced. Her blood type is AB negative.

1. How long, on average, would you expect her labor to continue?

_____

_____

_____

2. Using Table 15-1 in the textbook, list the information that is to be recorded on the monitoring board.

_____

_____

_____

3. During stage two, the fetal heart tones begin to slow and do not increase. The physician is notified and he orders a stat cesarean section. Why?

_____

_____

_____

_____

(continues)

CASE STUDY 1 (continued)

4. The mother is placed on the OR table. Describe her position. Why does she need a Foley catheter?

_____

_____

_____

_____

5. The surgeon makes an incision into the uterus and completes the delivery of the baby's head. How is the sterile field prepared for imminent delivery of the fetus? What is the first thing you will give the surgeon once the head is delivered?

_____

_____

_____

_____

_____

6. The umbilical cord is clamped and cut. The baby is passed off the field. What is done next?

_____

_____

_____

_____

7. After delivery of the placenta, the surgeon asks you to look at it. What are you looking for and why?

_____

_____

_____

_____

8. After the baby is born, the mother is given injections of RhoGAM and Pitocin. Why?

_____

_____

_____

_____

9. How many counts are taken during cesarean section and why?

_____

_____

_____

_____

CASE STUDY 2

Coretta has been admitted for a diagnostic laparoscopy for pelvic pain of unknown origin.

1. What equipment will be needed for the procedure?

2. What instruments will be needed for the procedure?

3. In what position will Coretta be placed?

4. Describe how the uterus will be manipulated during the procedure.

5. Describe the insufflation technique. What is used to establish the pneumoperitoneum? What are the pressure settings?

6. What are the common complications of laparoscopy?

CASE STUDY 3

Elaine is scheduled for a TAH.

1. What instrumentation will be needed for the procedure?

_____

_____

_____

_____

2. Name the ligaments to be transected. Describe the method and instrumentation used to perform the transection?

_____

_____

_____

_____

3. As the vaginal cuff is transected, you take special precautions with the instruments. Why?

_____

_____

_____

_____

4. Blunt dissection may be used to dissect the bladder free. What instrument will be used?

_____

_____

_____

_____

Lab 15: Obstetrics and Gynecology

Introduction

Obstetrics and gynecological (Ob-Gyn) surgery deals with the female reproductive organs and the unborn child. It is one of the most common surgery specialties that you will learn. These cases tend to the part of a large surgical specialty that is practiced just about everywhere, from large hospitals to small surgical centers. Learning the surgery step by step in lecture will help you in the lab portion. This is where you will learn the "hands-on" of the specialty and the instruments that will be used for each piece of the surgery.

Game: Ob-Gyn Surgery on Felt Mayo Stands

Time involved: 1–2 weeks setup

Instructors: Make a list of instruments you expect students to know as part of the Ob-Gyn surgery lab. Have the students trace the real instruments on the felt if possible; if not, have them find pictures that they can cut out and trace onto the felt or other material. I like felt because it tends to be very durable, but paper or cardboard can be substituted. There should be no need for multiple cutouts of the same instruments if students are given the chance to show how many of those instruments they would have on the Mayo using a numbered marker (a piece of paper with a number designation on it). The students are given a list of surgeries that they are expected to know. This can also be made easier if you have photos of these Mayo stand setups for the students to study.

Students: You will need several pieces of felt, paper, or cardboard. The largest piece should be cut to the size of a regular Mayo stand. You need to make the cutouts as close as possible to life-sized instruments using felt or some other material. Label them for easy reference on the backside of the cutouts.

Supplies: Felt, paper, or cardboard; real instruments, or pictures that have been printed and cut out from the computer; felt-tip marker; scissors; measuring tool

How the Game Is Played

The students are given a list of surgeries that they are expected to know. The instructor will then assign one of these surgeries to the student in the lab. The student will then be expected to complete a Mayo stand setup utilizing the instruments they have cut out in a specified time frame. Score the students according to placement of instruments, time needed for setup, correct instrumentation, and correct number of instruments.

Practical: Set Up Obstetrical or Gynecological Surgery Cases

Utilizing a full lab/OR setup, assign the students to learn different surgical cases. Given a number to learn, the students will then be expected to set up some of these cases under the supervision of the instructor. They should use as much of the OR equipment as needed including back table, Mayo stand, ring stands, instrument trays, and pans. The student should be scored on correct placement of supplies, practicing economy of time and motion (pick it up and place it one time), correct order of instruments, correct number of instruments, aseptic technique, time to set up, and order of use for instruments and supplies; a mock surgery should be performed so the student can practice anticipating the needs of the surgeon.

Skill Assessment 15-1

Student Name	
SKILL	**Gynecology Surgery**
Instructions	Instructor will demonstrate assembly. Practice procedure with your partner. When ready, notify instructor to schedule the check-off. Skills assessment must be completed satisfactorily by _____ (due date).
Supplies	• Policy/guidelines handout used by local facilities or physicians regarding D&C/hysteroscopy setup preferences • Simulated medications (vials or pictures of vials) • Basic D&C tray appropriate to local facility • Other GYN trays or instrument pictures as available

Note: Student must perform skill independently without prompting.

Practice with Partner Date:		Skills Testing Date:		
PROCEDURAL STEPS				**COMMENTS**
1. Assembles and prepares supplies and lab for practice.	Correct	Needs Review		
2. Identifies typical variants of vaginal diagnostic procedures; includes precautions to prevent contamination of specimen or possible seeding of cancerous tissue. Identifies precautions to take regarding laser ablation of condylomata.	Correct	Needs Review		
3. Identifies instruments correctly and precautions for use.	Correct	Needs Review		
4. Demonstrates adequate case preparation for D&C. Setup is organized with supplies and instrumentation in order of use according to local policy/guidelines.	Correct	Needs Review		
5. Identifies solutions that can be used during surgery, their use, and any precautions.	Correct	Needs Review		
6. Demonstrates anticipation of procedure sequence to setup closure clean setup.	Correct	Needs Review		
7. Maintains work area neat and organized.	Correct	Needs Review		
8. Breaks down setup and stores appropriately.	Correct	Needs Review		

Performance Evaluation Criteria		**Rating**
• Assembled necessary supplies and equipment.		
• Identified variations of vaginal diagnostic and therapeutic procedures including colposcopy, PAP smear, LEEP cone, cold conization, cryotherapy, D&C, hysteroscopy, laser ablation, and thermal ablation.		
• Demonstrated setup of a D&C including lubrication, dilation, and methods to obtain specimens.		
• Identifies procedure for hysteroscopy to insufflate uterus and precautions for solutions used.		
• Identifies solutions used including use and precautions for Monsel's solution, Lugol's solution, acetic acid, methylene blue, and dextran solutions (hysokan).		
• Anticipated correctly each step of D&C procedure.		

Skill Assessment 15-1 (*continued*)

	• Demonstrated attention to detail—work area is completed as instructed and maintained in an organized, clean, and safe manner. If not, needs improvement with: _____.	
	• Student prepared and performed procedure independently.	
	• Performed each step in appropriate sequence.	
	Overall Rating (Satisfactory; Must Redo; Fail):	
Instructor Comments		

Student Signature	*Date*
Instructor Signature	*Date*

CHAPTER 16

Ophthalmic Surgery

After studying this chapter, the reader should be able to:

A 1. Recognize the anatomy of the eye.

P 2. Summarize the pathology that prompts surgical intervention of the eye and related terminology.

3. Determine any special preoperative ophthalmic diagnostic procedures/tests.

O 4. Determine any special preoperative preparation procedures.

5. Indicate the names and uses of ophthalmic instruments, supplies, and drugs.

6. Indicate the names and uses of special equipment.

7. Determine the intraoperative preparation of the patient undergoing an ophthalmic procedure.

8. Summarize the surgical steps of ophthalmic procedures.

9. Interpret the purpose and expected outcomes of the ophthalmic procedures.

10. Recognize the immediate postoperative care and possible complications of the ophthalmic procedures.

S 11. Assess any specific variations related to the preoperative, intraoperative, and postoperative care of the ophthalmic patient.

Select Key Terms

Define the following, using your textbook glossary or a medical dictionary if necessary:

1. anterior chamber _____

_____

2. BSS _____

_____

3. cataract _____

_____

4. chalazion _____

_____

5. dacryo- _____

_____

6. diathermy _____

_____

7. enucleation _____

_____

8. extracapsular cataract extraction _____

_____

9. extrinsic muscles _____

_____

10. globe _____

_____

11. intracapsular cataract extraction _____

_____

12. iridotomy _____

_____

13. kerato- _____

_____

14. lacrimal _____

_____

15. ocutome _____

_____

16. posterior chamber _____

_____

17. retrobulbar _____

_____

18. strabismus _____

_____

19. trephine _____

_____

20. tunic _____

_____

Anatomy

1. Identify the structures of the eye shown in Figure 16-1.

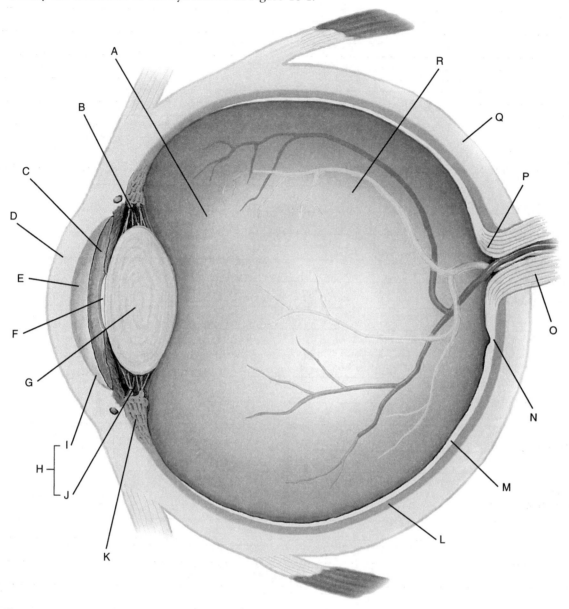

Figure 16-1

A. _____

B. _____

C. _____

D. _____

E. _____

F. _____

G. _____

H. _____

I. _____

J. _____

K. _____

L. _____

M. _____

N. _____

O. _____

P. _____

Q. _____

R. _____

2. Identify the extrinsic muscles of the eye, the eyelid muscle, and the function of each shown in Figure 16-2.

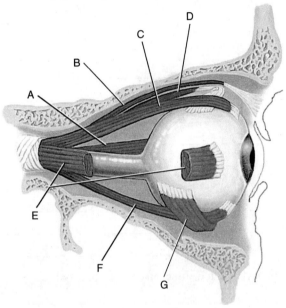

Figure 16-2

A. _____

B. _____

C. _____

D. _____

E. _____

F. _____

G. _____

3. Identify the structures of the lacrimal apparatus shown in Figure 16-3.

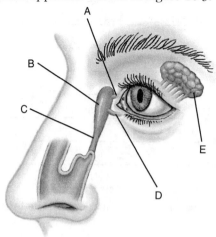

Figure 16-3

A. _____

B. _____

C. _____

D. _____

E. _____

4. What is the purpose of the lacrimal system?

_____

_____

_____

5. Identify and describe the function of each tunic or layer of the eye.

A. _____

B. _____

C. _____

6. Identify and describe the function of the two intrinsic muscles of the eye.

A. _____

B. _____

C. Define pupil: _____

7. Name the bones that form the orbit.

A. _____

B. _____

C. _____

D. _____

E. _____

F. _____

G. _____

8. Describe the location and function of the conjunctiva.

_____

_____

9. Complete this sentence: The cornea is continuous with the _____ .

10. Discuss the two cavities of the eye. Identify and describe the type of fluid found in each one.

_____

_____

_____

_____

11. Describe the location and function of the crystalline lens.

_____

_____

_____

_____

12. Analyze and describe the blind spot. Is this normal anatomy?

_____

_____

13. Describe the macula and fovea centralis. Why is this an important area of the eye?

_____

_____

14. Describe the function(s) of the rods and the cones. Where are they located?

_____

_____

_____

_____

Pathology

1. Glaucoma

   A. What fluid is affected and where?

   _____

   B. Why does the increase in IOP lead to blindness?

   _____

2. Describe three reasons for cataract formation.

   A. _____

   B. _____

   C. _____

3. Describe the formation of a cataract and the symptoms it causes.

   _____

   _____

   _____

   _____

4. Retina

   A. Describe what happens when a large retinal detachment occurs.

   _____

   _____

   B. Explain why a patient may see "spots" or "flashes of light" with the development of retinal detachment.

   _____

   _____

   _____

5. What visual defect will occur in a person who lacks cones in the retina?

   _____

   _____

   _____

6. Describe four causes of corneal clouding.

   A. _____

   B. _____

   C. _____

   D. _____

7. Analyze a chalazion. Describe what it is and identify what causes it.

   _____

   _____

   _____

8. The patient may be scheduled for excision of a pterygium. Describe what causes a pterygium and where it is found.

   _____

   _____

9. What condition causes dacryocystitis?

   _____

   _____

10. Strabismus _____

   A. Define diplopia.

   _____

   _____

   _____

   B. Explain the difference between comitant and incomitant strabismus. Which type is most likely to have diplopia?

   _____

   _____

   _____

11. List three indications for enucleation.

    A. _____

    B. _____

    C. _____

12. Describe the difference between ectropion and entropion.

    _____

    _____

    _____

13. Where is the limbus cornea?

    _____

    _____

    _____

14. The surgeon is dictating and you hear the word ptosis. What does it mean in ophthalmic cases?

    _____

    _____

    _____

Operation

Matching

Match the medication with the classification.

____ 1. Antibiotic

____ 2. Isotonic solution

____ 3. Cycloplegic

____ 4. Anesthetic

____ 5. Vitreous substitute

____ 6. Anti-inflammatory

____ 7. Vasoconstrictor

____ 8. Miotic

____ 9. Mydriatic

____ 10. Enzyme

A. Atropine

B. Pilocarpine

C. Celestone

D. Wydase

E. Tetracaine

F. Cyclogyl

G. Sodium hyaluronate

H. Balanced Salt Solution (BSS)

I. Gentamicin

J. Epinephrine

Match the medication or classification with the action.

____ 11. Infection treatment or prevention

____ 12. Dilates pupils

____ 13. Prevents sclera from collapsing

____ 14. Pain prevention

____ 15. Hormone additive slows absorption of anesthetic

A. Anti-inflammatory

B. Balanced Salt Solution (BSS)

C. Epinephrine

D. Gentamicin

E. Miotic

____ 16. Prevents swelling

____ 17. Enzyme additive disperses anesthetic uniformly

____ 18. Constricts pupils

____ 19. Prevents corneal dryness

____ 20. Paralyzes the ciliary muscle

F. Mydriacyl

G. Neo-Synephrine

H. Sodium hyaluronate

I. Tetracaine

J. Wydase

Short Answer

21. Surgical repair of the eyelid can be identified as a(n) _____ .

22. Two popular procedures to correct ptosis include _____

23. Glaucoma—Describe how each of these procedures relieve the ocular pressure:

    A. Iridectomy _____

    B. Trabeculoplasty _____

    C. What canal is blocked causing an increase in IOP? _____

24. Using the textbook, identify the following equipment and supplies used commonly in eye surgery.

    A. Describe the type of drape used to fit the eye.

    _____

    _____

    B. Describe a loupe.

    _____

    _____

    C. What is the purpose of Weck sponges?

    _____

    _____

    D. Why are powder free gloves typically used for eye surgery?

    _____

    _____

    E. What is a caliper used for?

    _____

    _____

25. Recession/resection is used for correcting what condition of the eye?

    _____

    _____

26. Retinal tear treatments

    A. Describe the common procedure used to treat retinal tears.

    _____

    _____

B. How is cryotherapy used to treat retinal detachment?

_____

_____

C. Identify why a gas bubble may be used during this procedure.

_____

_____

D. Describe what kind of gas is used and what a gas bubble means to the patient postop.

_____

_____

E. What treatment may be used if buckling or cryosurgery fails?

_____

_____

27. Lacrimal system:

A. What procedure is performed to open the blocked tear ducts of an infant?

_____

_____

B. The topical anesthetic cocaine is often used to prepare the nose, even if a general anesthetic is planned. Why?

_____

_____

28. Eye Excision:

A. Describe the difference between these two treatments. Identify which one allows better cosmetic results.

1. Enucleation _____

2. Evisceration _____

29. Cornea

A. Describe the purpose of the cornea.

_____

_____

B. What type of instrument is a trephine?

_____

C. In eye surgery, what procedure is a trephine used for?

_____

D. How long can the donor cornea be stored?

_____

_____

E. When might rejection occur?

_____

_____

30. Cataract treatment:

    A. Describe two methods for cataract extraction.

    _____

    _____

    B. Describe the incision made that is self healing.

    _____

    _____

    C. Phacoemulsification may be used. Describe how the machine works.

    _____

    _____

    D. What can acetylcholine be used for? What classification does that make acetylcholine?

    _____

    _____

31. What is a diathermy apparatus used to accomplish?

    _____

    _____

    _____

    _____

Matching

Match the ophthalmic instrument with the correct usage.

_____ 32. Measures intraocular pressure (IOP)   A. Barraquer

_____ 33. Dilating and probing   B. Beaver

_____ 34. Grasping and holding   C. Bishop-Harmon

_____ 35. Eye speculum   D. Castroviejo

_____ 36. Cutting scalpel handle   E. Desmarres chalazion forceps

_____ 37. Micro scissor   F. Stephens

_____ 38. Grasps lower eyelid to facilitate excision   G. Bowman

_____ 39. Micro needle holder   H. Jameson

_____ 40. Small scissors for blepharoplasty   I. Tonometer

_____ 41. Blunt muscle hook   J. Westcott

42. Vitrectomy:

    A. What can be used to replace the vitreous humor?

    _____

    B. What is the ocutome used for?

    _____

C. What is the purpose of applying fluorescein to the cornea? What tool must be used in conjunction with fluorescein? (Note: You may need to utilize information in the pharmacology chapter.)

_____

_____

_____

_____

Specific Variations

Student Name: _____ Date: _____

Instructor: _____

The student will be provided with basic patient information (real or simulated) and is expected to complete the following case study.

1. Procedure name:

_____

_____

_____

2. Definition of procedure:

_____

_____

_____

_____

_____

3. What is the purpose of the procedure?

_____

_____

_____

_____

_____

4. What is the expected outcome of the procedure?

_____

_____

_____

_____

5. Patient age: _____

6. Gender: _____

7. Additional pertinent patient information:

_____

_____

_____

_____

8. Probable preoperative diagnosis:

_____

_____

_____

_____

_____

_____

9. How was the diagnosis determined?

_____

_____

_____

_____

_____

_____

10. Discuss the relevant anatomy.

_____

_____

_____

_____

_____

_____

_____

11. List the general and procedure-specific equipment that will be needed for the procedure.

_____

_____

_____

_____

_____

12. List the general and procedure-specific instruments that will be needed for the procedure.

_____

_____

_____

_____

_____

_____

13. List the basic and procedure-specific supplies that will be needed for the procedure.

Pack _____

Basin _____

Gloves _____

Blades _____

Drapes _____

Drains _____

Dressings_____

Suture—Type of Suture, Needle (if applicable), and Anticipated Tissue Usage

_____

_____

_____

_____

_____

_____

_____

Pharmaceuticals

_____

_____

_____

_____

Miscellaneous

_____

_____

_____

_____

_____

14. Operative preparation:

_____

_____

_____

_____

_____

_____

_____

15. What type of anesthesia will likely be used? Why?

_____

_____

_____

_____

16. List any special anesthesia equipment that may be needed.

_____

_____

_____

_____

_____

17. Patient position during the procedure:

_____

_____

_____

_____

_____

18. What supplies will be necessary for positioning?

_____

_____

_____

_____

_____

19. What type of shave/skin preparation will be necessary (if any)?

_____

_____

_____

_____

_____

20. Define the anatomic perimeters of the prep.

_____

_____

_____

_____

_____

_____

21. List the order in which the drapes will be applied, and describe any specific variations.

_____

_____

_____

_____

_____

_____

_____

22. List any practical considerations.

_____

_____

_____

_____

_____

_____

_____

23. List the procedural steps, and describe the preparatory and supportive actions of the STSR during each step (use additional space if necessary).

_____

_____

_____

24. What is the postoperative diagnosis?

_____

_____

_____

_____

_____

25. Describe the immediate postoperative care.

_____

_____

_____

_____

_____

26. What is the patient's long-term prognosis?

_____

_____

_____

_____

_____

_____

27. What are the possible complications?

_____

_____

_____

_____

_____

_____

28. Comments or questions:

_____

_____

_____

_____

_____

_____

29. What is the most valuable information you obtained from preparing this surgical procedure case study?

_____

_____

_____

_____

_____

Case Studies

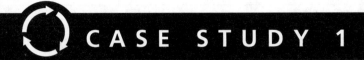

Susan is admitted to the hospital for eye surgery. She was diagnosed in childhood with diabetes and is now 50 years old. Susan also has been diagnosed with retinopathy, a frequently occurring condition in diabetic patients. Her vision has been deteriorating over the last several years. She has recently suffered a vitreous hemorrhage due to neovascularization of the eye, which is common in diabetic patients.

1. What procedure will be performed to resolve the problem?

_____

_____

_____

_____

2. Briefly describe the procedure, and explain how Susan will benefit.

_____

_____

_____

_____

3. What are the possible approaches that the surgeon may use to enter the eye? Which is preferred?

_____

_____

_____

_____

4. What piece of equipment is crucial to a vitrectomy?

_____

_____

_____

_____

5. What substance, if any, will be used to replace the vitreous humor?

_____

_____

_____

_____

CASE STUDY 2

Ronald has been having trouble with his stereoscopic vision. His wife says that he appears to have a "lazy eye." The amount of misalignment seems to stay the same no matter which direction his eyes are looking. Ronald has been admitted to the ambulatory care center for surgery.

1. What is the correct term for the condition that Ronald has?

_____

_____

_____

_____

2. Would this condition be considered "comitant" or "incomitant"?

_____

_____

_____

_____

3. What surgical procedure will be performed to correct this condition?

_____

_____

_____

_____

4. In which position will Ronald be placed for this procedure?

_____

_____

_____

_____

5. What are the anatomic boundaries for the prep?

_____

_____

_____

_____

Lab 16: Ophthalmic Surgery

Introduction

Ophthalmic surgery deals with the eye and surrounding structures. This specialty tends to be difficult to learn because so many of the instruments do not relate to other specialties and many physicians will employ private scrubs. Take to heart though that many of the surgeries tend to work in an almost factory-like step-by-step way. Once you learn to do a cataract extraction and lens replacement, you may only have to change a few instruments and their order to do many different surgeries. Learning the surgery step by step in lecture will help you in the lab portion. This is where you will learn the hands on of the specialty and the instruments that will be used for each piece of the surgery.

Game: Ophthalmic Surgery on Felt Mayo Stands

Time involved: 1-2 weeks setup.

Instructors: Make a list of instruments you expect students to know as part of the ophthalmic surgery lab. Have the students trace the real instruments onto the felt if possible; if not, have them find pictures they can cut out and trace onto the felt or other material. I like the felt because it tends to be very durable, but paper or cardboard can be substituted. There should be no need for multiple cut-outs of the same instruments if students are given the chance to show how many of those instruments they would have on the Mayo by way of a numbered marker (a piece of paper with a number designation on it). The students are given a list of surgeries that they are expected to know. Note: This can be made easier if you have photos of these Mayo stand setups for the students to study.

Students: You will need several pieces of felt, paper, or cardboard. The largest piece should be cut to the size of a regular Mayo stand. You should make cut outs of instruments as close as possible to life size using felt or some other material. Label them for easy reference on the backside of the cutout.

Supplies: Felt, paper, or cardboard; real instruments, or pictures that have been printed and cut out from the computer; felt-tip marker; scissors; measuring tool.

How the Game Is Played

The students are given a list of surgeries that they are expected to know. The instructor will then assign one of those surgeries to the student in the lab. The student will then be expected to complete a Mayo stand setup in a specified time frame using the instruments they have cut out. Score them according to placement of instruments, time needed for setup, correct instrumentation, and correct number of instruments.

Practical: Set Up Ophthalmic Surgery Cases

Utilizing a full lab/OR setup, assign the students to different surgical cases. The students will then be expected to set up some of these cases under the supervision of the instructor. They should use as much of the OR equipment as needed including backtable, Mayo stand, and ring stands and instrument trays and pans. The student should be scored on correct placement of supplies, practicing economy of time and motion (pick it up and place it one time), correct order of instruments, correct number of instruments, aseptic technique, time to set up, and order of use for instruments and supplies; a mock surgery should be performed so the student can work on anticipating the needs of the surgeon.

Skill Assessment 16-1

Student Name	
SKILL	**Ophthalmic Surgery—Application of Clean Concept**
Instructions	Instructor will demonstrate assembly. Practice procedure with your partner. When ready, notify instructor to schedule the check-off. Skills assessment must be completed satisfactorily by _____ (due date).
Supplies	• Simulated or donated ophthalmic supplies as available • BSS solution, irrigation cannula and syringe, disposable eye knife • Basic ophthalmic instrument tray if available (simulation using fine wire)

Note: Student must perform skill independently without prompting.

Practice with Partner Date:		**Skills Testing Date:**	
PROCEDURAL STEPS			**COMMENTS**
1. Assembles and prepares supplies and lab for practice.	Correct	Needs Review	
2. Identifies microscopic instruments correctly including which require specialized handling to prevent potential damage to tissue.	Correct	Needs Review	
3. Demonstrates knowledge of ophthalmic surgery case preparation. States care of microscopic instrumentation correctly. Identifies principles related to preventing lint or damage to instrument tips.	Correct	Needs Review	
4. Demonstrates knowledge of STSR's responsibilities including passing techniques and medications for ophthalmic surgery correctly.	Correct	Needs Review	
5. Demonstrates safe preparation, handling, and passing of micro instruments and supplies (if available).	Correct	Needs Review	
6. Demonstrates knowledge of ophthalmic surgery.	Correct	Needs Review	
7. Breaks down ophthalmic setup and stores appropriately.	Correct	Needs Review	

Performance Evaluation Criteria	**Rating**
• Assembled necessary supplies and equipment. • Identified microscopic instruments which require specialized handling such as Bishop Harmon iris forceps, eye knives such as diamond knife, and needle holders such as the tying forceps. Identified common ophthalmic instrumentation either by picture or instrument correctly. • Demonstrated knowledge of Mayo setup for instrumentation. ○ Stated or demonstrated inspection of instruments for damage before procedure. Delicate tips never laid on the Mayo stand. Propped or maintained with tips elevated. No towels or gauze that could bend delicate tips. ○ Weck-cel sponges (pressed cellulose) utilized to wipe blood and keep instruments clean and free of lint. Stated Weck-cel spears may be used for blotting by surgeon. ○ Bipolar or disposable DC/battery eye cautery or Gelfoam used for hemostasis.	

Skill Assessment 16-1 (*continued*)

	• Demonstrated knowledge of STSR's responsibilities including passing techniques and BSS irrigation with ophthalmic surgery. Identified correctly: Never pass instruments over eyes.
	   ○ Plain and chromic gut may be rinsed to remove preservative prior to use. Sharps are passed carefully as placed in surgeon's hand and removed to prevent distraction from microscope.
	   ○ Irrigation solution such as balanced salt solutions used to keep the cornea from drying out and must be on any setup where surgery includes exposure of the eye during the case.
	   ○ No lint or powder to prevent corneal irritation.
	   ○ Instillation of eye drops by pulling down on lower eyelid and placing drop in lower conjunctiva. Ensure tip does not come in contact with eye (contamination). Pressure can be placed on inner canthus to prevent systemic absorption from mucous membranes of nasolacrimal ducts.
	   ○ Traction sutures used to stabilize or position the eye (hemostat used to secure the free ends).
	   ○ Remove all air bubbles when priming infusion cannula of vitrectomy machine.
	   ○ Donor cornea buttons may be stored 30 days prior use. Donor medium is sent as specimen for culture.
	• Demonstrated knowledge of ophthalmic surgery environmental awareness. Maintains a quiet room with no loud noises or sudden movements. Does not touch OR table, patient, or microscope during surgical procedure while physician is working, which can result in movement and injury. (No injury to eyes.) Ophthalmic patients are not allowed to cough or strain since this increases IOP.
	• Demonstrated attention to detail—work area is completed as instructed and maintained in an organized, clean, and safe manner. If not, needs improvement with: _____
	• Student prepared and performed skill independently.	

	Overall Rating (Satisfactory; Must Redo; Fail):	
Instructor Comments		

Student Signature	**Date**
Instructor Signature	**Date**

CHAPTER 17

Otorhinolaryngologic Surgery

OBJECTIVES

After studying this chapter, the reader should be able to:

A 1. Recognize the relevant anatomy of the ear, nose, and upper aerodigestive tract.

P 2. Summarize the pathology that prompts otorhinolaryngologic surgical intervention and the related terminology.

3. Determine any preoperative otorhinolaryngologic diagnostic procedures/tests.

O 4. Determine any otorhinolaryngologic preoperative preparation procedures.

5. Indicate the names and uses of otorhinolaryngologic instruments, supplies, and drugs.

6. Indicate the names and uses of special otorhinolaryngologic equipment.

7. Summarize the surgical steps of the otorhinolaryngologic procedures.

8. Discuss the purpose and expected outcomes of the otorhinolaryngologic procedures.

9. Recognize the immediate postoperative care and possible complications of the otorhinolaryngologic procedures.

S 10. Assess any specific variations related to the preoperative, intraoperative, and postoperative care of the otorhinolaryngologic patient.

Select Key Terms

Define the following, using your textbook glossary or a medical dictionary:

1. aerodigestive tract _____

_____

2. apnea _____

_____

3. carina _____

_____

4. cholesteatoma _____

_____

5. chondroradionacrosis _____

_____

6. congenital _____

_____

7. dynamic equilibrium _____

_____

8. epiglottis _____

_____

9. epistaxis _____

_____

10. Gelfoam _____

_____

11. glottis _____

_____

12. hydrops _____

_____

13. hypertrophy _____

_____

14. laryngo- _____

_____

15. myringo- _____

_____

16. olfaction _____

_____

17. oropharynx _____

_____

18. oto- _____

_____

19. pharyngotympanic tube _____

_____

20. polyp_____

_____

21. polysomnography _____

_____

22. rhino- _____

_____

23. –sclerosis _____

_____

24. SMR _____

_____

25. T&A _____

_____

26. UPPP _____

_____

Anatomy

1. Identify the structures of the ear shown in Figure 17-1. Refer to Anatomy Plate #4 in textbook appendix.

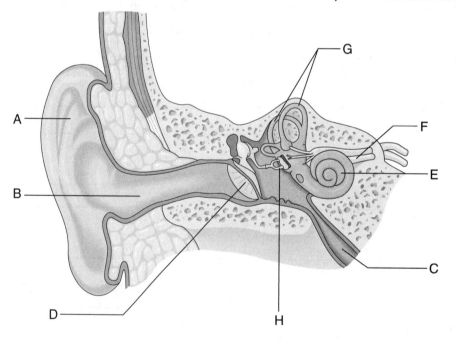

Figure 17-1

A. _____   E. _____

B. _____   F. _____

C. _____   G. _____

D. _____   H. _____

2. Identify the structures of the upper aerodigestive tract shown in Figure 17-2. Refer to Figure 17-25 in your textbook.

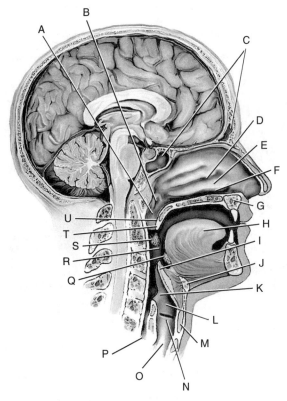

Figure 17-2

A. _____

B. _____

C. _____

D. _____

E. _____

F. _____

G. _____

H. _____

I. _____

J. _____

K. _____

L. _____

M. _____

N. _____

O. _____

P. _____

Q. _____

R. _____

S. _____

T. _____

U. _____

3. Identify the structures of the larynx shown in Figure 17-3. Refer to Figures 17-26 and 17-27 in your textbook.

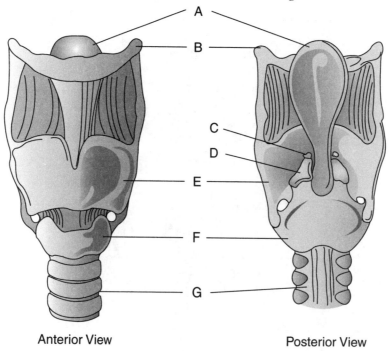

Anterior View   Posterior View

Figure 17-3

A. Leaf-like structure that protects the opening to the larynx: _____

B. Only bone in the body that does not articulate with another: _____

C. Smaller pyramid shaped, laterally attached to the epiglottis: _____

D. Larger pyramid shaped, more medial cartilage: _____

E. Base of epiglottis is attached inferiorly to this area: _____

F. The only complete cartilage located at the base of the larynx: _____

G. Extends from the larynx to the bronchus with C-shaped hyaline cartilage: _____

4. List two functions of the nose. (Nasal functions are not located in the textbook; see your instructor or anatomy textbook for assistance.)

A. _____

B. _____

5. Which bone houses the mastoid sinus?

_____

_____

_____

6. Name the three sections of the pharynx.

A. _____

B. _____

C. _____

7. Which of the tonsils are removed during a tonsillectomy?

_____

_____

_____

8. Name the four pairs of paranasal sinuses, and give their locations.

    A. _____

    B. _____

    C. _____

    D. _____

9. Provide the scientific and common names for the ossicles in their proper sequence, moving from lateral to medial.

    _____

    _____

    _____

10. What are nasal conchae? Describe their function.

    _____

    _____

    _____

11. What is the main source of arterial blood to the nose, and from which vessel is it derived?

    _____

    _____

    _____

12. Where are the adenoids located?

    _____

    _____

    _____

Pathology

1. Can tonsillitis affect the palatine tonsils?

    _____

    _____

    _____

    _____

2. Which nerve is affected in a patient with sensorineural deafness?

    _____

    _____

    _____

3. What is the cause of hypertrophied turbinates?

    _____

    _____

    _____

    _____

4. What is the cause of obstructive sleep apnea?

_____

_____

_____

_____

5. What is the most common cause of otitis media?

_____

_____

_____

_____

6. What causes the nasal septum to deviate from the midline?

_____

_____

_____

_____

7. Where is a Zenker's diverticulum located, and which diagnostic examination will be helpful in determining the diagnosis?

_____

_____

_____

_____

8. List the symptoms of Ménière's syndrome.

_____

_____

_____

9. List several reasons for nasal septal perforation.

_____

_____

_____

_____

10. What are some of the causes of nasal obstruction?

_____

_____

_____

11. What is the usual cause of a vocal cord nodule?

_____

_____

_____

_____

_____

12. Define deafness.

_____

_____

_____

_____

13. What is the origin of a polyp?

_____

_____

_____

_____

Operation

1. What is the name of the procedure used to remove nasal polyps, and what special instrument may be used to perform the procedure?

_____

_____

_____

_____

2. What is the unique feature of the #12 knife blade?

_____

_____

_____

_____

3. Describe the differences between rhinoplasty and septoplasty.

_____

_____

_____

_____

4. What are the reasons for reversing the operating table during ear surgery?

_____

_____

_____

_____

5. Is sinus endoscopy a diagnostic or a functional procedure? Why?

_____

_____

_____

_____

6. What source of energy will be needed to operate the rotating drill?

_____

_____

_____

7. What is intranasal antrostomy, and what special instrument may be needed to facilitate the procedure?

_____

_____

_____

8. What is the most common autologous site for securing a graft for myringoplasty?

_____

_____

_____

9. What are the classifications for tympanoplasty, and how are they determined?

_____

_____

_____

_____

10. Where is the incision made to facilitate drainage of the frontal sinus?

_____

_____

_____

11. What is the pillar dissector used for?

_____

_____

_____

12. Describe panendoscopy, and list any special equipment that may be required.

_____

_____

_____

Specific Variations

Student Name: _____ Date: _____

Instructor: _____

The student will be provided with basic patient information (real or simulated) and is expected to complete the following case study.

1. Procedure name:

   _____

   _____

   _____

   _____

2. Definition of procedure:

   _____

   _____

   _____

   _____

3. What is the purpose of the procedure?

   _____

   _____

   _____

   _____

4. What is the expected outcome of the procedure?

   _____

   _____

   _____

   _____

5. Patient age: _____

6. Gender: _____

7. Additional pertinent patient information:

   _____

   _____

   _____

   _____

8. Probable preoperative diagnosis:

   _____

   _____

   _____

   _____

9. How was the diagnosis determined?

_____

_____

_____

_____

10. Discuss the relevant anatomy.

_____

_____

_____

_____

11. List the general and procedure-specific equipment that will be needed for the procedure.

_____

_____

_____

_____

12. List the general and procedure-specific instruments that will be needed for the procedure.

_____

_____

_____

_____

13. List the basic and procedure-specific supplies that will be needed for the procedure.

    Pack _____

    Basin _____

    Gloves _____

    Blades _____

    Drapes _____

    Drains _____

    Dressings _____

    Suture—Type of Suture, Needle (if applicable), and Anticipated Tissue Usage

    _____

    _____

    _____

    _____

    Pharmaceuticals

    _____

    _____

    _____

    _____

Miscellaneous

_____

_____

_____

_____

14. Operative preparation:

_____

_____

_____

_____

15. What type of anesthesia will likely be used? Why?

_____

_____

_____

_____

16. List any special anesthesia equipment that may be needed.

_____

_____

_____

_____

17. What is the patient position during the procedure?

_____

_____

_____

_____

18. What supplies will be necessary for positioning?

_____

_____

_____

_____

19. What type of shave/skin preparation will be necessary (if any)?

_____

_____

_____

_____

20. Define the anatomic perimeters of the prep.

_____

_____

_____

_____

21. List the order in which the drapes will be applied, and describe any specific variations.

_____

_____

_____

22. List any practical considerations.

_____

_____

_____

23. List the procedural steps, and describe the preparatory and supportive actions of the STSR during each step (use additional space if necessary).

_____

_____

_____

_____

24. What is the postoperative diagnosis?

_____

_____

_____

_____

25. Describe the immediate postoperative care.

_____

_____

_____

_____

26. What is the patient's long-term prognosis?

_____

_____

_____

_____

27. What are the possible complications?

_____

_____

_____

_____

28. Comments or questions:

_____

_____

_____

_____

29. What is the most valuable information you obtained from preparing this surgical procedure case study?

_____

_____

_____

_____

_____

Case Studies

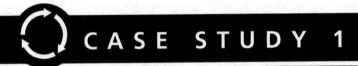

CASE STUDY 1

Stan, a 46-year-old male, is about to spend the night in the "sleep lab." After numerous complaints from his wife that his heavy snoring is keeping her awake, Stan visited his primary care physician. Following a complete physical, Stan was diagnosed with hypertension and obesity, and he was referred to an otorhinolaryngologist.

1. What tests will Stan undergo in the "sleep lab"?

_____

_____

_____

_____

2. What diagnosis do you think that the otorhinolaryngologist is considering?

_____

_____

_____

_____

3. What are Stan's conservative treatment options?

_____

_____

_____

_____

4. If Stan's condition eventually requires surgery, which procedure will be performed, and what structures will be removed?

_____

_____

_____

_____

CASE STUDY 2

Fred, a 4-year-old male, has been placed in respite foster care because of his uncontrollable temper tantrums, which include long bouts of screaming. The foster family noticed that Fred's voice was hoarse and that it did not improve over time. He was seen by an otorhinolaryngologist, who determined that Fred has developed nodules on his vocal cords.

1. Is Fred's condition life-threatening?

   _____

   _____

   _____

   _____

2. How was Fred's condition diagnosed?

   _____

   _____

   _____

   _____

3. What action will be necessary to treat Fred's condition?

   _____

   _____

   _____

   _____

4. If surgery is required, what type of procedure will be necessary, and how will it be accomplished?

   _____

   _____

   _____

   _____

5. If surgery is necessary, will the foster parents have the legal authority to sign his operative consent?

   _____

   _____

   _____

   _____

Lab 17: Otorhinolaryngologic Surgery

Introduction

Otorhinolaryngologic surgery deals with the ears, nose, and throat. This specialty tends to be difficult to learn because so many of the instruments do not relate to other specialties and many physicians will employ private scrubs. The instruments may look very similar to each other with only subtle changes between each. It will take a lot of concentration and studying to learn many of the micro ear instruments. Learning the surgery step by step in lecture will help you in the lab portion. This is where you will learn the hands on of the specialty and the instruments that will be used for each piece of the surgery.

Game: Otorhinolaryngologic Surgery on Felt Mayo Stands

Time involved: 1–2 weeks setup

Instructors: Make a list of instruments you expect students to know as part of the otorhinolaryngologic surgery lab. Have the students trace the real instruments onto the felt if possible; if not, have them find pictures they can cut out and trace onto the felt or other material. I like felt because it tends to be very durable, but paper or cardboard can be substituted. There should be no need for multiple cutouts of the same instruments if students are given the chance to show how many of those instruments they would have on the Mayo by way of a numbered marker (a piece of paper with a number designation on it). The students are given a list of surgeries that they are expected to know. **Note:** This can also be made easier if you have photos of the Mayo stand setups for the students to study.

Students: You will need several pieces of felt, paper, or cardboard. The largest piece should be cut to the size of a regular Mayo stand. You will make cutouts of instruments as close as possible to life size using felt or some other material. Label the back of the cutouts for easy reference.

Supplies: Felt, paper, or cardboard; real instruments, or pictures that have been printed and cut out from the computer; felt tip marker; scissors; measuring tool

How the Game is Played

The students are given a list of surgeries that they are expected to know. The instructor will assign one of those surgeries to the student in the lab. The student will then be expected to complete a Mayo stand setup in a specified time frame utilizing the instruments they have cut out. Score the students according to placement of instruments, time needed for setup, correct instrumentation, and correct number of instruments.

Practical: Set Up General Surgery Cases

Utilizing a full lab/OR setup, assign the students different surgical cases to learn. The students will then be expected to set up some of these cases under the supervision of the instructor. They should utilize as much of the OR equipment as needed including back table, Mayo stand, ring stands, instrument trays, and pans. The student should be scored on correct placement of supplies, practicing economy of time and motion (pick it up and place it one time), correct order of instruments, correct number of instruments, aseptic technique, time to set up, and order of use for instruments and supplies; a mock surgery should be performed so the student can practice anticipating the needs of the surgeon.

CHAPTER 18

Oral and Maxillofacial Surgery

OBJECTIVES

After studying this chapter, the reader should be able to:

A 1. Recognize the anatomy relevant to oral and maxillofacial surgery.

P 2. Summarize the pathology that prompts oral and maxillofacial surgery, and the related terminology.

3. Determine any special preoperative diagnostic procedures/tests pertaining to oral and maxillofacial surgery.

O 4. Determine special preoperative preparation procedures related to oral and maxillofacial surgery.

5. Indicate the names and uses of oral and maxillofacial instruments, supplies, and drugs.

6. Indicate the names and uses of special equipment used for oral and maxillofacial surgery.

7. Determine the intraoperative preparation of the patient undergoing an oral or maxillofacial procedure.

8. Summarize the surgical steps of oral and maxillofacial procedures.

9. Interpret the purpose and expected outcomes of oral and maxillofacial procedures.

10. Recognize the immediate postoperative care and possible complications of oral and maxillofacial procedures.

S 11. Assess any specific variations related to the preoperative, intraoperative, and postoperative care of the oral and maxillofacial surgical patient.

Select Key Terms

Define the following, using your textbook glossary or a medical dictionary:

1. alveolar process _____

_____

2. arthroscopy _____

_____

3. calvarial _____

_____

4. condyle _____

_____

5. coronal flap _____

_____

6. craniosynostosis _____

_____

7. dentition _____

_____

8. glenoid fossa _____

_____

9. gnath- _____

_____

10. labia _____

_____

11. malar bone _____

_____

12. malocclusion _____

_____

13. maxillofacial _____

_____

14. meniscus _____

_____

15. mouth prop _____

_____

16. orbicular _____

_____

17. osteotomy _____

_____

18. pan- _____

_____

19. ramus _____

_____

20. reduction _____

_____

21. sagittal _____

_____

22. symphysis _____

_____

23. TMJ _____

_____

Anatomy

1. Identify the bones of the anterior skull shown in Figure 18-1.Refer to Anatomy Plate #7 in your textbook appendix.

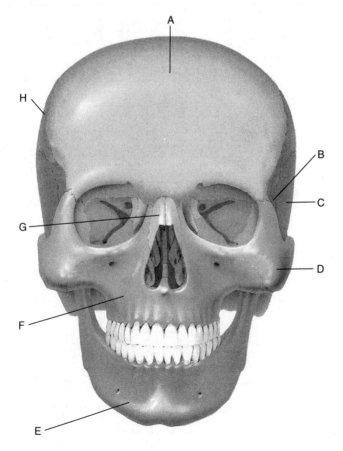

Figure 18-1

A. _____

B. _____

C. _____

D. _____

E. _____

F. _____

G. _____

H. _____

2. Identify the structures of the lateral skull shown in Figure 18-2. Refer to Anatomy Plate #7 in your textbook appendix.

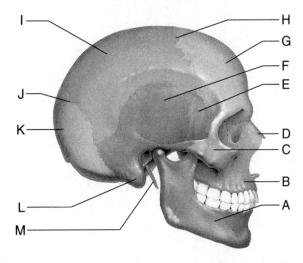

Figure 18-2

A. _____

B. _____

C. _____

D. _____

E. _____

F. _____

G. _____

H. _____

I. _____

J. _____

K. _____

L. _____

M. _____

3. Identify the structures of the mouth shown in Figure 18-3. Refer to Anatomy Plate #6 in your textbook appendix.

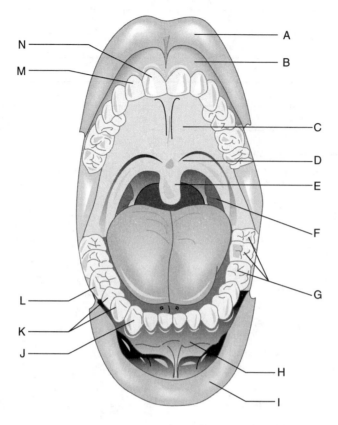

Figure 18-3

A. _____

B. _____

C. _____

D. _____

E. _____

F. _____

G. _____

H. _____

I. _____

J. _____

K. _____

L. _____

M. _____

N. _____

4. Identify the structures of the orbit shown in Figure 18-4. Refer to Figure 18-4 located at the Online Companion website. (Go to www.delmarlearning.com\companions, click on 'Allied Health,' then the textbook title and edition.)

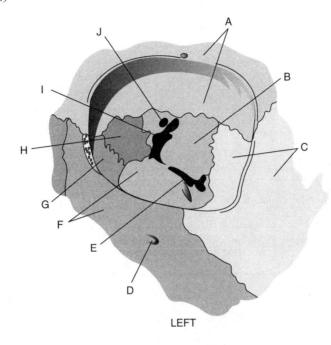

LEFT

Figure 18-4

A. _____

B. _____

C. _____

D. _____

E. _____

F. _____

G. _____

H. _____

I. _____

J. _____

5. The anterior portion of the palate is referred to as the _____ palate.

6. What is the location and function of the soft palate?

_____

_____

_____

_____

7. The malar bone is also referred to as the _____ bone.

8. What is the vomer and where is it located?

_____

_____

_____

9. What is another name for the facial nerve? Which facial muscles are innervated by the facial nerve?

_____

_____

_____

_____

10. Which four muscles control movement of the lower jaw?

_____

_____

_____

_____

11. When does embryologic development of the face occur?

_____

_____

_____

_____

12. Where is the orbicularis oris muscle situated? What is its function?

_____

_____

_____

_____

13. Describe the components and features of the TMJ.

_____

_____

_____

_____

14. What is the ramus of the mandible?

_____

_____

_____

_____

15. What are the two main functions of the orbit?

_____

_____

_____

_____

Pathology

1. What are dental caries, and what is their cause?

   _____

   _____

   _____

   _____

2. What is meant by the term malocclusion? List two causes.

   _____

   _____

   _____

   _____

3. How does Paget's disease affect facial anatomy?

   _____

   _____

   _____

   _____

4. Describe a tri-malar fracture.

   _____

   _____

   _____

   _____

5. List the four categories of mandibular fractures.

   A. _____

   B. _____

   C. _____

   D. _____

6. What type of midfacial fracture is the most common?

   _____

   _____

   _____

   _____

7. What is laterognathism? List two causes.

   A. _____

   B. _____

8. What specific radiographic view is used to detect a fracture of the frontal bone?

   _____

   _____

_____

_____

9. Define cerebrospinal rhinorrhea.

_____

_____

_____

_____

10. List three methods for diagnosing a zygomatic fracture.

_____

_____

_____

_____

11. List three visual findings that could indicate the presence of a zygomatic fracture.

A. _____

B. _____

C. _____

12. Premature closure of the sutures of the skull is called _____.

13. Name and describe the four categories of tooth fractures.

A. _____

B. _____

C. _____

D. _____

14. List two advantages of three-dimensional imaging.

A. _____

B. _____

15. In addition to radiographic studies (including three-dimensional imaging), what other items may be useful to the surgeon during facial reconstruction surgery?

_____

_____

_____

_____

Operation

1. What is the importance of having the X-rays in the operating room prior to and during the surgical procedure?

_____

_____

_____

_____

2. What is accomplished by inserting a mouth prop during certain oral surgical procedures?

_____

_____

_____

_____

3. What is the purpose of inserting a throat pack? How is it inserted?

_____

_____

_____

_____

4. When is the throat pack removed? Why?

_____

_____

_____

_____

5. List two options for sealing an intranasal dural tear.

    A. _____

    B. _____

6. Define autogenous, and list two possible donor sites for autogenous bone grafts

_____

_____

_____

_____

    A. _____

    B. _____

7. Why is a local anesthetic with epinephrine often injected at the operative site preoperatively when the patient is under general anesthesia?

_____

_____

_____

_____

8. Describe the location of a coronal incision.

_____

_____

_____

_____

9. List two methods for securing and positioning a soft tissue flap.

    A. _____

    B. _____

10. In what position will the patient be placed for a posterior cranial expansion?

_____

_____

_____

_____

11. What type of procedure is performed to treat orthognathia?

_____

_____

_____

_____

12. What can be done during lengthy oral procedures to prevent drying and cracking of the lips?

_____

_____

_____

_____

13. Why is it important to assure that all metal implants are of the same type?

_____

_____

_____

_____

14. If a bone graft is needed during a procedure in which the patient has a coronal incision, what type of bone will be considered as the first choice? Why?

_____

_____

_____

15. In what situation(s) is arch bar fixation employed?

_____

_____

_____

_____

Specific Variations

Student Name: _____ Date: _____

Instructor: _____

The student will be provided with basic patient information (real or simulated) and is expected to complete the following case study.

1. Procedure name:

   _____

   _____

   _____

   _____

2. Definition of procedure:

   _____

   _____

   _____

   _____

3. What is the purpose of the procedure?

   _____

   _____

   _____

   _____

4. What is the expected outcome of the procedure?

   _____

   _____

   _____

   _____

5. Patient age: _____

6. Gender: _____

7. Additional pertinent patient information:

   _____

   _____

   _____

   _____

8. Probable preoperative diagnosis:

   _____

   _____

   _____

   _____

9. How was the diagnosis determined?

_____

_____

_____

_____

10. Discuss the relevant anatomy.

_____

_____

_____

_____

11. List the general and procedure-specific equipment that will be needed for the procedure.

_____

_____

_____

_____

12. List the general and procedure-specific instruments that will be needed for the procedure.

_____

_____

_____

_____

13. List the basic and procedure-specific supplies that will be needed for the procedure.

Pack _____

Basin _____

Gloves _____

Blades _____

Drapes _____

Drains _____

Dressings _____

Suture—Type of Suture, Needle (if applicable), and Anticipated Tissue Usage

_____

_____

_____

Pharmaceuticals

_____

_____

_____

Miscellaneous

_____

_____

_____

_____

14. Operative preparation:

_____

_____

_____

_____

15. What type of anesthesia will likely be used? Why?

_____

_____

_____

_____

16. List any special anesthesia equipment that may be needed.

_____

_____

_____

_____

17. Patient position during the procedure:

_____

_____

_____

_____

18. What supplies will be necessary for positioning?

_____

_____

_____

_____

19. What type of shave/skin preparation will be necessary (if any)?

_____

_____

_____

_____

20. Define the anatomic perimeters of the prep.

_____

_____

_____

_____

21. List the order in which the drapes will be applied, and describe any specific variations.

_____

_____

_____

_____

22. List any practical considerations.

_____

_____

_____

_____

23. List the procedural steps, and describe the preparatory and supportive actions of the STSR during each step (use additional space if necessary).

_____

_____

_____

_____

24. What is the postoperative diagnosis?

_____

_____

_____

_____

25. Describe the immediate postoperative care.

_____

_____

_____

_____

26. What is the patient's long-term prognosis?

_____

_____

_____

_____

27. What are the possible complications?

_____

_____

_____

_____

28. Comments or questions:

_____

_____

_____

_____

29. What is the most valuable information you obtained from preparing this surgical procedure case study?

_____

_____

_____

_____

_____

Case Studies

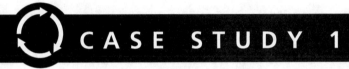

CASE STUDY 1

Lucricia is a 14-year-old female patient with cerebral palsy and epilepsy. She is scheduled for dental restoration, including gingivectomy for hyperplasia of her gums, under general anesthesia.

1. What procedures may be performed during dental restoration?

_____

_____

_____

_____

2. What is the wound classification for this procedure?

_____

_____

_____

_____

3. Describe how to prepare the dental mirror for use. Why does the mirror require preparation?

_____

_____

_____

_____

4. The surgeon asks for a Wieder. What is it used for?

_____

_____

_____

_____

CASE STUDY 2

Roberto experienced a severe blow to his left cheek when he accidentally struck the corner of the wall as he was rushing through a dark hallway during the night, on his way to the bathroom. He has severe pain, and it appears to him that his face no longer has a symmetrical appearance.

1. What type of injury do you suspect that Roberto has incurred?

_____

_____

_____

_____

2. What type of examination(s) will be performed by the maxillofacial surgeon to confirm the diagnosis?

_____

_____

_____

_____

3. How will Roberto's problem be corrected?

_____

_____

_____

_____

Lab 18: Oral and Maxillofacial Surgery

Introduction

Oral and maxillofacial surgery deals with surgery of the facial structures and the mouth. This section will be very similar to the orthopedic lab. Learning the surgery step by step in lecture will help you in the lab portion. This is where you will learn the hands on of the specialty and the instruments that will be used for each piece of the surgery.

Game: Oral and Maxillofacial Surgery on Felt Mayo Stands

Time involved: 1-2 weeks setup

Instructors: Make a list of instruments you expect students to know as part of the Oral and Maxillofacial Surgery Lab; this list will be similar to that for the orthopedic lab. Have the students trace the real instruments onto felt if possible; if not, have them find pictures they can cut out and trace onto the felt or other material. I like the felt because it tends to be very durable, but paper or cardboard can be substituted. There should be no need for multiple cutouts of the same instruments if students are given the chance to show how many of those instruments they would have on the Mayo by way of a numbered marker (a piece of paper with a number designation on it). The students are given a list of surgeries that they are expected to know. Note: This can also be made easier if you have photos of these Mayo stand setups for the students to study.

Students: You will need several pieces of felt, paper, or cardboard. The largest piece should be cut to the size of a regular Mayo stand. You will proceed to make cutouts of instruments as close as possible to life size using felt or some other material. Label the backsides of the cutouts for easy reference.

Supplies: Felt, paper, or cardboard; real instruments, or pictures that have been printed and cut out from the computer; felt-tip marker; scissors; measuring tool

How the Game is Played

The students are given a list of surgeries that they are expected to know. The instructor will then assign one of those surgeries to the student in the lab. The student will then be expected to complete a Mayo stand setup in a specified time frame utilizing the instruments they have cut out. Score the students according to placement of instruments, time needed for set-up, correct instrumentation, and correct number of instruments.

Practical: Set Up Oral/Maxilofacial Surgery Cases

Utilizing a full lab/OR setup, assign the students different surgical cases to learn. The students will then be expected to set up some of these cases under the supervision of the instructor. They should utilize as much of the OR equipment as needed including backtable, Mayo stand, ring stands, instrument trays, and pans. The student should be scored on correct placement of supplies, practicing economy of time and motion (pick it up and place it one time), correct order of instruments, correct number of instruments, aseptic technique, time to set up, and order of use for instruments and supplies; a mock surgery should be performed so the student can practice anticipating the needs of the surgeon.

CHAPTER 19

Plastic and Reconstructive Surgery

OBJECTIVES

After studying this chapter, the reader should be able to:

A 1. Recognize the relevant anatomy and physiology of the skin and its underlying tissues.

P 2. Summarize the pathology that prompts plastic/reconstructive surgical intervention and the related terminology.

3. Determine any special preoperative plastic/reconstructive diagnostic procedures/tests.

O 4. Determine any special preoperative preparation procedures related to plastic/reconstructive surgical procedures.

5. Indicate the names and uses of plastic/reconstructive instruments, supplies, and drugs

6. Indicate the names and uses of special equipment related to plastic/ reconstructive surgery.

7. Determine the intraoperative preparation of the patient undergoing a plastic/reconstructive procedure.

8. Summarize the surgical steps of the plastic/reconstructive procedure.

9. Interpret the purpose and expected outcomes of the plastic/reconstructive procedure.

10. Recognize the immediate postoperative care and possible complications of the plastic/reconstructive procedure.

S 11. Assess any specific variations related to the preoperative, intraoperative, and postoperative care of the plastic/reconstructive patient.

Select Key Terms

Define the following, using your textbook glossary or a medical dictionary:

1. aesthetic _____

_____

2. arthrodesis _____

_____

3. augmentation _____

_____

4. carpal tunnel _____

_____

5. cheilo _____

_____

6. cleft _____

_____

7. dermatome _____

_____

8. elliptical _____

_____

9. ganglion cyst _____

_____

10. gynecomastia _____

_____

11. integumentary _____

_____

12. MPJ _____

_____

13. poly- _____

_____

14. radial hypoplasia _____

_____

15. replantation _____

_____

16. rhinoplasty _____

_____

17. schisis _____

_____

18. sebum _____

_____

19. STSG _____

_____

20. syndactyly _____

_____

21. synthesis _____

_____

22. xenograft _____

_____

Anatomy

1. Identify the structures shown in Figure 19-1. Refer to Figure 19-1 in your textbook.

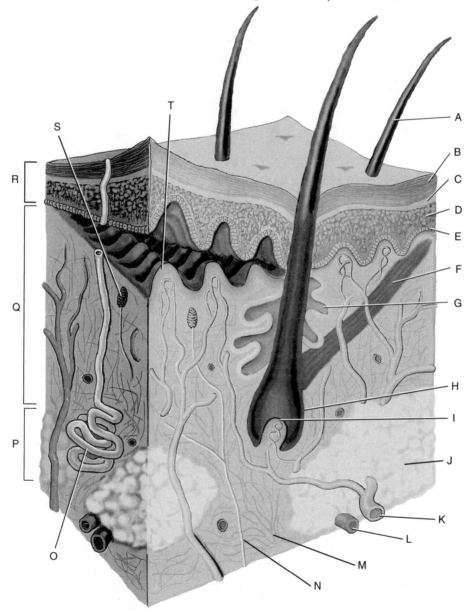

Figure 19-1

A. _____

B. _____

C. _____

D. _____

E. _____

F. _____

G. _____

H. _____

I. _____

J. _____

K. _____

L. _____

M. _____

N. _____

O. _____

P. _____

Q. _____ .

R. _____ .

S. _____ .

T. _____

2. Identify the bones of the dorsal hand shown in Figure 19-2. Refer to Figure 19-3 in your textbook.

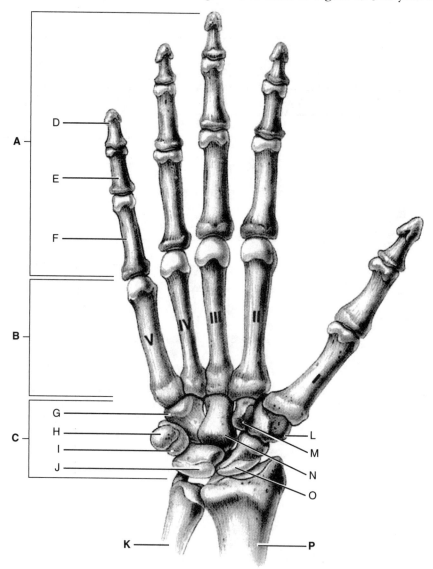

Figure 19-2

A. _____

B. _____

C. _____

D. _____

E. _____

F. _____

G. _____

H. _____

I. _____

J. _____

K. _____

L. _____

M. _____

N. _____

O. _____

P. _____

3. Identify the structures of the breast shown in Figure 19-3. Refer to Figure 19-3 located at the Online Companion website. (Go to www.delmarlearning.com/companions, click on 'Allied Health,' then the text-book title and edition.)

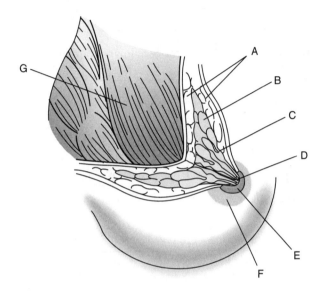

Figure 19-3

A. _____

B. _____

C. _____

D. _____

E. _____

F. _____

G. _____

4. Name the two major layers of the integumentary system.

A. _____

B. _____

5. List the major functions of the skin.

A. _____

B. _____

C. _____

D. _____

E. _____

F. _____

G. _____

6. Sweat glands are also known as the _____ glands.

7. Name and briefly describe the three types of sudoriferous glands.

    A. _____

    _____

    B. _____

    _____

    C. _____

    _____

8. Name the structures that are contained in the anterior (palmar) compartment of the hand.

    _____

    _____

    _____

    _____

9. In utero, the development of the lip and palate is complete by the _____.

10. Name the five layers of the epidermis in sequence from the outermost to innermost layer.

    A. _____

    B. _____

    C. _____

    D. _____

    E. _____

11. Name the three functions of the subcutaneous tissue layer.

    A. _____

    B. _____

    C. _____

12. Name the two divisions of the dermis, and briefly describe them.

    A. _____

    B. _____

13. Name the secretion that is produced in the sebaceous glands. What is the purpose of the secretion?

    _____

    _____

    _____

    _____

14. What is the function of the palate?

    _____

    _____

    _____

    _____

Pathology

1. Which tissue layer(s) is/are affected by a second-degree burn?

   _____

   _____

   _____

   _____

2. Use the Rule of Nines to determine the percentage of the body surface area affected by a third-degree burn of the chest, back, and left arm.

   _____

   _____

   _____

   _____

3. Name the bacteria that are the main causative agents of acne vulgaris.

   A. _____

   B. _____

   C. _____

4. Only 20% of cleft deformities are genetic. What is/are the cause(s) of the remaining 80%?

   _____

   _____

   _____

   _____

5. What is the most common type of polydactyly?

   _____

   _____

   _____

   _____

6. What is a ganglion cyst?

   _____

   _____

   _____

   _____

7. What causes the formation of a ganglion cyst?

   _____

   _____

   _____

   _____

8. Name three treatment options for a ganglion cyst.

   A. _____

   B. _____

   C. _____

9. What is the cause of ptosis of the eyelid?

_____

_____

_____

_____

10. Define neoplasm. Is a neoplasm malignant?

_____

_____

_____

_____

11. Give three examples of common malignant neoplasms of the skin.

A. _____

B. _____

C. _____

12. What is the cause of cheiloschisis and palatoschisis?

_____

_____

_____

_____

13. Name two diseases of the hand that are caused by stenosing tenosynovitis.

A. _____

B. _____

14. List three manifestations of palmar fascia contraction (Dupuytren's disease).

A. _____

B. _____

C. _____

15. What is the cause of rheumatoid arthritis (RA)?

_____

_____

_____

_____

Operation

1. Describe the difference between nasal and rhinoplasty instrumentation.

_____

_____

_____

_____

2. What is the purpose/function of a dermatome?

_____

_____

_____

_____

3. List two possible power sources for the oscillating-blade-type dermatome.

   A. _____

   B. _____

4. What is the purpose of a mesh graft device?

_____

_____

_____

_____

5. What is the purpose of a tacking suture used during a rhytidectomy?

_____

_____

_____

_____

6. What is the advantage of tumescent liposuction over the traditional method?

_____

_____

_____

_____

7. What is the common name for the umbilical template used during abdominoplasty? What is its purpose?

_____

_____

_____

_____

8. How is sterile mineral oil used during procurement of an STSG?

_____

_____

_____

_____

9. How is the recipient site prepared prior to placement of an STSG? Why?

_____

_____

_____

_____

10. Why is palatoplasty considered a clean, rather than sterile, procedure?

_____

_____

_____

_____

11. What anatomic area is prepped prior to draping for hand surgery?

_____

_____

_____

12. Why is the extremity wrapped with an Esmarch bandage prior to tourniquet inflation?

_____

_____

_____

_____

13. Provide two indications for joint replacement in the hand.

A. _____

B. _____

14. Replantation of a digit begins with the attachment of which structure(s)?

_____

_____

_____

_____

15. List four incision options for augmentation mammoplasty that produce a minimal or completely hidden scar.

A. _____

B. _____

C. _____

D. _____

Specific Variations

Student Name: _____ Date: _____

Instructor: _____

The student will be provided with basic patient information (real or simulated) and is expected to complete the following case study.

1. Procedure name:

   _____

   _____

   _____

   _____

2. Definition of procedure:

   _____

   _____

   _____

   _____

3. What is the purpose of the procedure?

   _____

   _____

   _____

   _____

4. What is the expected outcome of the procedure?

   _____

   _____

   _____

   _____

5. Patient age: _____

6. Gender: _____

7. Additional pertinent patient information:

   _____

   _____

   _____

   _____

8. Probable preoperative diagnosis:

   _____

   _____

   _____

   _____

9. How was the diagnosis determined?

_____

_____

_____

_____

10. Discuss the relevant anatomy.

_____

_____

_____

_____

11. List the general and procedure-specific equipment that will be needed for the procedure.

_____

_____

_____

_____

12. List the general and procedure-specific instruments that will be needed for the procedure.

_____

_____

_____

_____

13. List the basic and procedure-specific supplies that will be needed for the procedure.

Pack _____

Basin _____

Gloves _____

Blades _____

Drapes _____

Drains _____

Dressings_____

_____

Suture—Type of Suture, Needle (if applicable), and Anticipated Tissue Usage

_____

_____

_____

_____

Pharmaceuticals

_____

_____

_____

_____

Miscellaneous

_____

_____

_____

_____

14. Operative preparation:

_____

_____

_____

_____

15. What type of anesthesia will likely be used? Why?

_____

_____

_____

_____

16. List any special anesthesia equipment that may be needed.

_____

_____

_____

_____

17. Patient position during the procedure:

_____

_____

_____

_____

18. What supplies will be necessary for positioning?

_____

_____

_____

_____

19. What type of shave/skin preparation will be necessary (if any)?

_____

_____

_____

_____

20. Define the anatomic perimeters of the prep.

_____

_____

_____

_____

21. List the order in which the drapes will be applied, and describe any specific variations.

_____

_____

_____

_____

22. List any practical considerations.

_____

_____

_____

_____

23. List the procedural steps, and describe the preparatory and supportive actions of the STSR during each step (use additional space if necessary).

_____

_____

_____

_____

24. What is the postoperative diagnosis?

_____

_____

_____

_____

25. Describe the immediate postoperative care.

_____

_____

_____

_____

26. What is the patient's long-term prognosis?

_____

_____

_____

_____

27. What are the possible complications?

_____

_____

28. Comments or questions:

_____

_____

_____

_____

29. What is the most valuable information you obtained from preparing this surgical procedure case study?

_____

_____

_____

_____

Case Studies

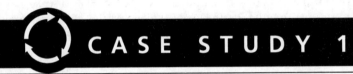

CASE STUDY 1

Three-year-old Bobby accidentally pulled on the tablecloth, causing his mother's scalding coffee to spill on his left neck, shoulder, and chest. It has been determined that Bobby has suffered second- and third-degree burns over 9% of his body. The accident occurred three weeks ago, and Bobby is now scheduled for an STSG.

1. How was the extent of Bobby's injury determined?

_____

_____

_____

_____

2. What was the biggest risk that Bobby faced with these third-degree burns?

_____

_____

_____

_____

3. What is "STSG," and what special instrument will be required to obtain the graft?

_____

_____

_____

_____

(contiunes)

CASE STUDY 1 *(continued)*

4. From which anatomic site is the graft most likely to be procured?

_____

_____

_____

_____

CASE STUDY 2

Sven is a 62-year-old dairy farmer. He has been diagnosed with Dupuytren's disease. The disease has progressed to the point where Sven is unable to use his right hand effectively to connect the milking machine to his cows. He has put off surgery as long as possible, but now the inevitable has arrived.

1. What is Dupuytren's disease?

_____

_____

_____

_____

2. Is the condition painful?

_____

_____

_____

_____

3. What procedure will be necessary to treat Sven's condition?

_____

_____

_____

_____

4. Can Sven expect to regain full function and normal appearance?

_____

_____

_____

_____

Lab 19: Plastics and Reconstructive Surgery

Introduction

Plastic and reconstructive surgery deals with surgery utilized to reconstruct or help with aesthetics. Instruments and sutures in this area tend to be very fine and very delicate. Asymmetry and the aesthetics of the finished product is how we gauge most of these surgeries. Learning the surgery step by step in lecture will help you in the lab portion. This is where you will learn the hands on of the specialty and the instruments that will be used for each piece of the surgery.

Game: Plastics and Reconstructive Surgery on Felt Mayo Stands

Time involved: 1–2 weeks setup

Instructors: Make a list of instruments you expect students to know as part of the plastic and reconstructive surgery lab. Have the students trace the real instruments onto the felt if possible, if not have them find pictures they can cut out and trace onto the felt or other material. I like felt because it tends to be very durable, but paper or cardboard can be substituted. There should be no need for multiple cutouts of the same instruments if students are given the chance to show how many of those instruments they would have on the Mayo by way of a numbered marker (a piece of paper with a number designation on it). The students are given a list of surgeries that they are expected to know. **Note:** This can also be made easier if you have photos of these Mayo stand setups for the students to study.

Students: You will need several pieces of felt, paper, or cardboard. The largest piece should be cut to the size of a regular Mayo stand. You will then cut out instruments as close to life size as possible using felt or some other material. Label the backsides of the cutouts for easy reference.

Supplies: Felt, paper, or cardboard; real instruments, or pictures that have been printed and cut out from the computer; felt-tip marker; scissors; measuring tool

How the Game is Played

The students are given a list of surgeries that they are expected to know. The instructor will then assign one of those surgeries to the student in the lab. The student will then be expected to complete a Mayo stand setup in a specified time frame utilizing the instruments they have cut out. Score the students according to placement of instruments, time needed for setup, correct instrumentation, and correct number of instruments.

Practical: Set Up General Surgery Cases

Utilizing a full lab/OR setup, assign the students different surgical cases to learn. The students will then be expected to set up some of these cases under the supervision of the instructor. They should utilize as much of the OR equipment as needed including backtable, Mayo stand, ring stands, instrument trays, and pans. The student should be scored on correct placement of supplies, practicing economy of time and motion (pick it up and place it one time), correct order of instruments, correct number of instruments, aseptic technique, time to set up, and order of use for instruments and supplies; a mock surgery should be performed so the student can work on anticipating the needs of the surgeon.

CHAPTER 20

Genitourinary Surgery

OBJECTIVES

After studying this chapter, the reader should be able to:

A 1. Recognize the relevant anatomy of the genitourinary system.

P 2. Recognize the pathology that prompts genitourinary system surgical intervention and the related terminology.

3. Assess any special preoperative genitourinary diagnostic procedures/tests.

O 4. Assess any special preoperative genitourinary preparation procedures.

5. Indicate the names and uses of genitourinary instruments, supplies, and drugs.

6. Indicate the names and uses of special genitourinary equipment.

7. Determine the intraoperative preparation of the patient undergoing the genitourinary procedure.

8. Summarize the steps of the genitourinary procedure.

9. Determine the purpose and expected outcomes of the genitourinary procedures.

10. Assess the immediate postoperative care and possible complications of the genitourinary procedure.

S 11. Recognize any specific variations related to the preoperative, intraoperative, and postoperative care of the genitourinary patient.

Select Key Terms

Define the following, using your textbook glossary or a medical dictionary:

1. ACTH _____

_____

2. afferent _____

_____

3. calculi _____

_____

4. conduit _____

_____

5. cortex _____

_____

6. ESWL _____

_____

7. Gerota's fascia _____

_____

8. Gibson incision _____

_____

9. hilum _____

_____

10. hirsutism _____

_____

11. hypertrophy _____

_____

12. hypospadias _____

_____

13. incontinence _____

_____

14. intravenous urogram (IVU) _____

_____

15. medulla _____

_____

16. prepuce _____

_____

17. retroperitoneal _____

_____

18. stoma _____

_____

19. suprarenal glands _____

_____

20. torsion _____

_____

21. TURP _____

_____

22. UTI _____

_____

23. vesical trigone _____

_____

Anatomy

1. Identify the main structures shown in Figure 20-1. Refer to Figure 20-1 in your textbook.

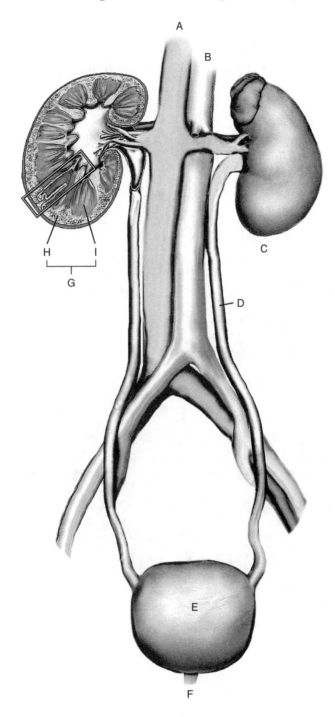

Figure 20-1

A. _____

B. _____

C. _____

D. _____

E. _____

F. _____

G. _____

H. _____

I. _____

2. Identify the structures shown in Figure 20-2. Refer to Figure 20-2 located at the Online Companion website. (Go to www.delmarlearning.com/companions, click on 'Allied Health,' then the textbook title and edition.)

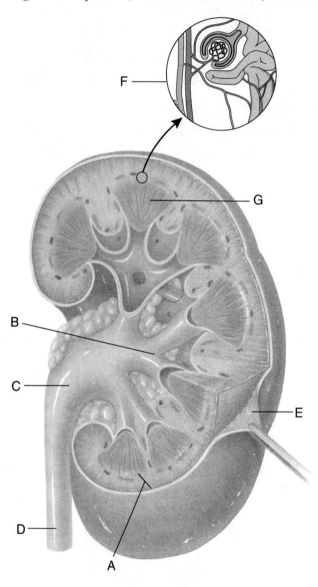

Figure 20-2

A. _____

B. _____

C. _____

D. _____

E. _____

F. _____

G. _____

3. Identify the structures shown in Figure 20-3. Refer to Figure 20-3 located at the Online Companion website.

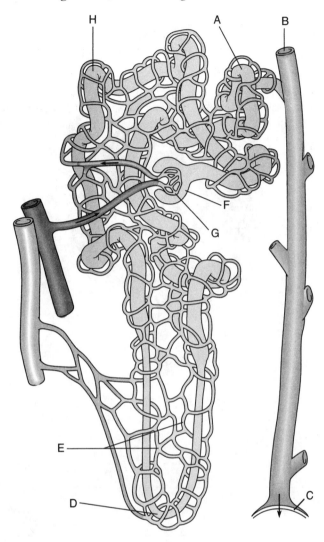

Figure 20-3

A. _____

B. _____

C. _____

D. _____

E. _____

F. _____

G. _____

H. _____

4. Identify the structures shown in Figure 20-4. Refer to Figure 20-3 in your textbook.

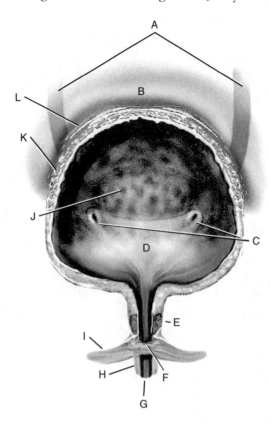

Figure 20-4

A. _____

B. _____

C. _____

D. _____

E. _____

F. _____

G. _____

H. _____

I. _____

J. _____

K. _____

L. _____

5. Identify the structures shown in Figure 20-5. Refer to Anatomy plate #10 in your textbook appendix.

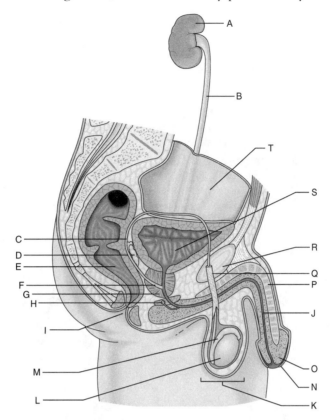

Figure 20-5

A. _____

B. _____

C. _____

D. _____

E. _____

F. _____

G. _____

H. _____

I. _____

J. _____

K. _____

L. _____

M. _____

N. _____

O. _____

P. _____

Q. _____

R. _____

S. _____

T. _____

6. Identify the structures shown in Figure 20-6. Refer to Figure 20-4 in your textbook.

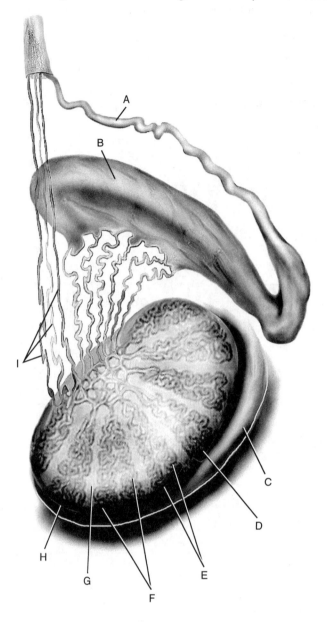

Figure 20-6

A. _____

B. _____

C. _____

D. _____

E. _____

F. _____

G. _____

H. _____

I. _____

7. Using the numbers 1–5, trace the pathway of sperm cells from the site of meiosis through the ducts of the male reproductive system as they exit the body by placing the following elements in the correct order.

   A. _____ Ductus deferens

   B. _____ Ejaculatory duct

   C. _____ Epididymis

   D. _____ Seminiferous tubules (testis)

   E. _____ Urethra

8. Using the numbers 1–13, trace the pathway of fluid from the time it leaves the circulatory system until it leaves the body as urine by placing the following elements in the correct order.

   A. _____ Afferent arteriole

   B. _____ Bladder

   C. _____ Bowman's capsule

   D. _____ Calyx

   E. _____ Collecting tubule

   F. _____ Distal convoluted tubule

   G. _____ Glomerulus

   H. _____ Loop of Henle

   I. _____ Proximal convoluted tubule

   J. _____ Renal artery

   K. _____ Renal pelvis

   L. _____ Ureter

   M. _____ Urethra

9. Name the two portions of the adrenal gland and the function of each.

   A. _____

   B. _____

10. Describe the location of the kidneys.

    _____

    _____

    _____

    _____

11. Peristalsis conducts urine from the kidney to the bladder. Why does the ureter run obliquely through the bladder wall?

    _____

    _____

    _____

    _____

12. What are the anatomic boundaries of the trigone of the bladder?

    _____

    _____

    _____

    _____

13. Name the three cavernous structures of the penis.

    A. _____

    B. _____

    C. _____

14. What is the function of the detrusor muscle?

    _____

    _____

    _____

    _____

15. What are the functional units of the kidney, and approximately how many are located within each kidney?

    _____

    _____

    _____

    _____

Pathology

1. List two possible causes for Cushing's syndrome and the possible treatments for each.

    A. _____

    B. _____

2. What is pheochromocytoma? List the classic symptoms.

    _____

    _____

    _____

    _____

3. List the four basic chemical types of urinary calculi and their causes.

    A. _____

    B. _____

    C. _____

    D. _____

4. What is the recurrence rate of urinary calculi? What can be done to reduce the possibility of recurrence?

    _____

    _____

    _____

    _____

5. Why is family history an important factor in the diagnosis of PKD?

    _____

    _____

_____

_____

6. Name two conditions of the kidney that often lead to ESRD.

   A. _____

   B. _____

7. What are the two treatment options for a patient with ESRD?

   A. _____

   B. _____

8. What age group is most commonly affected by BPH? Why?

   _____

   _____

   _____

   _____

9. Is it possible for hypospadias to occur in a female patient?

   _____

   _____

   _____

   _____

10. List two complications that may occur if cryptorchidism is undiagnosed or untreated.

    A. _____

    B. _____

11. What is the normal blood level of PSA? Does an elevated PSA indicate the presence of a malignant process?

    _____

    _____

    _____

    _____

12. An IVU has been unsuccessful in demonstrating a ureteral obstruction. What diagnostic exam may be recommended as the next step?

    _____

    _____

    _____

    _____

13. Table 20-6 in the textbook lists the abnormal constituents of urine. If a patient exhibits an increase in leukocytes, what condition(s) could this indicate?

    _____

    _____

    _____

    _____

14. What condition is the MIBG nuclear medicine study designed to detect?

_____

_____

_____

_____

15. What is KUB? What information may be provided during this type of exam?

_____

_____

_____

_____

Operation

1. A retrograde urogram is considered a diagnostic radiographic procedure. Why is it often performed in the operating room rather than the radiology department?

_____

_____

_____

_____

2. List at least three features of the Cysto room that may not be found in the general OR.

_____

_____

_____

_____

3. What is the function of a deflecting mechanism?

_____

_____

_____

_____

4. What is the purpose of an O'Connor shield?

_____

_____

_____

_____

5. What specific structure is the Gibson incision designed to access?

_____

_____

_____

_____

6. In which position is the patient placed when use of a flank incision is anticipated?

   _____

   _____

   _____

   _____

7. List the three flank incision options, and give a brief description of the location of each.

   A. _____

   B. _____

   C. _____

8. What is the purpose of renal cooling?

   _____

   _____

   _____

   _____

9. Why is it important for the STSR to have a chest tube, insertion supplies, and a water-seal drainage system readily available during a nephrectomy?

   _____

   _____

   _____

   _____

10. List the three sources from which kidneys are obtained for transplant.

    A. _____

    B. _____

    C. _____

11. What is the purpose of suprapubic cystostomy?

    _____

    _____

    _____

    _____

12. Will the surgical technologist be scrubbed in for cystoscopy? What is the main function of the surgical technologist during cystoscopy?

    _____

    _____

    _____

    _____

13. List four procedures that may be performed transurethrally.

    A. _____

    B. _____

    C. _____

    D. _____

14. Why is it necessary for the assistant to change the gloves (and possibly the gown) during MMK?

_____

_____

_____

_____

15. What is the purpose of repeatedly introducing the cystoscope during a Stamey procedure?

_____

_____

_____

_____

Specific Variations

Student Name: _____ Date: _____

Instructor: _____

Surgical Procedure—Student Case Study Report

The student will be provided with basic patient information (real or simulated) and is expected to complete the following case study.

1. Procedure name:

   _____

   _____

   _____

   _____

2. Definition of procedure:

   _____

   _____

   _____

   _____

3. What is the purpose of the procedure?

   _____

   _____

   _____

   _____

4. What is the expected outcome of the procedure?

   _____

   _____

   _____

   _____

5. Patient age: _____

6. Gender: _____

7. Additional pertinent patient information:

   _____

   _____

   _____

   _____

8. Probable preoperative diagnosis:

   _____

   _____

   _____

   _____

9. How was the diagnosis determined?

_____

_____

_____

_____

10. Discuss the relevant anatomy.

_____

_____

_____

_____

11. List the general and procedure-specific equipment that will be needed for the procedure.

_____

_____

_____

_____

12. List the general and procedure-specific instruments that will be needed for the procedure.

_____

_____

_____

_____

13. List the basic and procedure-specific supplies that will be needed for the procedure.

Pack _____

Basin _____

Gloves _____

Blades _____

Drapes _____

Drains _____

Dressings_____

Suture—Type of Suture, Needle (if applicable), and Anticipated Tissue Usage

_____

_____

_____

_____

Pharmaceuticals

_____

_____

_____

Miscellaneous

_____

_____

_____

_____

14. Operative preparation:

_____

_____

_____

_____

15. What type of anesthesia will likely be used? Why?

_____

_____

_____

_____

16. List any special anesthesia equipment that may be needed.

_____

_____

_____

_____

17. Patient position during the procedure:

_____

_____

_____

_____

18. What supplies will be necessary for positioning?

_____

_____

_____

_____

19. What type of shave/skin preparation will be necessary (if any)?

_____

_____

_____

_____

20. Define the anatomic perimeters of the prep.

_____

_____

_____

_____

21. List the order in which the drapes will be applied, and describe any specific variations.

_____

_____

_____

_____

22. List any practical considerations.

_____

_____

_____

_____

23. List the procedural steps, and describe the preparatory and supportive actions of the STSR during each step (use additional space if necessary).

_____

_____

_____

_____

24. What is the postoperative diagnosis?

_____

_____

_____

_____

25. Describe the immediate postoperative care.

_____

_____

_____

_____

26. What is the patient's long-term prognosis?

_____

_____

_____

_____

27. What are the possible complications?

_____

_____

_____

_____

28. Comments or questions:

_____

_____

_____

_____

29. What is the most valuable information you obtained from preparing this surgical procedure case study?

_____

_____

_____

_____

Case Studies

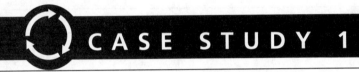

CASE STUDY 1

Patricia has been experiencing several seemingly unrelated symptoms that include weight loss, headache, "heartburn," sweating, trembling, rapid heart rate, heat intolerance, and a feeling of anxiousness. Patricia's daughter finally convinced her to see her primary care physician, who has determined that Patricia has a tumor of the adrenal medulla.

1. What diagnostic studies are needed to confirm the diagnosis?

_____

_____

_____

_____

2. What is the name of Patricia's tumor, and how serious is it? Why?

_____

_____

_____

_____

3. What is the necessary treatment for Patricia's condition? What type of procedure will most likely be performed?

_____

_____

_____

_____

CASE STUDY 2

Six-year-old Belinda has been suffering from chronic urinary tract infections. The appearance of blood in her urine led to further testing that produced a diagnosis of PKD. Belinda's condition has nearly destroyed both kidneys. Belinda, her parents, and her twin sister, Melinda, are all extremely concerned about Belinda's future.

1. What does PKD mean, and what type of PKD does Belinda have?

   _____

   _____

   _____

   _____

2. Was invasive testing necessary to determine Belinda's diagnosis?

   _____

   _____

   _____

   _____

3. What course is the disease expected to follow?

   _____

   _____

   _____

   _____

4. What will be the most likely outcome for Belinda?

   _____

   _____

   _____

5. Several years have passed; Belinda has been scheduled for a renal transplant. She is receiving a cadaver kidney since her twin sister has developed PKD herself. How will the kidney be preserved until it is reimplanted in Belinda's pelvis?

   _____

   _____

   _____

   _____

Lab 20: Genitourinary Surgery

Introduction

Genitourinary surgery deals with surgery of the urinary tract and with male reproductive structures. In this unit you will find many open procedures along with many procedures that are done with endoscopes. Learning the surgeries step by step in lecture will help you in the lab portion. This is where you will learn the hands on of the specialty and the instruments that will be used for each piece of the surgery.

Game: Genitourinary Surgery on Felt Mayo Stands

Time involved: 1–2 weeks setup

Instructors: Make a list of instruments you expect students to know as part of the genitourinary surgery lab. Have the students trace the real instruments onto felt if possible; if not, have them find pictures they can cut out and trace onto the felt or other material. I like felt because it tends to be very durable, but paper or cardboard can be substituted. There should be no need for multiple cutouts of the same instruments if students are given the chance to show how many of those instruments they would have on the Mayo by way of a numbered marker (a piece of paper with a number designation on it). The students are given a list of surgeries that they are expected to know.
Note: This can be made easier if you have photos of these Mayo stand setups for the students to study.

Students: You will need several pieces of felt, paper, or cardboard. The largest piece should be cut to the size of a regular Mayo stand. The student will proceed to cut out instruments as close to life size as possible using felt or some other material. Label the backside of the cutouts for easy reference.

Supplies: Felt, paper, or cardboard; real instruments, or pictures that have been printed and cut out from the computer; felt-tip marker; scissors; measuring tool

How the Game is Played

The students are given a list of surgeries that they are expected to know. The instructor will then assign one of those surgeries to the student in the lab. The student will then be expected to complete a Mayo stand setup in a specified time frame using the instruments they have cut out. Score the students according to placement of instruments, time needed for setup, correct instrumentation, and correct number of instruments.

Practical: Set Up General Surgery Cases

Utilizing a full lab/OR setup, assign the students to different surgical cases to learn. The students will then be expected to set up some of these cases under the supervision of the instructor. They should use as much of the OR equipment as needed including backtable, Mayo stand, ring stands, instrument trays, and pans. The student should be scored on correct placement of supplies, practicing economy of time and motion (pick it up and place it one time), correct order of instruments, correct number of instruments, aseptic technique, time to set up, and order of use for instruments and supplies; a mock surgery should be performed so the student can work on anticipating the needs of the surgeon.

CHAPTER 21

Orthopedic Surgery

OBJECTIVES

After studying this chapter, the reader should be able to:

A 1. Recognize the relevant anatomy and physiology of the musculoskeletal system.

P 2. Summarize the pathology of the musculoskeletal system that prompts surgical intervention, and the related terminology.

3. Determine any special preoperative orthopedic diagnostic procedures/tests.

O 4. Determine any special preoperative preparation related to orthopedic procedures.

5. Indicate the names and uses of orthopedic instruments, supplies, and drugs.

6. Indicate the names and uses of special equipment related to orthopedic procedures.

7. Determine the intraoperative preparation of the patient undergoing an orthopedic procedure.

8. Summarize the surgical steps of the orthopedic procedures.

9. Interpret the purpose and expected outcomes of the orthopedic procedures.

10. Recognize the immediate postoperative care and possible complications of the orthopedic procedures.

S 11. Assess any specific variations related to the preoperative, intraoperative, and postoperative care of the orthopedic patient.

Select Key Terms

Define the following, using your textbook glossary or a medical dictionary if necessary:

1. abduction _____

   _____

2. AC joint _____

   _____

3. adduction _____

   _____

4. amphiarthrosis _____

   _____

5. avascular necrosis _____

   _____

6. cancellous bone _____

   _____

7. cartilage _____

   _____

8. comminuted _____

   _____

9. compartmental syndrome _____

   _____

10. compound fracture _____

    _____

11. cortical bone _____

    _____

12. delayed union _____

    _____

13. diarthrosis _____

    _____

14. distraction _____

    _____

15. epiphysis _____

    _____

16. flexion _____

17. ligament _____

_____

18. malunion _____

_____

19. marrow _____

_____

20. nonunion _____

_____

21. osteogenesis _____

_____

22. pedicle _____

_____

23. proximal _____

_____

24. shoulder joint _____

_____

25. splint _____

_____

26. valgus _____

_____

Anatomy

1. Identify the skeletal bones shown in Figure 21-1. Refer to Anatomy Plate #11 in your textbook appendix.

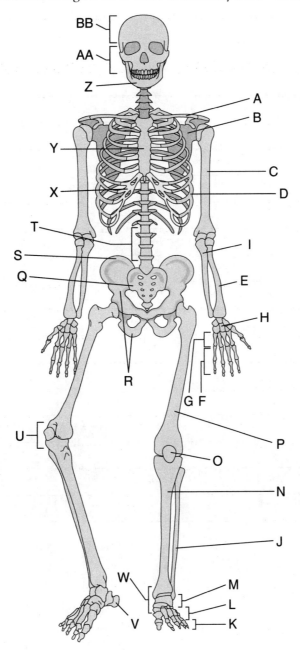

Figure 21-1

A. _____

B. _____

C. _____

D. _____

E. _____

F. _____

G. _____

H. _____

I. _____

J. _____

K. _____

L. _____

M. _____

N. _____

O. _____

P. _____

Q. _____

R. _____

S. _____

T. _____

U. _____

V. _____

W. _____

X. _____

Y. _____

Z. _____

AA. _____

BB. _____

2. Identify the structures of the vertebral column shown in Figure 21-2. Refer to Figure 21-2 located at the Online Companion website. (Go to www.delmarlearning.com/companions, click on 'Allied Health,' then on the textbook title and edition.)

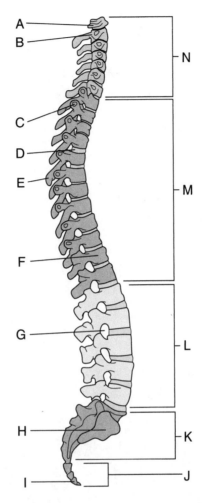

Figure 21-2

A. _____

B. _____

C. _____

D. _____

E. _____

F. _____

G. _____

H. _____

I. _____

J. _____

K. _____

L. _____

M. _____

N. _____

3. Identify the vertebral structures shown in Figure 21-3. Refer to Figure 21-3 located at the Online Companion website.

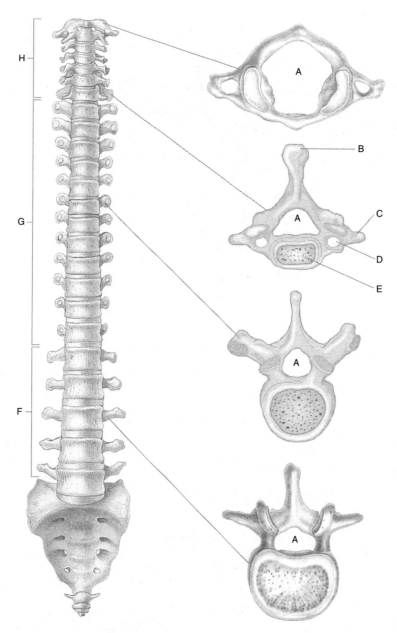

Figure 21-3

A. _____

B. _____

C. _____

D. _____

E. _____

F. _____

G. _____

H. _____

4. Identify the structures shown in Figure 21-4. Refer to Figure 21-4 located at the Online Companion website.

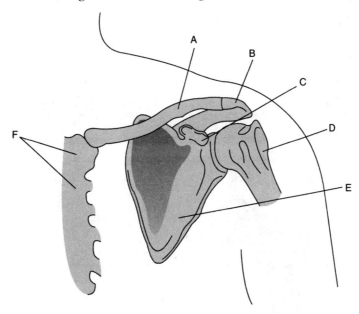

Figure 21-4

A. _____

B. _____

C. _____

D. _____

E. _____

F. _____

5. Identify the bones of the pelvic girdle shown in Figure 21-5. Refer to Figure 21-5 located at the Online Companion website.

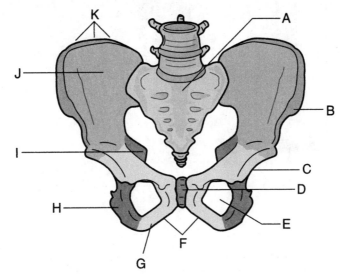

Figure 21-5

A. _____

B. _____

C. _____

D. _____

E. _____

F. _____

G. _____

H. _____

I. _____

J. _____

K. _____

6. Identify the elements of a long bone as shown in Figure 21-6. Refer to Figure 21-4 in your textbook.

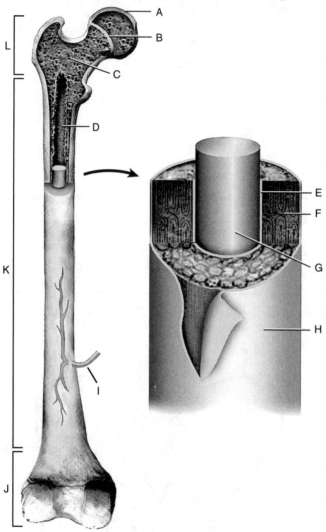

Figure 21-6

A. _____

B. _____

C. _____

D. _____

E. _____

F. _____

G. _____

H. _____

I. _____

J. _____

K. _____

L. _____

7. Identify the elements of the fractures as shown in Figure 21-7. Refer to Table 21-3 in your textbook.

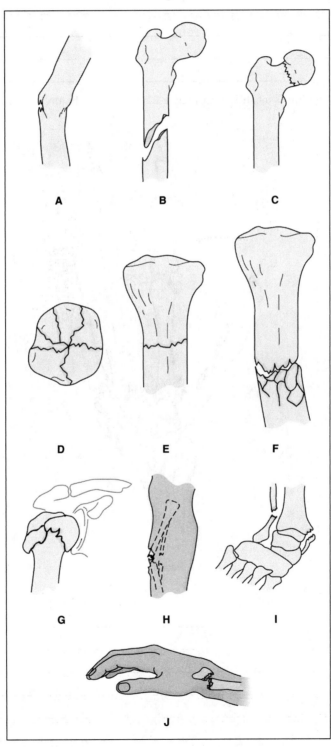

Figure 21-7

A. _____

B. _____

C. _____

D. _____

E. _____

F. _____

G. _____

H. _____

I. _____

J. _____

8. Identify the hand and wrist joints as shown in Figure 21-8. Refer to Figure 21-13 in your textbook.

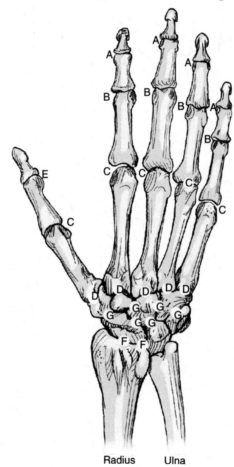

Radius   Ulna

Figure 21-8

A. _____

B. _____

C. _____

D. _____

E. _____

F. _____

G. _____

9. List the five functions of the skeletal system.

   A. _____

   B. _____

   C. _____

   D. _____

   E. _____

10. List four factors that affect bone growth.

    A. _____

    B. _____

    C. _____

    D. _____

11. Define the term sesamoid, and give two examples of sesamoid bones.

    _____

    _____

12. What are the two main divisions of the skeleton? Briefly describe each division.

    A. _____

    B. _____

13. List the eight bones of the cranium.

    A. _____

    B. _____

    C. _____

    D. _____

    E. _____

    F. _____

    G. _____

    H. _____

14. Name the three bones that comprise the knee joint.

    A. _____

    B. _____

    C. _____

15. Describe the function of a gliding joint, and provide an example of a gliding joint.

    _____

    _____

    _____

    _____

    _____

    _____

16. Define circumduction, and give an example of a joint that is capable of circumduction.

_____

_____

_____

_____

_____

_____

17. In addition to calcium, name four other minerals that are stored within bone.

A. _____

B. _____

C. _____

D. _____

Pathology

1. What is ankylosis, and what is its cause?

_____

_____

_____

_____

_____

_____

2. How does vitamin D help to prevent osteomalacia?

_____

_____

_____

_____

3. Describe a greenstick fracture.

_____

_____

_____

_____

_____

4. Does a patient who has subluxation have a fracture? Explain your answer.

_____

_____

_____

_____

5. Describe nonunion, and provide two reasons why nonunion may occur.

_____

_____

_____

_____

6. What is the cause of compartment syndrome? How is compartment syndrome manifested?

_____

_____

_____

_____

7. What is the main complication of osteoporosis?

_____

_____

_____

_____

8. What bone is affected by a Colles' fracture?

_____

_____

_____

_____

9. A tumor of the cartilage is called a(n) _____

10. What is the most common type of meniscal tear? Describe the defect.

_____

_____

_____

_____

11. _____ is an inflammation of the bone and bone marrow.

12. An elevated erythrocyte sedimentation rate (ESR) is an indicator of what type of condition?

_____

_____

_____

_____

13. What muscles comprise the rotator cuff? How will a tear of one or more of these muscles or their tendinous attachments affect the shoulder?

_____

_____

_____

_____

_____

_____

14. An arthrogram is an X-ray of what specific structure(s)?

_____

_____

_____

_____

_____

Operation

1. What is meant by the term exsanguination? How does this apply to extremity surgery with the use of a tourniquet?

_____

_____

_____

_____

_____

2. What is the maximum recommended time that tourniquet pressure may be applied to an upper extremity? Why?

_____

_____

_____

_____

_____

3. What are two advantages to postoperative use of the continuous passive motion (CPM) machine?

A. _____

B. _____

4. What precautions must be taken when the use of a C-arm is anticipated?

_____

_____

_____

_____

5. Describe the direction of the blade motion of a reciprocating saw.

_____

_____

_____

_____

_____

_____

6. What is bone wax, and how is it used?

_____

_____

_____

_____

7. List two situations in which a bone graft may be required.

A. _____

B. _____

8. What is the reason for application of irrigation fluid to the wound when sawing or drilling bone?

_____

_____

_____

_____

9. When using methyl methacrylate (MMA) cement, what is the importance of using a closed mixing system?

_____

_____

_____

_____

10. What information must be documented following prosthesis insertion?

A. _____

B. _____

C. _____

D. _____

11. List two reasons why arthroscopy may be performed.

A. _____

B. _____

12. What is a reamer used to accomplish?

_____

_____

_____

_____

13. What are the three main advantages of maintaining laminar airflow in the OR during a surgical procedure?

A. _____

B. _____

C. _____

14. Following closed reduction, what method of immobilization is commonly employed?

_____

_____

_____

_____

_____

_____

15. List the three types of traction.

   A. _____

   B. _____

   C. _____

Specific Variations

Student Name _____ Date _____

Instructor _____

The student will be provided with basic patient information (real or simulated) and is expected to complete the following case study.

1. Procedure name:

   _____

   _____

   _____

2. Definition of procedure:

   _____

   _____

   _____

   _____

   _____

3. What is the purpose of the procedure?

   _____

   _____

   _____

   _____

   _____

4. What is the expected outcome of the procedure?

   _____

   _____

   _____

   _____

5. Patient age: _____

6. Gender: _____

7. Additional pertinent patient information:

   _____

   _____

   _____

   _____

8. Probable preoperative diagnosis:

   _____

   _____

   _____

   _____

_____

_____

9. How was the diagnosis determined?

_____

_____

_____

_____

_____

_____

10. Discuss the relevant anatomy.

_____

_____

_____

_____

_____

_____

11. List the general and procedure-specific equipment that will be needed for the procedure.

_____

_____

_____

_____

_____

_____

12. List the general and procedure-specific instruments that will be needed for the procedure.

_____

_____

_____

_____

_____

_____

13. List the basic and procedure-specific supplies that will be needed for the procedure.

Pack _____

Basin _____

Gloves _____

Blades _____

Drapes _____

_____

Drains _____

Dressings _____

Suture—Type of Suture, Needle (if applicable), and Anticipated Tissue Usage

_____

_____

_____

_____

_____

_____

Pharmaceuticals

_____

_____

_____

_____

Miscellaneous

_____

_____

_____

_____

_____

14. Operative preparation:

_____

_____

_____

_____

_____

15. What type of anesthesia will likely be used? Why?

_____

_____

_____

_____

16. List any special anesthesia equipment that may be needed.

_____

_____

_____

_____

_____

_____

17. Patient position during the procedure:

_____

_____

_____

_____

_____

18. What supplies will be necessary for positioning?

_____

_____

_____

_____

_____

19. What type of shave/skin preparation will be necessary (if any)?

_____

_____

_____

_____

_____

20. Define the anatomic perimeters of the prep.

_____

_____

_____

_____

_____

21. List the order in which the drapes will be applied, and describe any specific variations.

_____

_____

_____

_____

_____

22. List any practical considerations.

_____

_____

_____

_____

_____

_____

23. List the procedural steps, and describe the preparatory and supportive actions of the STSR during each step (use additional space if necessary).

_____

_____

_____

_____

_____

24. What is the postoperative diagnosis?

_____

_____

_____

_____

_____

_____

25. Describe the immediate postoperative care.

_____

_____

_____

_____

26. What is the patient's long-term prognosis?

_____

_____

_____

_____

_____

27. What are the possible complications?

_____

_____

_____

_____

_____

_____

_____

28. Comments or questions:

_____

_____

_____

_____

_____

_____

29. What is the most valuable information you obtained from preparing this surgical procedure case study?

_____

_____

_____

_____

_____

_____

_____

_____

Case Studies

CASE STUDY 1

Ellenor is a 65-year-old female who was admitted to the hospital for a total hip arthroplasty.

1. Describe a routine draping procedure for this case.

    _____

    _____

    _____

    _____

2. What kind of incision is used?

    _____

    _____

    _____

    _____

(continues)

CASE STUDY 1 (continued)

3. After the femoral osteotomy guide is placed over the lateral femur and neck, what should the STSR plan to do next?

_____

_____

_____

_____

4. Will the incision be drained?

_____

_____

_____

_____

5. Describe the immediate postoperative care the patient will receive.

_____

_____

_____

_____

CASE STUDY 2

Leroy was admitted to the emergency department with a fracture of the left tibia and fibula. The fracture was reduced, the leg placed in a cast, and Leroy was sent home.

1. Why are casts placed on limbs with reduced fractures?

_____

_____

_____

_____

2. What is the meaning of the term distraction? What complications can be caused by distraction?

_____

_____

_____

_____

(continues)

⟳ C A S E   S T U D Y   2   (*continued*)

3. What is the most important factor in bone healing?

_____

_____

_____

_____

4. To what does the term "delayed union" refer?

_____

_____

_____

_____

Lab 21: Orthopedic Surgery

Introduction

Orthopedic surgery deals with surgery of the bones and supportive structures. In this unit you will find many open procedures along with many procedures that are done with endoscopes. Learning the surgeries step by step in lecture will help you in the lab portion. This is where you will learn the "hands-on" of the specialty and the instruments that will be used for each piece of the surgery.

Game: Orthopedic Surgery on Felt Mayo Stands

Time involved: 1-2 weeks setup

Instructors: Make a list of instruments you expect students to know as part of the orthopedic surgery lab. Have the students trace the real instruments onto felt if possible; if not, have them find pictures they can cut out and trace onto the felt or other material. I like felt because it tends to be very durable, but paper or cardboard can be substituted. There should be no need for multiple cutouts of the same instruments if students are given the chance to show how many of those instruments they would have on the Mayo by way of a numbered marker (a piece of paper with a number designation on it). The students are given a list of surgeries that they are expected to know. **Note:** This can also be made easier if you have photos of these Mayo stand setups for the students to study.

Students: You will need several pieces of felt, paper, or cardboard. The largest piece should be cut to the size of a regular Mayo stand. You will proceed to cut out instruments as close as possible to life size using felt or some other material. Label the backside of these cutouts for easy reference.

Supplies: Felt, paper, or cardboard; real instruments, or pictures that have been printed and cut out from the computer; felt-tip marker; scissors; measuring tool

How the Game is Played

The students are given a list of surgeries that they are expected to know. The instructor will then assign one of those surgeries to the student in the lab. The student will then be expected to complete a Mayo stand setup in a specified time frame using the instruments they have cut out. Score the students according to placement of instruments, time needed for setup, correct instrumentation, and correct number of instruments.

Practical: Set Up Orthopedic Surgery Cases

Utilizing a full lab/OR setup, assign the students different surgical cases to learn. The students will then be expected to set up some of these cases under the supervision of the instructor. They should utilize as much of the OR equipment as needed including backtable, Mayo stand, ring stands, instrument trays, and pans. The student should be scored on correct placement of supplies, practicing economy of time and motion (pick it up and place it one time), correct order of instruments, correct number of instruments, aseptic technique, time to set up, and order of use for instruments and supplies; a mock surgery should be performed so the student can work on anticipating the needs of the surgeon.

CHAPTER 22

Cardiothoracic Surgery

OBJECTIVES

After studying this chapter, the reader should be able to:

A 1. Recognize the relevant anatomy of the cardiovascular and respiratory systems.

P 2. Summarize the pathology that prompts cardiac or thoracic surgical intervention, and the related terminology.

3. Determine any special preoperative diagnostic procedures/tests for the patient undergoing cardiac or thoracic surgery.

O 4. Determine any special preoperative preparation procedures.

5. Indicate the names and uses of cardiovascular and thoracic instruments, supplies, and drugs.

6. Indicate the names and uses of special equipment for the cardiac or thoracic procedure.

7. Determine the intraoperative preparation of the patient undergoing a cardiac or thoracic procedure.

8. Summarize the surgical steps of the cardiac and thoracic procedures.

9. Interpret the purpose and expected outcomes of the cardiac and thoracic procedures.

10. Recognize the immediate postoperative care and possible complications of the cardiac and thoracic procedures.

S 11. Assess any specific variations related to the preoperative, intraoperative, and postoperative care of the patient undergoing a cardiac or thoracic procedure.

Select Key Terms

Define the following using your textbook glossary or a medical dictionary:

1. alveoli _____

_____

2. aneurysm _____

_____

3. arrhythmia _____

_____

4. atria _____

_____

5. bradycardia _____

_____

6. cardiac cycle _____

_____

7. ductus arteriosus _____

_____

8. hyaline cartilage _____

_____

9. infarction _____

_____

10. infiltrate _____

_____

11. mediastinum _____

_____

12. myocardium _____

_____

13. oxygenated _____

_____

14. pericardium _____

_____

15. pleura _____

_____

16. prolapse _____

_____

17. PVC _____

_____

18. regurgitation _____

_____

19. stent _____

_____

20. systole _____

_____

21. tachycardia _____

_____

22. tamponade _____

_____

23. ventricles _____

_____

Anatomy

1. Identify the structures shown in Figure 22-1. Refer to Figure 22-4 in your textbook.

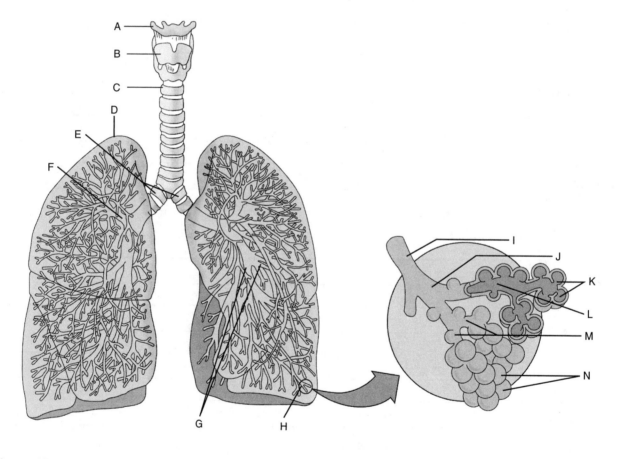

Figure 22-1

A. _____

B. _____

C. _____

D. _____

E. _____

F. _____

G. _____

H. _____

I. _____

J. _____

K. _____

L. _____

M. _____

N. _____

2. Identify the structures shown in Figure 22-2. Refer to the figures in Chapter 22 of your textbook.

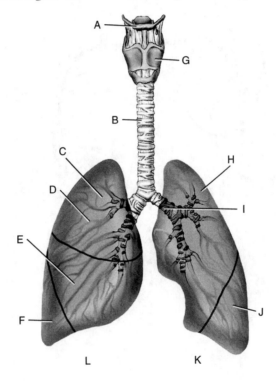

Figure 22-2

A. _____

B. _____

C. _____

D. _____

E. _____

F. _____

G. _____

H. _____

I. _____

J. _____

K. _____

L. _____

3. Identify the structures shown in Figure 22-3. Refer to Figure 22-2 in your textbook.

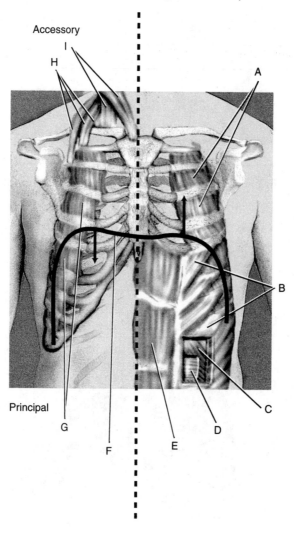

Figure 22-3

A. _____

B. _____

C. _____

D. _____

E. _____

F. _____

G. _____

H. _____

I. _____

4. Identify the structures shown in Figure 22-4. Refer to Figure 22-8 in your textbook.

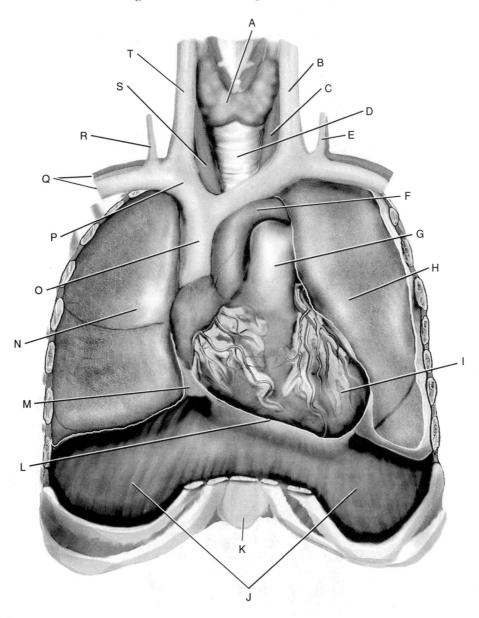

Figure 22-4

A. _____

B. _____

C. _____

D. _____

E. _____

F. _____

G. _____

H. _____

I. _____

J. _____

K. _____

L. _____

M. _____

N. _____

O. _____

P. _____

Q. _____

R. _____

S. _____

T. _____

5. Identify the cardiac valves shown in Figure 22-5. Refer to Figure 22-10 in your textbook.

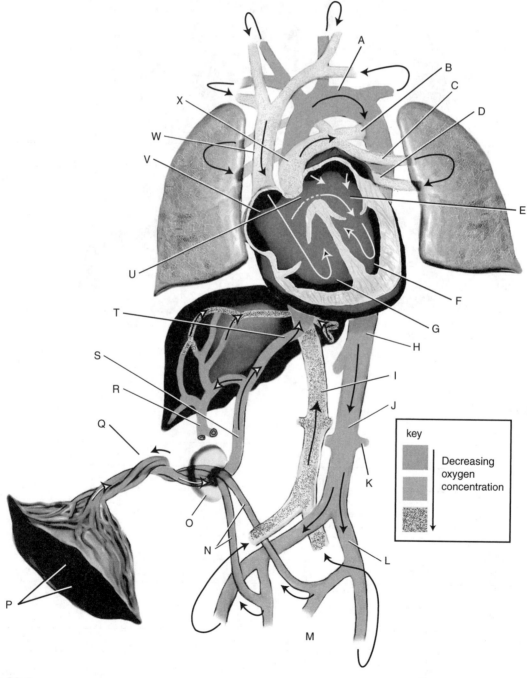

Figure 22-5

A. _____

B. _____

C. _____

D. _____

E. _____

F. _____

G. _____

H. _____

I. _____

J. _____

K. _____

L. _____

M. _____

N. _____

O. _____

P. _____

Q. _____

R. _____

S. _____

T. _____

U. _____

V. _____

W. _____

X. _____

6. Using the numbers 1–8, list the following events in the proper chronological sequence to complete the cardiac cycle.

   A. _____ Atria contract

   B. _____ AV node stimulated

   C. _____ Impulse moves through right and left bundles branches

   D. _____ Impulse transmitted to bundle of His

   E. _____ Impulse travels via internodal atrial pathways

   F. _____ Purkinje fibers stimulated

   G. _____ SA node generates initial impulse

   H. _____ Ventricles contract

7. Using the numbers 1–13, trace the flow of blood from the time it leaves the venae cavae to the time it enters the aorta by placing the following elements in the correct order.

   A. _____ Aorta

   B. _____ Aortic (semilunar) valve

   C. _____ Bicuspid (mitral) valve

D. _____ Left atrium

E. _____ Left ventricle

F. _____ Lungs

G. _____ Pulmonary arteries

H. _____ Pulmonary valve

I. _____ Pulmonary veins

J. _____ Right atrium

K. _____ Right ventricle

L. _____ Tricuspid (right AV) valve

M. _____ Venae cavae

8. Name the three layers of the heart wall.

A. _____

B. _____

C. _____

9. Name the four cardiac valves and describe their locations.

A. _____

B. _____

C. _____

D. _____

10. Define cardiac output.

_____

_____

_____

_____

11. What is the function of the bundle of His?

_____

_____

_____

_____

12. Name and describe the two layers of the pleura.

A. _____

_____

B. _____

_____

13. What structures are contained within the mediastinum?

_____

_____

_____

_____

_____

14. Name the principal muscles of inspiration.

    A. _____

    B. _____

Pathology

1. List three methods used to detect lung tumors.

    A. _____

    B. _____

    C. _____

2. Describe the condition known as flail chest.

    _____

    _____

    _____

    _____

3. Penetrating chest trauma will result in which condition? What treatment is necessary?

    _____

    _____

    _____

    _____

    _____

4. What is cardiac tamponade? What treatment is necessary?

    _____

    _____

    _____

    _____

    _____

5. List the three types of thoracic outlet syndrome and the cause of each.

    A. _____

    B. _____

    C. _____

6. Describe a Type II dissecting aneurysm of the thoracic aorta. What does dissecting mean in reference to an aneurysm?

    _____

    _____

    _____

7. What is the composition of an atheroma? What causes formation of an atheroma?

   _____

   _____

   _____

   _____

8. Which cardiac enzyme levels rise following myocardial infarction?

   A. _____

   B. _____

   C. _____

9. List three complications of myocardial infarction.

   A. _____

   B. _____

   C. _____

10. What effect does alcohol have on cardiac tissue?

    _____

    _____

    _____

11. Describe the condition known as patent ductus arteriosus, list the symptoms, and provide treatment options.

    _____

    _____

    _____

    _____

12. List the four cardiac defects seen in the classic form of tetralogy of Fallot.

    A. _____

    B. _____

    C. _____

    D. _____

13. List two variables and two inherited risk factors for coronary atherosclerosis.

    A. _____

    B. _____

    C. _____

    D. _____

14. What is/are the cause(s) of mitral regurgitation?

    _____

    _____

_____

_____

15. A commissurotomy is performed to treat which condition?

_____

_____

_____

_____

Operation

1. List the two types of mediastinoscopy, and provide a brief description of each.

    A. _____

    B. _____

2. Is bronchoscopy strictly a diagnostic procedure? Explain your answer.

    _____

    _____

    _____

3. In which position will the patient be placed in order to accomplish a posterolateral thoracotomy?

    _____

    _____

    _____

4. Explain the difference between lobectomy and pneumonectomy.

    _____

    _____

    _____

    _____

5. What is the purpose of inserting a double-lumen endotracheal tube during a thoracotomy?

    _____

    _____

    _____

    _____

6. In which position will the patient be placed to accomplish a median sternotomy?

    _____

    _____

    _____

    _____

7. What is empyema? What procedure is performed to treat empyema?

_____

_____

_____

_____

8. Which body functions are taken over by the pump oxygenator during open-heart surgery?

_____

_____

_____

_____

9. Describe the placement of the cannulas necessary for a cardiopulmonary bypass.

_____

_____

_____

_____

10. Name two blood vessels that are most commonly used as the graft during CABG procedures.

   A. _____

   B. _____

11. List the two basic types of materials that are used for cardiac valve replacement.

   A. _____

   B. _____

12. What are the two main components of a pacemaker?

   A. _____

   B. _____

13. Why is it important to have an open-heart team on "standby" during PTCA?

_____

_____

_____

14. Is cardiopulmonary bypass necessary for closure of a patent ductus arteriosus in an infant?

_____

_____

_____

15. What is the purpose of administering potassium cardioplegia solution during open-heart procedures?

_____

_____

_____

_____

Specific Variations

Student Name _____ Date _____

Instructor _____

The student will be provided with basic patient information (real or simulated) and is expected to complete the following case study.

1. Procedure name:

   _____

   _____

   _____

2. Definition of procedure:

   _____

   _____

   _____

   _____

3. What is the purpose of the procedure?

   _____

   _____

   _____

   _____

   _____

4. What is the expected outcome of the procedure?

   _____

   _____

   _____

5. Patient age: _____

6. Gender: _____

7. Additional pertinent patient information:

   _____

   _____

   _____

   _____

8. Probable preoperative diagnosis:

   _____

   _____

   _____

   _____

   _____

9. How was the diagnosis determined?

_____

_____

_____

_____

_____

_____

10. Discuss the relevant anatomy.

_____

_____

_____

_____

_____

_____

_____

11. List the general and procedure-specific equipment that will be needed for the procedure.

_____

_____

_____

_____

_____

_____

12. List the general and procedure-specific instruments that will be needed for the procedure.

_____

_____

_____

_____

_____

_____

13. List the basic and procedure-specific supplies that will be needed for the procedure.

Pack _____

Basin _____

Gloves _____

Blades _____

Drapes _____

_____

Drains _____

Dressings _____

_____

Suture—Type of Suture, Needle (if applicable), and Anticipated Tissue Usage

_____

_____

_____

_____

_____

_____

Pharmaceuticals

_____

_____

_____

_____

_____

Miscellaneous

_____

_____

_____

_____

_____

_____

14. Operative preparation:

_____

_____

_____

_____

_____

_____

15. What type of anesthesia will likely be used? Why?

_____

_____

_____

_____

16. List any special anesthesia equipment that may be needed.

_____

_____

_____

_____

_____

_____

_____

17. Patient position during the procedure:

_____

_____

_____

_____

18. What supplies will be necessary for positioning?

_____

_____

_____

_____

19. What type of shave/skin preparation will be necessary (if any)?

_____

_____

_____

_____

_____

_____

20. Define the anatomic perimeters of the prep.

_____

_____

_____

_____

_____

21. List the order in which the drapes will be applied, and describe any specific variations.

_____

_____

_____

_____

22. List any practical considerations.

_____

_____

_____

_____

_____

_____

23. List the procedural steps, and describe the preparatory and supportive actions of the STSR during each step (use additional space if necessary).

_____

_____

_____

_____

_____

24. What is the postoperative diagnosis?

_____

_____

_____

_____

_____

_____

_____

25. Describe the immediate postoperative care.

_____

_____

_____

_____

_____

_____

26. What is the patient's long-term prognosis?

_____

_____

_____

_____

_____

27. What are the possible complications?

_____

_____

_____

_____

_____

_____

_____

28. Comments or questions:

_____

_____

_____

_____

_____

_____

_____

29. What is the most valuable information you obtained from preparing this surgical procedure case study?

_____

_____

_____

_____

Case Studies

CASE STUDY 1

Elroy has been transported to the emergency department following a motor vehicle accident (MVA). He was the unrestrained driver of one of the vehicles, and his body hit the steering wheel on impact. Elroy has dyspnea, tachypnea, and tachycardia, appears extremely anxious, and is showing signs of shock. Upon examination, the emergency physician notes distant heart sounds, hypotension, and jugular venous distension. A Swan-Ganz catheter placed by the physician reveals equal RA and pulmonary capillary wedge pressures and an elevated CVP.

1. What type of injury is suspected as a result of the blunt chest trauma?

_____

_____

_____

_____

2. What diagnostic exams are indicated?

_____

_____

_____

_____

(continues)

CASE STUDY 1 (continued)

3. What is the treatment for this condition?

_____
_____
_____
_____

CASE STUDY 2

Timothy, a 49-year-old construction worker, fell from a scaffold and was rushed to the emergency department, where he was evaluated by the trauma team. Timothy complained of chest pain, and severe respiratory distress was noted by the physician. Chest x-ray revealed fractures of the fifth and sixth ribs on the right and absence of lung markings over the affected area.

1. In addition to Timothy's fractured ribs, what other condition is affecting him?

_____
_____
_____
_____

2. What treatment will be provided?

_____
_____
_____
_____

3. What type of wound drainage system will be needed? Why?

_____
_____
_____
_____

4. Will a wound dressing be necessary? If so, what type and why?

_____
_____
_____
_____

Lab 22: Cardiothoracic Surgery

Introduction

Cardiothoracic surgery deals with surgery of the heart and thoracic structures. It can be one of the harder specialties to learn because so many instruments tend to do the same thing but have subtle changes that make them better for one area or another. It will be of some help that there will also be some orthopedic instruments that are going to be used. In this unit you will find many open procedures along with many procedures that are done with endoscopes. Learning the surgeries step by step in lecture will help you in the lab portion. This is where you will learn the "hands-on" of the specialty and the instruments that will be used for each piece of the surgery.

Game: Cardiothoracic Surgery on Felt Mayo Stands

Time involved: 1-2 weeks setup

Instructors: Make a list of instruments you expect students to know as part of the cardiothoracic surgery lab. Have the students trace the real instruments onto the felt if possible; if not, have them find pictures they can cut out and trace onto the felt or other material. I like felt because it tends to be very durable, but paper or cardboard can be substituted. There should be no need for multiple cutouts of the same instruments if students are given the chance to show how many of those instruments they would have on the Mayo by way of a numbered marker (a piece of paper with a number designation on it). The students are given a list of surgeries that they are expected to know. **Note:** This can also be made easier if you have photos of these Mayo stand setups for the students to study.

Students: You will need several pieces of felt, paper, or cardboard. The largest piece should be cut to the size of a regular Mayo stand, although a larger overhead or over-the-bed table may be used. In this case utilize a large table or backtable to take its place. You should make cutouts of instruments as close as possible to life size using felt or some other material. Label the backsides of the cutouts for easy reference.

Supplies: Felt, paper, or cardboard; real instruments, or pictures that have been printed and cut out from the computer; felt-tip marker; scissors; measuring tool

How the Game is Played

The students are given a list of surgeries that they are expected to know. The instructor will then assign one of those surgeries to the student in the lab. The student will then be expected to complete a Mayo stand setup in a specified time frame using the instruments they have cut out. Score the students according to placement of instruments, time needed for setup, correct instrumentation, and correct number of instruments.

Practical: Set Up General Surgery Cases

Utilizing a full lab/OR setup, assign the students different surgical cases to learn. The students will then be expected to set up some of these cases under the supervision of the instructor. They should utilize as much of the OR equipment as needed including backtable, Mayo stand, ring stands, instrument trays, and pans. The student should be scored on correct placement of supplies, practicing economy of time and motion (pick it up and place it one time), correct order of instruments, correct number of instruments, aseptic technique, time to set up, and order of use for instruments and supplies; a mock surgery should be performed so the student can work on anticipating the needs of the surgeon.

Peripheral Vascular Surgery

OBJECTIVES

After studying this chapter, the reader should be able to:

A 1. Recognize the relevant anatomy of the peripheral vascular system.

P 2. Summarize the pathology that prompts surgical intervention of the peripheral vascular system, and the related terminology.

3. Determine any special preoperative peripheral vascular diagnostic procedures.

4. Determine any special preoperative preparation procedures.

O 5. Indicate the names and uses of peripheral vascular instruments, supplies, and drugs.

6. Indicate the names and uses of special equipment.

7. Determine the intraoperative preparation of the patient undergoing the peripheral vascular procedure.

8. Summarize the surgical steps of the peripheral vascular procedures.

9. Interpret the purpose and expected outcomes of the peripheral vascular procedures.

10. Recognize the immediate postoperative care and possible complications of the peripheral vascular procedures.

S 11. Assess any specific variations related to the preoperative, intraoperative, and postoperative care of the patient undergoing peripheral vascular surgery.

Select Key Terms

Define the following using your textbook glossary or a medical dictionary:

1. adventitia _____

_____

2. bifurcation _____

_____

3. capillary _____

_____

4. claudication_____

_____

5. contralateral _____

_____

6. diastole_____

_____

7. embolus _____

_____

8. Fogarty catheter _____

_____

9. in situ _____

_____

10. innominate _____

_____

11. intima _____

_____

12. ischemia_____

_____

13. mitigate _____

_____

14. morbidity_____

_____

15. mortality _____

_____

16. occlusion _____

_____

17. papaverine _____

_____

18. patency_____

_____

19. phrenic _____

_____

20. pledget _____

_____

21. plethysmography _____

_____

22. sinus _____

_____

23. thrombus _____

_____

24. valve _____

_____

Anatomy

1. Identify the parts of the capillary bed shown in Figure 23-1. Refer to Figure 23-1 in your textbook.

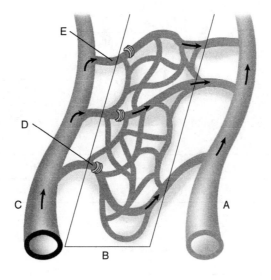

Figure 23-1

A. _____

B. _____

C. _____

D. _____

E. _____

2. Identify the blood circuits shown in Figure 23-2. Refer to Figure 23-2 in your textbook.

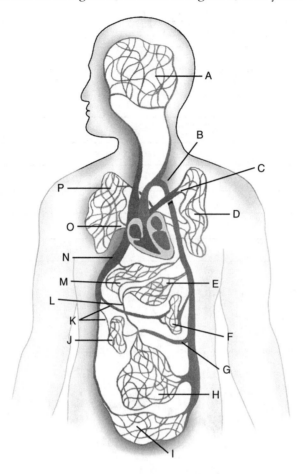

Figure 23-2

A. _____

B. _____

C. _____

D. _____

E. _____

F. _____

G. _____

H. _____

I. _____

J. _____

K. _____

L. _____

M. _____

N. _____

O. _____

P. _____

3. Identify the blood vessel types and structures shown in Figure 23-3. Refer to Figure 23-3 in your textbook.

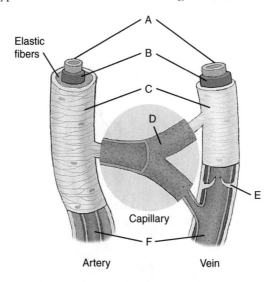

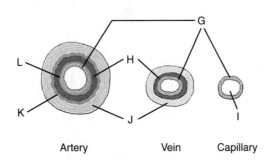

Figure 23-3

A. _____

B. _____

C. _____

D. _____

E. _____

F. _____

G. _____

H. _____

I. _____

J. _____

K. _____

L. _____

4. Identify the parts of the abdominal aortic aneurysm shown in Figure 23-4. Refer to Figure 23-7 in your text-book.

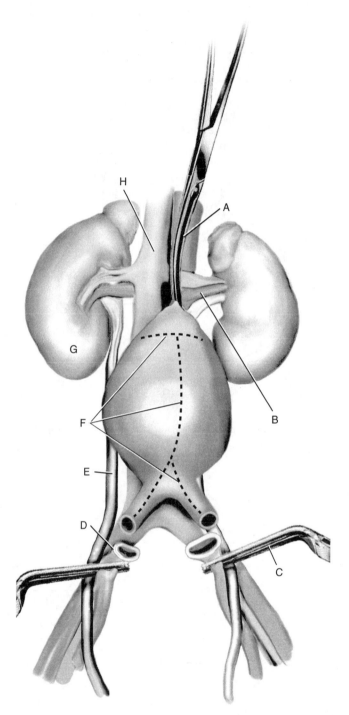

Figure 23-4

A. _____

B. _____

C. _____

D. _____

E. _____

F. _____

G. _____

H. _____

5. List the three tunics of a blood vessel wall, and briefly describe the composition and function of each structure.

    A. _____

    B. _____

    C. _____

6. What structures receive arterial blood from the brachiocephalic artery?

    _____

    _____

    _____

    _____

7. Which artery or arteries, if any, branch off the ascending aorta?

    _____

    _____

    _____

    _____

    _____

8. Each common carotid artery bifurcates into two sections. Provide the names of the two branches and the structures supplied with arterial blood from each.

    A. _____

    B. _____

9. What effect does the autonomic nervous system have on vasoconstriction?

    _____

    _____

    _____

    _____

10. Which is larger, the lumen of an artery or the lumen of a vein in a similar location?

    _____

    _____

    _____

    _____

11. What effect does vasodilation have on blood pressure?

    _____

    _____

_____

_____

12. What is blood pressure?

_____

_____

_____

_____

13. List three factors that affect arterial blood pressure.

   A. _____

   B. _____

   C. _____

14. What does the term resistance describe within the cardiovascular system? How does increased resistance affect blood pressure?

_____

_____

_____

_____

15. List the three main branches of the common hepatic artery, and name the structure(s) served by each.

   A. _____

   B. _____

   C. _____

Pathology

1. What causes claudication?

_____

_____

_____

_____

2. List the four signs/symptoms of acute arterial occlusion.

   A. _____

   B. _____

   C. _____

   D. _____

3. There are several types of emboli. Name two.

   A. _____

   B. _____

4. List three types of treatment for embolism.

    A. _____

    B. _____

    C. _____

5. What is the shape of a fusiform aneurysm? What portion of the aorta is most often involved?

    _____

    _____

    _____

    _____

6. What are the symptoms of an atherosclerotic aneurysm of the femoral or popliteal artery?

    _____

    _____

    _____

    _____

    _____

7. What term is used to describe inflammation of a vein?

    _____

    _____

    _____

    _____

    _____

8. What is the cause of a TIA (transient ischemic attack)?

    _____

    _____

    _____

    _____

    _____

9. What is plaque? (Note: Use a medical dictionary to define.)

    _____

    _____

    _____

    _____

10. What examinations may be performed to identify a lesion of the common carotid artery?

    _____

    _____

    _____

    _____

11. What is the difference between ischemia and necrosis?

_____

_____

_____

_____

_____

12. What are the signs/symptoms associated with a TIA?

_____

_____

_____

_____

_____

13. List four risk factors associated with the development of peripheral vascular disease.

    A. _____

    B. _____

    C. _____

    D. _____

14. How is the establishment of collateral blood flow encouraged in patients with vascular insufficiency of the lower extremity?

_____

_____

_____

_____

_____

15. List three physical signs of vascular insufficiency of the lower extremity.

    A. _____

    B. _____

    C. _____

Operation

1. In what situation will contrast solution (e.g., Conray, Hypaque) be needed on the sterile field?

_____

_____

_____

2. List three hemostatic agents that are typically used during peripheral vascular surgical procedures.

   A. _____

   B. _____

   C. _____

3. What is a Fogarty catheter used to accomplish?

   _____

   _____

   _____

   _____

4. What is the purpose of an intraluminal stent?

   _____

   _____

   _____

   _____

5. Vascular grafts are available in several configurations. Name two.

   A. _____

   B. _____

6. Why do some types of vascular graft material have rigid rings (exoskeleton) built into the graft? In which location are the reinforced grafts commonly implanted?

   _____

   _____

   _____

   _____

7. What is the primary indication for carotid endarterectomy?

   _____

   _____

   _____

   _____

8. During carotid endarterectomy, is the use of a shunt necessary? Why?

   _____

   _____

   _____

   _____

9. Vascular grafts are available in several materials. Name two.

   A. _____

   B. _____

10. What instruments are typically used to perform an arteriotomy?

_____

_____

_____

_____

11. What is the purpose of creating a tunnel during a femoral popliteal bypass?

_____

_____

_____

_____

12. List two complications that may arise following implantation of a composite graft.

A. _____

B. _____

13. Why is it necessary to pre-clot a vascular graft that is made of knitted polyester?

_____

_____

_____

_____

_____

14. What is a patch suture? How is it prepared?

_____

_____

_____

_____

15. Why is it important for the STSR to remain sterile and keep the back table and Mayo stand intact until the patient has been transported to the PACU?

_____

_____

_____

_____

_____

_____

Specific Variations

Student Name _____ Date _____

Instructor _____

The student will be provided with basic patient information (real or simulated) and is expected to complete the following case study.

1. Procedure name:

   _____

   _____

   _____

2. Definition of procedure:

   _____

   _____

   _____

   _____

   _____

3. What is the purpose of the procedure?

   _____

   _____

   _____

   _____

   _____

4. What is the expected outcome of the procedure?

   _____

   _____

   _____

   _____

5. Patient age: _____

6. Gender: _____

7. Additional pertinent patient information:

   _____

   _____

   _____

   _____

8. Probable preoperative diagnosis:

   _____

   _____

   _____

   _____

   _____

9. How was the diagnosis determined?

_____

_____

_____

_____

_____

_____

10. Discuss the relevant anatomy.

_____

_____

_____

_____

_____

_____

_____

11. List the general and procedure-specific equipment that will be needed for the procedure.

_____

_____

_____

_____

_____

_____

12. List the general and procedure-specific instruments that will be needed for the procedure.

_____

_____

_____

_____

_____

_____

13. List the basic and procedure-specific supplies that will be needed for the procedure.

Pack _____

Basin _____

Gloves _____

Blades _____

Drapes _____

Drains _____

Dressings _____

Suture—Type of Suture, Needle (if applicable), and Anticipated Tissue Usage

_____

_____

_____

_____

_____

_____

Pharmaceuticals

_____

_____

_____

_____

_____

Miscellaneous

_____

_____

_____

_____

_____

14. Operative preparation:

_____

_____

_____

_____

_____

_____

15. What type of anesthesia will likely be used? Why?

_____

_____

_____

_____

16. List any special anesthesia equipment that may be needed.

_____

_____

_____

_____

_____

_____

_____

17. Patient position during the procedure:

_____

_____

_____

_____

_____

18. What supplies will be necessary for positioning?

_____

_____

_____

_____

_____

19. What type of shave/skin preparation will be necessary (if any)?

_____

_____

_____

_____

_____

_____

20. Define the anatomic perimeters of the prep.

_____

_____

_____

_____

_____

21. List the order in which the drapes will be applied, and describe any specific variations.

_____

_____

_____

_____

_____

_____

22. List any practical considerations.

_____

_____

_____

_____

_____

_____

23. List the procedural steps, and describe the preparatory and supportive actions of the STSR during each step (use additional space if necessary).

_____

_____

_____

_____

_____

24. What is the postoperative diagnosis?

_____

_____

_____

_____

_____

_____

25. Describe the immediate postoperative care.

_____

_____

_____

_____

26. What is the patient's long-term prognosis?

_____

_____

_____

_____

_____

27. What are the possible complications?

_____

_____

_____

_____

_____

_____

_____

28. Comments or questions:

_____

_____

_____

_____

_____

_____

29. What is the most valuable information you obtained from preparing this surgical procedure case study?

_____

_____

_____

_____

Case Studies

CASE STUDY 1

Joe is a 50-year-old male who was brought to the emergency department in hemorrhagic shock due to a ruptured abdominal aneurysm. The surgeon called the surgery department to alert them that he is in transit with the patient for immediate intervention. The OR team leader, in turn, has notified the STSR and circulator who are assigned to the case. The surgical team springs into action.

1. What supplies will the STSR open onto the sterile field first?

_____

_____

_____

_____

_____

2. What instrument sets will be needed?

_____

_____

_____

_____

_____

(*continues*)

CASE STUDY 1 *(continued)*

3. What instruments will be needed first?

_____

_____

_____

_____

_____

CASE STUDY 2

Wayne, a 67-year-old male, presented to the emergency department with the following symptoms: cold extremity of the right foot and ankle, complaining of severe pain, pale right foot and ankle, and no pedal pulse of the right foot or ankle.

1. What is the preliminary diagnosis?

_____

_____

_____

_____

_____

_____

2. What diagnostic examination(s) will be done?

_____

_____

_____

_____

_____

_____

3. Will surgical intervention be necessary? If so, what procedure will be scheduled?

_____

_____

_____

_____

_____

_____

Lab 23: Peripheral Vascular Surgery

Introduction

Peripheral vascular surgery deals with surgery of the vascular system within the appendages and axiom of the body not within the thoracic region. You will be dealing with smaller vascular structures that may necessitate very delicate instruments. It can be one of the harder specialties to learn because so many instruments tend to do the same thing but have subtle differences that make them better for one area or another. In this unit you will find many open procedures along with many procedures that are done with endoscopes. Learning the surgeries step by step in lecture will help you in the lab portion. This is where you will learn the hands on of the specialty and the instruments that will be used for each piece of the surgery.

Game: Peripheral Vascular Surgery on Felt Mayo stands

Time involved: 1–2 weeks setup

Instructors: Make a list of instruments you expect students to know as part of the peripheral vascular surgery lab. Have the students trace the real instruments onto the felt if possible; alternatively have them find pictures they can cut out and trace onto the felt or other material. I like felt because it tends to be very durable, but paper or cardboard can be substituted. There should be no need for multiple cutouts of the same instruments if students are given the chance to show how many of the instruments they would have on the Mayo by way of a numbered marker (a piece of paper with a number designation on it). The students are given a list of surgeries that they are expected to know. **Note:** This can also be made easier if you have photos of the Mayo stand setups for the students to study.

Students: You will need several pieces of felt, paper, or cardboard. The largest piece should be cut to the size of a regular Mayo stand. You will then make cutouts of instruments as close as possible to life size using felt or some other material. Label the backsides of the cutouts for easy reference.

Supplies: Felt, paper, or cardboard; real instruments, or pictures that have been printed and cut out from the computer; felt-tip marker; scissors; measuring tool

How the Game is Played

The students are given a list of surgeries that they are expected to know. The instructor will then assign one of those surgeries to the student in the lab. The student will then be expected to complete a Mayo stand setup in a specified time frame using the instruments they have cut out. Score the students according to placement of instruments, time needed for setup, correct instrumentation, and correct number of instruments.

Practical: Set Up General Surgery Cases

Utilizing a full lab/OR setup, assign the students different surgical cases to learn. The students will then be expected to set up some of these cases under the supervision of the instructor. They should utilize as much of the OR equipment as needed including backtable, Mayo stand, ring stands, instrument trays, and pans. The student should be scored on correct placement of supplies, practicing economy of time and motion (pick it up and place it one time), correct order of instruments, correct number of instruments, aseptic technique, time to set up, and order of use for instruments and supplies; a mock surgery should be performed so the student can practice anticipating the needs of the surgeon.

CHAPTER 24

Neurosurgery

OBJECTIVES

After studying this chapter, the reader should be able to:

A 1. Recognize the relevant anatomy and physiology of the neurological system.

P 2. Summarize the pathology that prompts surgical intervention of the neurological system, and the related terminology.

3. Determine any special preoperative neurological diagnostic procedures/tests.

4. Determine any special preoperative preparation procedures related to neurosurgery.

O 5. Indicate the names and uses of neurosurgical instruments, supplies, and drugs.

6. Indicate the names and uses of special equipment related to neurosurgery.

7. Determine the intraoperative preparation of the patient undergoing the neurosurgical procedure.

8. Summarize the surgical steps of the neurosurgical procedures.

9. Interpret the purpose and expected outcomes of the neurosurgical procedures.

10. Recognize the immediate postoperative care and possible complications of the neurosurgical procedures.

S 11. Assess any specific variations related to the preoperative, intraoperative, and postoperative care of the neurosurgical patient.

12. Summarize recent advances in neurosurgery.

Select Key Terms

Define the following using your textbook glossary or a medical dictionary:

1. abscess _____

   _____

2. acute _____

   _____

3. autonomic nervous system _____

   _____

4. cerebellum_____

   _____

5. cerebrum _____

   _____

6. circle of Willis _____

   _____

7. CNS _____

   _____

8. decompress _____

   _____

9. dysraphism _____

   _____

10. epidural _____

    _____

11. extruded _____

    _____

12. glioma _____

    _____

13. hematoma _____

    _____

14. ICP _____

    _____

15. integration _____

    _____

16. meninges_____

    _____

17. osteophyte _____

    _____

18. parasympathetic nervous system _____

    _____

19. PNS _____

    _____

20. radiculopathy _____

    _____

21. somatic nervous system _____

    _____

22. sympathetic nervous system _____

_____

23. TIA _____

_____

24. transsphenoidal _____

_____

Anatomy

1. Identify the major divisions of the autonomic nervous system shown in Figure 24-1. Refer to Figure 24-2 in your textbook.

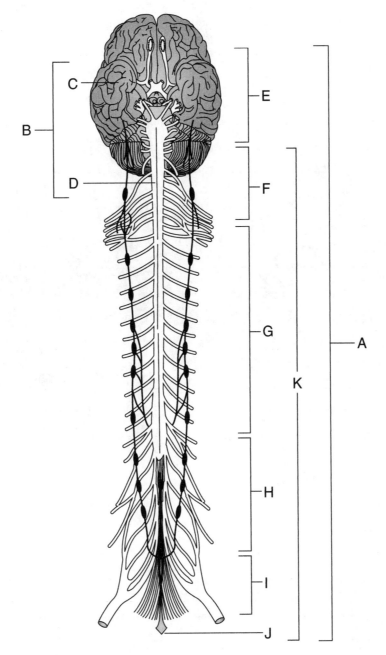

Figure 24-1

A. _____

B. _____

C. _____

D. _____

E. _____

F. _____

G. _____

H. _____

I. _____

J. _____

K. _____

2. Identify the structures of the external surface of the brain shown in Figure 24-2. Refer to Figure 24-4 in your textbook.

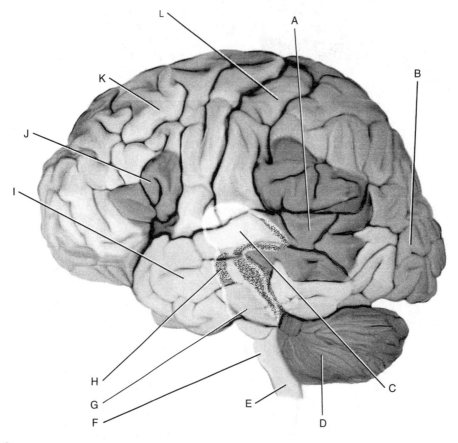

Figure 24-2

A. _____

B. _____

C. _____

D. _____

E. _____

F. _____

G. _____

H. _____

I. _____

J. _____

K. _____

L. _____

3. Identify the meninges and related structures shown in Figure 24-3. Refer to Figure 24-3 in your textbook.

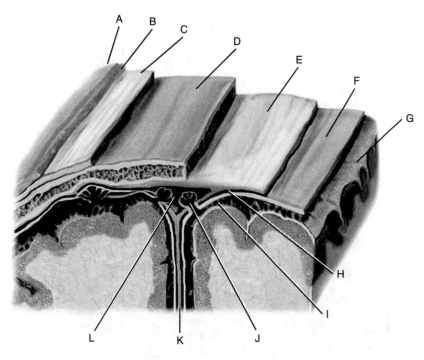

Figure 24-3

A. _____

B. _____

C. _____

D. _____

E. _____

F. _____

G. _____

H. _____

I. _____

J. _____

K. _____

L. _____

4. Identify the cranial nerves and other structures shown in Figure 24-4. Refer to Figure 24-11 in your textbook.

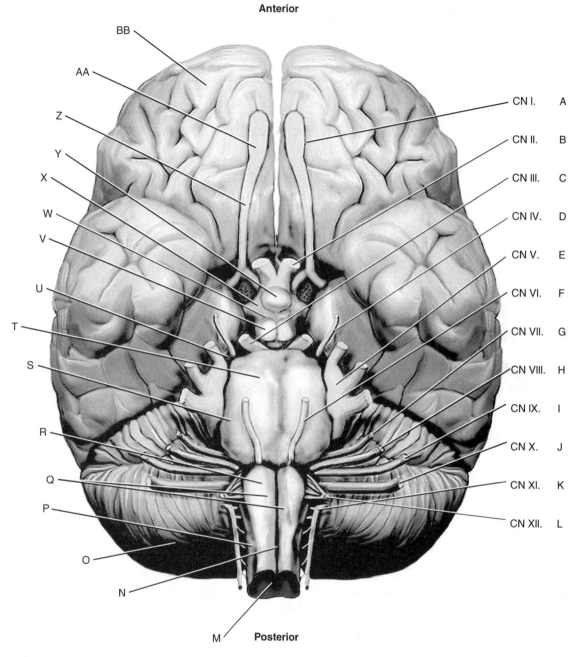

Figure 24-4

A. _____

B. _____

C. _____

D. _____

E. _____

F. _____

G. _____

H. _____

I. _____

J. _____

K. _____

L. _____

M. _____

N. _____

O. _____

P. _____

Q. _____

R. _____

S. _____

T. _____

U. _____

V. _____

W. _____

X. _____

Y. _____

Z. _____

AA. _____

BB. _____

5. Identify the ventricles of the brain and related structures shown in Figure 24-5. Refer to Figure 24-7 in your textbook.

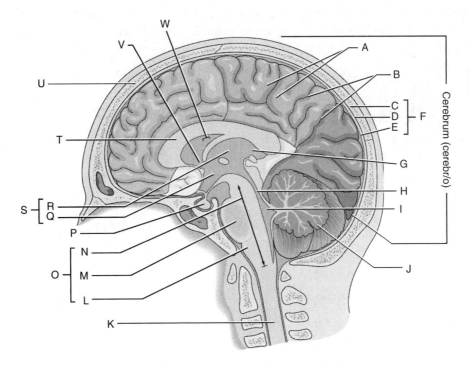

Figure 24-5

A. _____

B. _____

C. _____

D. _____

E. _____

F. _____

G. _____

H. _____

I. _____

J. _____

K. _____

L. _____

M. _____

N. _____

O. _____

P. _____

Q. _____

R. _____

S. _____

T. _____

U. _____

V. _____

W. _____

6. Identify the pathway of impulses (reflex arc) and related structures shown in Figure 24-6. Refer to Figure 24-8 in your textbook.

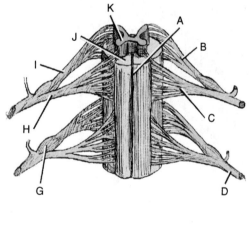

A

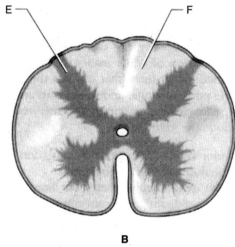

B

Figure 24-6

A. _____

B. _____

C. _____

D. _____

E. _____

F. _____

G. _____

H. _____

I. _____

J. _____

K. _____

7. Name the bones and structures of the cranium shown in Figure 24-7. Refer to Figure 24-2 in your textbook.

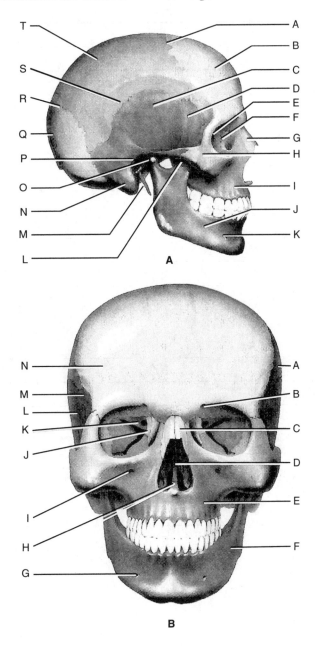

Figure 24-7

(A)

A. _____

B. _____

C. _____

D. _____

E. _____

F. _____

G. _____

H. _____

I. _____

J. _____

K. _____

L. _____

M. _____

N. _____

O. _____

P. _____

Q. _____

R. _____

S. _____

T. _____

(B)

A. _____

B. _____

C. _____

D. _____

E. _____

F. _____

G. _____

H. _____

I. _____

J. _____

K. _____

L. _____

M. _____

N. _____

8. Name the three meningeal layers in sequence from outermost to innermost.

   A. _____

   B. _____

   C. _____

9. Where is CSF formed? How is it formed?

   _____

   _____

   _____

   _____

10. Name the three branches of the trigeminal nerve, and describe the functions of the target tissue(s) innervated by each branch.

    A. _____

    B. _____

    C. _____

11. What are the three primary functions of the nervous system?

    A. _____

    B. _____

    C. _____

12. What are the two subdivisions of the autonomic nervous system (ANS), and what is the basic function of each subdivision?

    A. _____

    B. _____

13. What is the circle of Willis?

    _____

    _____

    _____

    _____

    _____

14. The auditory processing area of the brain is located in the _____ lobe of the brain.

15. The vital centers of the brain (respiratory, cardiac, and vasomotor) are contained in which portion of the brainstem?

    _____

    _____

    _____

    _____

    _____

Pathology

1. Hydrocephalus has several causes. List three.

   A. _____

   B. _____

   C. _____

2. List three types of obstruction of the aqueducts between the ventricles that can lead to hydrocephalus.

   A. _____

   B. _____

   C. _____

3. Describe the condition known as spondylosis.

   _____

   _____

   _____

   _____

   _____

4. Name two radiographic techniques that may be used to identify spinal disorders, and describe how each is used.

   A. _____

   B. _____

5. What is the difference between a subdural hematoma and an epidural hematoma?

   _____

   _____

   _____

   _____

6. Define craniosynostosis, and describe the method(s) for diagnosing the condition.

   _____

   _____

   _____

   _____

   _____

7. Describe spina bifida.

   _____

   _____

   _____

   _____

   _____

8. List the three classifications (locations) of spinal cord tumors and the symptoms of each.

   A. _____

   B. _____

   C. _____

9. Carpal tunnel syndrome affects which nerve at what level?

_____

_____

_____

_____

10. What is the underlying cause of growth hormone (GH) overproduction?

_____

_____

_____

_____

_____

11. Describe two symptoms that a patient with herniated nucleus pulposus may experience.

    A. _____

    B. _____

12. What is the most common type of brain tumor?

_____

_____

_____

_____

13. What symptoms are associated with acoustic neuroma? Which nerve is affected?

_____

_____

_____

_____

14. If the patient presents with pain in the ring and small finger of the affected hand with weakness, what is the probable diagnosis? What procedure(s) is/are completed to relieve the symptoms?

_____

_____

_____

_____

15. List and describe the three types of subdural hematoma.

    A. _____

    B. _____

    C. _____

Operation

1. What is the Mayfield pin-fixation device used to accomplish?

   _____

   _____

   _____

   _____

2. How do Raney clips differ from aneurysm clips?

   _____

   _____

   _____

3. Access to the occipital lobe of the brain may be accomplished with the patient in either of two positions. Name the two possible positions.

   A. _____

   B. _____

4. What supplies may be necessary to remove scalp hair in the operating room?

   _____

   _____

   _____

   _____

5. List three options for treatment of a cerebral aneurysm.

   A. _____

   B. _____

   C. _____

6. It is important to restrict movement in and around the sterile field at all times, but why is this especially true during procedures near the cerebellopontine angle?

   _____

   _____

   _____

7. List the four main components of the ventriculoperitoneal shunt.

   A. _____

   B. _____

   C. _____

   D. _____

8. Name two approaches that can be used for surgery of the pituitary.

   A. _____

   B. _____

9. List two materials that can be implanted during cranioplasty and that can be molded to fit the cranial defect.

   A. _____

   B. _____

10. List two methods by which the bone flap is secured to the cranium following a craniotomy.

    A. _____

    B. _____

11. Why are two separate Mayo stands needed for transsphenoidal procedures?

    _____

    _____

    _____

    _____

12. What is papaverine used for during arterial intracranial surgery?

    _____

    _____

    _____

    _____

13. What is the ideal temperature for irrigation fluid that will be used intracranially?

    _____

    _____

    _____

14. What is the CUSA, and how is it used?

    _____

    _____

    _____

    _____

15. What is ICP? What procedure is completed to place an ICP monitor?

    _____

    _____

    _____

    _____

Specific Variations

Student Name _____ Date _____

Instructor _____

The student will be provided with basic patient information (real or simulated) and is expected to complete the following case study.

1. Procedure name:

    _____

    _____

    _____

2. Definition of procedure:

    _____

    _____

    _____

    _____

    _____

3. What is the purpose of the procedure?

    _____

    _____

    _____

    _____

    _____

4. What is the expected outcome of the procedure?

    _____

    _____

    _____

    _____

5. Patient age: _____

6. Gender: _____

7. Additional pertinent patient information:

    _____

    _____

    _____

8. Probable preoperative diagnosis:

    _____

    _____

    _____

_____

_____

9. How was the diagnosis determined?

_____

_____

_____

_____

10. Discuss the relevant anatomy.

_____

_____

_____

_____

_____

_____

_____

11. List the general and procedure-specific equipment that will be needed for the procedure.

_____

_____

_____

_____

_____

_____

12. List the general and procedure-specific instruments that will be needed for the procedure.

_____

_____

_____

_____

_____

13. List the basic and procedure-specific supplies that will be needed for the procedure.

Pack _____

Basin _____

Gloves _____

Blades _____

Drapes _____

Drains _____

Dressings _____

Suture—Type of Suture, Needle (if applicable), and Anticipated Tissue Usage

_____

_____

_____

_____

_____

Pharmaceuticals

_____

_____

_____

_____

Miscellaneous

_____

_____

_____

_____

_____

_____

14. Operative preparation:

_____

_____

_____

_____

15. What type of anesthesia will likely be used? Why?

_____

_____

_____

_____

16. List any special anesthesia equipment that may be needed.

_____

_____

_____

_____

_____

_____

17. Patient position during the procedure:

_____

_____

_____

_____

18. What supplies will be necessary for positioning?

_____

_____

_____

_____

19. What type of shave/skin preparation will be necessary (if any)?

_____

_____

_____

_____

20. Define the anatomic perimeters of the prep.

_____

_____

_____

_____

21. List the order in which the drapes will be applied, and describe any specific variations.

_____

_____

_____

_____

_____

_____

22. List any practical considerations.

_____

_____

_____

_____

_____

_____

_____

23. List the procedural steps, and describe the preparatory and supportive actions of the STSR during each step (use additional space if necessary).

_____

_____

_____

_____

_____

24. What is the postoperative diagnosis?

_____

_____

_____

_____

_____

_____

25. Describe the immediate postoperative care.

_____

_____

_____

_____

_____

_____

26. What is the patient's long-term prognosis?

_____

_____

_____

_____

_____

27. What are the possible complications?

_____

_____

_____

_____

_____

_____

28. Comments or questions:

_____

_____

_____

_____

_____

_____

_____

29. What is the most valuable information you obtained from preparing this surgical procedure case study?

_____

_____

_____

_____

Case Studies

CASE STUDY 1

Dr. Roberts was summoned to the emergency department to see a 34-year-old male who was brought in complaining of a severe headache of sudden onset. The patient described the headache as "violent, bursting, and explosive." He stated that it was the worst headache that he has ever experienced. The patient is nauseous, photophobic, and complaining of pain in the lower back. A lumbar puncture revealed blood within the cerebrospinal fluid.

1. What is the preliminary diagnosis?

    _____

    _____

    _____

    _____

2. What diagnostic test will reveal the condition, exact size, and location?

    _____

    _____

    _____

    _____

(continues)

CASE STUDY 1 *(continued)*

3. What are the treatment options?

_____

_____

_____

_____

CASE STUDY 2

Jamma, a 43-year-old female secretary for a law firm, presents to Dr. Michaels with complaints of numbness, tingling, and pain in the right hand. Dr. Michaels notes during the examination that the symptoms are localized to the thumb, index finger, long finger, and medial aspect of the ring finger. He also notes that pain occasionally radiates up the arm into the shoulder. Jamma states that the pain awakens her at night.

1. What is the diagnosis?

_____

_____

_____

_____

2. What is the etiology of the syndrome?

_____

_____

_____

_____

3. How is the condition treated? List the conservative and surgical options.

_____

_____

_____

_____

Lab 24: Neurosurgery

Introduction

Neurosurgery deals with surgery of the nervous system of the body. This will include both the central nervous system and the peripheral nervous system. You will be dealing with small and large nerve structures that may necessitate very delicate instruments and possibly the use of microscopes. It can be one of the harder specialties to learn because so many instruments tend to do the same thing but have subtle differences that make them better for one area or another. In this unit you will find many open procedures along with many procedures that are done with endoscopes and microscopes. Learning the surgeries step by step in lecture will help you in the lab portion. This is where you will learn the "hands-on" of the specialty and the instruments that will be used for each piece of the surgery.

Game: Neurosurgery on Felt Mayo Stands

Time involved: 1–2 weeks setup

Instructors: Make a list of instruments you expect students to know as part of the neurosurgery lab. Have the students trace the real instruments onto felt if possible; alternatively, have them find pictures they can cut out and trace onto felt or other material. I like felt because it tends to be very durable, but paper or cardboard can be substituted. There should be no need for multiple cutouts of the same instruments if students are given the chance to show how many of those instruments they would have on the Mayo by way of a numbered marker (a piece of paper with a number designation on it). The students are given a list of surgeries that they are expected to know.(**Note:** This can also be made easier if you have photos of these Mayo stand setups for the students to study.

Students: You will need several pieces of felt, paper, or cardboard. The largest piece should be cut to the size of a regular Mayo stand but many neurological surgery cases require use of a larger table such as a Mayfield overhead table. Utilize a backtable or a regular table to meet this need. You will then proceed to make cutouts of instruments as close as possible to life size using felt or some other material. Label the backsides of the cutouts for easy reference.

Supplies: Felt, paper, or cardboard; real instruments, or pictures that have been printed and cut out from the computer; felt-tip marker; scissors; measuring tool

How the Game Is Played

The students are given a list of surgeries that they are expected to know. The instructor will then assign one of those surgeries to the student in the lab. The student will then be expected to complete a Mayo stand setup in a specified time frame using the instruments they have cut out. Score the students according to placement of instruments, time needed for setup, correct instrumentation, and correct number of instruments.

Practical: Set Up General Surgery Cases

Utilizing a full lab/OR setup, assign the students different surgical cases to learn. The students will then be expected to set up some of these cases under the supervision of the instructor. They should utilize as much of the OR equipment as needed including backtable, Mayo stand, ring stands, instrument trays, and pans. The student should be scored on correct placement of supplies, practicing economy of time and motion (pick it up and place it one time), correct order of instruments, correct number of instruments, aseptic technique, time to set up, and order of use for instruments and supplies; a mock surgery should be performed so the student can practice anticipating the needs of the surgeon.